Forensic Aspects of Chemical and Biological Terrorism

Edited by
Cyril H. Wecht, M.D., J.D.

L&J® Lawyers & Judges Publishing Company, Inc.
Tucson, Arizona

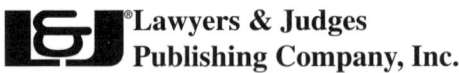

Lawyers & Judges Publishing Company, Inc.

P.O. Box 30040 • Tucson, AZ 85751-0040
(800) 209-7109 • FAX (800) 330-8795
e-mail: sales@lawyersandjudges.com

Library of Congress Cataloging-in-Publication Data

Forensic aspects of chemical and biological terrorism / edited by Cyril H. Wecht.
p. cm.
Includes bibliographical references and index.
ISBN 1-930056-67-2 (hardcover)
1. Chemical terrorism. 2. Bioterrorism. I. Wecht, Cyril H., 1931-
HV6431.F665 2004
614'.1--dc22

2004019767

ISBN 1-930056-67-2
Printed in the United States of America
10 9 8 7 6 5 4 3 2 1

online
www.lawyersandjudges.com

Contents

Foreword

In an era in which the FBI Director and Homeland Security Secretary are predicting attacks on U.S. soil by al-Qa'eda, Dr. Cyril Wecht has provided a comprehensive roadmap on identifying and responding to chemical and biological terrorism. This book would be useful at any time, but it's vital today.

Dr. Wecht has assembled a compelling lineup of distinguished experts in medicine, public health, psychology and law enforcement to provide practical advice on how to deal with the scourge of terrorism in a variety of forms. The experts tackle smallpox, chemical warfare agents, bombings and aviation attacks, among others.

This book will be helpful to the U.S. Senate and House of Representatives as we reorganize many governmental agencies and appropriate billions of dollars for homeland security. As a member of the Senate Appropriations Subcommittees on Defense and Homeland Security, and as a former Chairman of the Senate Intelligence Committee, I know I will refer repeatedly to this text in my own efforts to advance the fight against terrorism and defend our nation. It is must-reading for first responders to better prepare for potentially devastating chemical and biological attacks.

Dr. Cyril Wecht has brought to this book the same thoroughness and insight that have made him one of the nation's foremost medical experts. I have worked with and sparred with Dr. Wecht many times over many years, and always found him a skilled researcher and gifted debater and writer. Readers will appreciate those skills and talents in this important and well-crafted text.

—Arlen Specter
U.S. Senator, Pennsylvania

Introduction

An overwhelming majority of politically aware and socially concerned adults in the United States, whether they be right wing Republican conservatives or left wing Democratic liberals, would agree that the actuality and continuing threat of global terrorism is the most formidable, complex, and serious problem confronting western civilization at this time. No other singular issue or endeavor has impacted so dramatically on our every day lives and activities—parking your car in a large office building, entering a major league ballpark, checking in at an airport, picking up a document at a local or federal government building. Our world today is far different from what it was a generation ago. In fact, it can be reasonably contended that even World War II did not result in so much governmental freneticism and public warnings, direct physical intrusions on private citizens, and official societal limitations of speech and movement. To an unpleasant and uncomfortable degree, although perhaps understandably necessary, our routine existence has been dramatically altered because of terrorism.

This perplexing matter is not as freshly acute as many people may believe. In fact, terrorists killed far more Americans during the 1980s than during the 1990s. In 1983, Hezbollah suicide bombers attacked the U.S. Embassy in Beirut, killing sixty-three people. Later that year, in October, a 12,000 – pound bomb destroyed the Marine barracks in that same city, killing 241 Americans, the most deadly terrorist strike against the United States prior to the infamous event of September 11, 2001. In March 1984, Islamic terrorists kidnapped and subsequently executed a CIA officer. The following month, Hezbollah killed eighteen American soldiers in an attack on a restaurant near an airbase in Spain. Two U.S. military personnel were killed by another truck bombing in Beirut in September 1984. Terrorists hijacked an airline flight, TWA 847, in July 1985 and killed one American, Navy diver Robert Stethem, whose corpse was thrown out of the plane onto the runway. There followed the *Achille Lauro* incident in

October, in which Palestinian terrorists commandeered a cruise ship and executed Leon Klinghoffer, a wheelchair-bound American tourist. In December, Abu Nidal terrorists attacked travelers simultaneously at airports in Rome and Vienna. In March 1986, terrorists killed four Americans in Greece. In April, Libyans bombed a West Berlin disco, killing two American soldiers and injuring dozens more.

It is by now a well-established fact that Saddam Hussein used chemical weapons against Kurds in the northern Iraq town of Halabja on March 16, 1998, killing more than 5,000. Numerous journalists, various government delegations, and several international human rights groups who have investigated this matter have further concluded that Halabja was the first horrendous act of Saddam's notorious "Anfal" campaign, a genocide that resulted in the deaths of approximately 100,000 Kurds.

And so this reign of terror has continued unabated through the 1990s and into the twenty-first century. Regrettably, but not really unpredictably, terrorists have added biological and chemical modalities to their armamentarium with increasing frequency in recent years. As frightening and worrisome as physical destruction is, there is something much more ominous and viscerally disturbing about virulent microorganisms and highly toxic gases and other poisonous compounds. The knowledge that simply opening a letter could lead to your death; or that you could be waiting for a subway and find that you are suddenly unable to breathe, is enough to make the bravest amongst us shudder at the thought.

Terrorists who formerly relied largely on bombs and firearms are now in a position to exploit the effects of novel weapons that can be used against people, livestock, crops and water supplies. An added and almost entirely new factor is that some terrorists may seek their own death in the process—and so they are not deterred by the risk of contracting a fatal disease themselves. The threat may come from single-issue groups, religious groups or hostile states. The spectrum of attacks may extend from an individual spreading infectious agents in a crowded tube train to state-sponsored operations involving the introduction of human or livestock epidemics or crop pathogens. The last two could wreak havoc on a nation's economy.

In October 2001, the treat of bioterrorism became real for many people when contact with anthrax killed five unrelated individuals and sickened twelve others under highly suspicious circumstances. Since that time, the focus of resources at the Centers for Disease Control and Prevention and other public health agencies has been shifted to bioterrorism.

Simulations have provided dramatic evidence of a lack of preparedness for an attack involving smallpox. At the same time, some fear the consequences of overreaction. For example, vaccination against these agents likely to be used as biological weapons will often carry risks to recipients.

The Centers for Disease Control and Prevention and state and local public health authorities confirmed twenty-two cases of bioterrorism-related anthrax associated with the tainted mailings of fall 2001: eleven inhalation cases with five deaths and eleven confirmed or suspected cases of cutaneous anthrax.

The threat of a smallpox attack by terrorists is of particular concern. Germ warfare as a form of terrorism has a long and deadly history. Ancient armies tainted water supplies of entire cities with various fungi and herbs. One such germ warfare assault in the fourteenth century reportedly precipitated a bubonic plague epidemic that decimated the population of Europe. During World War I, German agents organized an anthrax factory in Washington, D.C. In World War II, anthrax experiments conducted by British and American scientists left Gruinard Island off the coast of Scotland uninhabitable for almost fifty years. The fifth plague that befell the Egyptians (*Exodus* 9:3) is believed to have been an anthrax epidemic that killed all the cattle in that country.

Anthrax, a disease caused by *Bacillus anthracis*, has a long association with human history. Anthrax can occur in three forms: cutaneous, gastrointestinal, and inhalational, the most lethal form. Such a pathogen possesses properties that make it an ideal terrorist weapon: ease of procurement, simplicity of production in large quantities at minimal expense, ease of dissemination with simple technology, and potential to overwhelm the medical system with a large number of casualties. Difficulty in tracing the source would be added to this list, as has been demonstrated by the inability of our governmental authorities to track down the perpetrators of the directed attacks of October and November 2001.

More than 100 hostages were killed in October, 2002 after Russian authorities used an unidentified gas to incapacitate terrorists holding 750 people in a Moscow theater. Nearly all of the deaths were due to the highly toxic gas, which Russian authorities have so far refused to identify. The 1997 Weapons Convention permits the production and use of riot-control agents for law enforcement purposes. Until the Russians inform us of the agent used, whether they were in violation of the Weapons Convention will remain uncertain. It is believed that Russia retains some 40,000 tons of chemical warfare blister agents and nerve gas.

Recent scientific developments have greatly expanded the spectrum and effectiveness of both biological and chemical devices, representing a quantum leap in military potential. The distinction between chemical and biological weapons has now become blurred. For instance, some toxins may now be synthesized in the laboratory and tailored for particular purposes. Thus, both types of weapons may be conveniently grouped as CB (chemical/biological). Of particular concern is the utility of such weapons in the hands of third-world states and terrorist organizations, where they can be a force multiplier, producing a disproportionate effect by spreading panic and overwhelming the available medical and logistic services. In response to such a threat, it has been suggested that the target nations, principally the western democracies, should continue the study of terrorist techniques and develop early-warning programs. Most importantly, they should formulate clear national biochemical warfare policies.

The Chemical Weapons Convention is a global treaty with more than 170 signatory nations. It bans the production, acquisition, stockpiling, transfer and use of chemical weapons—the first arms-control treaty to outlaw an entire class of so-called weapons of mass destruction. It also requires the signatories to declare and destroy, by certain deadlines, the chemical weapons they possess. Since the 1925 Geneva Protocol prohibiting the use of chemical and biological weapons in war—a reaction to gas attacks in World War I—the world has struggled to ban these weapons. In part, this is because of their indiscriminate nature. After September 11, 2001, it seems all the more important to eliminate stocks of such weapons because access to them could confer much uncontrollable and unpredictable power to terrorists. In a world with 70,000 metric tons of chemical weapon-materials, some of which may be vulnerable to terrorist theft, the verified elimination of these weapons would be a step toward greater security for all the civilized world.

In formulating a biochemical defense policy, hazard assessment is an essential factor. Thus, the utility and advantages and disadvantages of CB weapons require careful consideration. In general war, the use of CB weapons would do little harm to the infrastructure of a territory to be occupied—an advantage for the user. The fact that they may incapacitate rather then kill outright is an important consideration. This is because they could overwhelm the medical and casualty services, whereas the dead have no need of either. However, at present, weaponization and dispersion of CB weapons present difficulties. Accurate targeting is seldom possible and collateral adverse effects may occur among the attacker's own troops;

moreover, retribution in kind might also follow. In CB attacks on civilian populations, the fear factor works to the advantage of the terrorist. The use of anthrax letters illustrates this point. Additionally, this method allows for a delayed onset of infection, enabling the perpetrators to move away and attack elsewhere. CB agents many be used as weapons of mass destruction by spreading epidemics among human or animal populations or commercial crops while avoiding collateral damage to the infrastructure. It is not generally recognized that, although many CB agents are easy and cheap to produce, effective detection and countermeasures are as yet inadequate to meet a large-scale challenge. Little progress has been made on antivirals and vaccine research, and development requires further input.

On Wednesday, July 21, 2004, President Bush signed into law a bill to develop and stockpile vaccines and other antidotes to the effects of biological and chemical weapons. The $5.6 billion, ten-year Project BioShield program is intended to expand public and private research incentives to develop treatments, antidotes and vaccines that would otherwise not be developed by companies. Homeland Security now costs U.S. taxpayers approximately $37 billion a year.

The BioShield legislation will guarantee a market by having the federal government buy and stockpile drugs and vaccines to treat or protect people against such diseases as anthrax, smallpox and plague, and such poisons as ricin.

The U.S. federal statute defines terrorism as "violent acts or acts dangerous to human life that . . . appear . . . to be intended (i) to intimidate or coerce a civilian population; (ii) to influence the policy of a government by intimidation or coercion; or (iii) to affect the conduct of a government by assassination or kidnapping." It is overwhelmingly apparent that the use of chemical and biological agents to effectuate any political goal falls within this definition. It is therefore incumbent upon the government of the United States to do whatever is necessary, within the bounds of constitutional rights and laws, to protect our citizens from such acts of terrorism. In order to accomplish this objective, it is essential that the medical, scientific, public health, legal, and military experts and authorities who deal with the various aspects of chemical and biological weaponry be fully cognizant of their respective roles and responsibilities.

This reference book has been designed to provide appropriate information to such key individuals, as well as the general public. Each chapter has been written by an outstanding expert in his or her particular field. A working familiarity with the wealth of current knowledge set forth in this volume will contribute immeasurable to the enhancement of public health and safety in the potentially dangerous period in which we live, and perhaps the even more dangerous years that lie ahead.

Chapter 1

Definitions and Identification of Chemical and Biological Weapons Used in Terrorism

Maurice G. Rogev, M.D.

Synopsis

This chapter is dedicated to Gabriella, without whose infinite patience and encouragement I would have despaired of ever being able to complete the task. I also acknowledge the encouragement received from editor-in-chief Dr. Cyril H. Wecht, the assistance of Mr. Maurice Ostroff in editing, correcting and setting out this manuscript and in honor of the memory of the late Mrs. Marcia Ostroff of Raanana.

1.1 Introduction

The global menace of terrorism has taken on a frightening new dimension with the introduction of chemical and biological weapons (CBW) to the terrorist armory. Until recently terrorists used conventional explosives, gunfire and simple person to person violence using sharp instruments.

The potential and actual dangers associated with CBW in the hands of rogue states or terrorists has created an increased fear of the unknown. While military medical and technical personnel are generally trained to meet the challenges of possible CBW attacks, this chapter aims to provide some useful information to civilian forensic medical experts, forensic scientists and law enforcement agencies who have not yet received such training.

1.2 Definitions

terror. An act or acts of violence on civilians who are innocent or uninvolved in order to achieve political, religious or ideological objectives. The means used can be high explosives, toxic chemicals, or biological including microbiological agents. These means are employed by individuals or organizations.

clinical forensic medical examination. The examination of an individual who complains of having suffered an injury to his person by an act of violence. This will include individuals who are not conscious on arrival at the medical facility and cannot provide any information.

forensic autopsy. Examination of a cadaver performed by a qualified or certified forensic pathologist in circumstances that arouse suspicion that death resulted from an act of violence or that the death occurred in an unusual or unexpected manner. When the forensic pathologist has reason to believe that the death may have followed the exposure of the individual to a weapon of mass destruction his function is to confirm or deny this cause of death. The autopsy protocol must include all the relevant pathological details, both macroscopic and microscopic and the results of all the biological, toxicological and microbiological examinations that were carried out.

biological terror agent. A microbiological organism or a toxic substance that can be derived from members of the plant or animal kingdoms and is capable of causing severe illness following incapacity and leading to death. These substances can be used as weapons of mass destruction.

chemical terror agent. A toxic chemical substance capable of causing incapacity, severe illness or death.

Simpson K.G. in 1965[1] applied the following criteria:

- There must be symptoms suggesting poisoning.
- Autopsy findings must exclude any other cause of death but not pathological processes that of themselves would not cause death.

- Analytical findings must confirm the presence of a "noxious thing" or person.

  At that time the available chemical warfare agents were being used from time to time as war weapons but their use as weapons of terror was not yet contemplated.

  The "noxious thing" as described by Simpson only came to include the microbiological and biological agents in respect of their use as terror or war weapons at a much later date.

high-risk autopsy.[2] An autopsy performed on an individual whose death followed exposure to microorganisms that are classified by the European community standards as group 3 and 4 microorganisms. These are the microorganisms are readily transmitted from human to human. Autopsies on such bodies constitute a danger to autopsy personnel and to the environment. The strictest precautions must be taken to prevent such transmission.

LCt50. In the case of airborne dispersal of chemical agents, LCt50 is the concentration of a toxic chemical that is inhaled by a population over a specified time and is lethal in 50 percent of any given population

LD50. A measure of the short-term lethal toxicity of a substance, represented by the amount of the substance administered at one time, which causes the death of 50 percent of a group of test animals.

The CDC (Centers for Disease Control and Prevention) divides biological agents into three categories:[3]

high priority. Anthrax, smallpox, plague, tularemia, botulism, viral hemorrhagic fever.

second priority. Q fever, brucellosis, burkholderia, Mallei, alpha virus, ricin, toxin C1, perfringes, salmonella, shigella, coli, cholera.[4]

low priority. Hanta virus, multidrug resistant tuberculosis, Nipah virus, yellow fever virus.

Immunological procedures used to detect microbiological agents:

IgM. A macromolecule whose presence indicates an infection by a specific pathogen.

IgG. A gamma globulin that protects against bacteria viruses and toxins
RT PCR. Reverse transcription polymerase chain reaction test.
ELISA. The antigen detection enzyme-linked immunosorbent assay.

1.3 Historical Uses of CBW

The following examples of actual past terror attacks using CBW, demonstrate the variety of circumstances in which these attacks can occur.

A. Sarin

Morita et al.[5] and Jortani et al.[6] reported the incident in Matsumoto City, Japan in 1994 when a population was exposed to sarin. This is the first reported case of terrorist use of a nerve gas.

The second recorded incident in which sarin was used as a terror weapon occurred in the Tokyo subway system in March 1995. The terrorists carried the sarin solution, diluted in plastic bags, into the subway trains and punctured the bags with sharpened umbrella tips.[7]

B. Salmonella bacillus

The bacillus was deliberately introduced into salad bars by members of the religious cult Rajneeshee. Seven hundred and fifty-one cases of a gastrointestinal disease were recorded; there were no deaths.[8]

C. Anthrax

Anthrax bacillus spores were sent in an envelope addressed to random addresses in the United States in 2001. The spores were in the form of a white powder. Eleven people exposed to this powder suffered from inhalation anthrax; eleven cases of cutaneous anthrax were recorded; there were five deaths.[9]

D. Ricin

On January 5, 2003, six men suspected of producing ricin in their north London apartment were arrested following arrests of other radicals in Rome, Paris, and London, suspected of planning to carry out terrorist attacks using poisons.

Ricin, generally used in the form of a white powder is extremely toxic and presents a particular threat because of the wide availability of its source material, the castor plant, and the fact that the manufacturing techniques have been described in readily available literature.

Ricin was used in an attempted assassination of a U.S. marshal in 1991. In this case, ricin in a solvent was smeared onto the closed door handle of the marshal's vehicle. No injury was caused.

In 1995, ricin, in the form of a white powder, was found on a man as he entered Canada on his way to the United States. He was also in possession of several weapons.[10]

In September 1978, a pellet containing ricin was shot into the back of Vladimir Kostov in Paris; complete penetration was apparently prevented by Kostov's heavy sweater. No symptoms were noted. The pellet was removed surgically from Vladimir Kostov and found to be intact.[11]

Ten days later, a pellet containing ricin was "shot" through the modified ferrule of an umbrella that functioned as a weapon, into the leg of a Bulgarian exile Georgi Markov, in London. This time the wound was rapidly fatal.[12]

1.4 CBW Agents Available to Terrorists

The criteria by which the type of chemical, biological or microbiological agent can be identified will be the combination of the clinical, pathological and toxicological characteristics of each agent. There are a wide variety of agents that are available to the terrorist.[13]

Table 1.1 lists probable available agents. They are classified according to nature.[14,15]

Cohen and others reported an outbreak of *Giardia lamblia* in Edinburgh, Scotland caused by the deliberate introduction of fecal material into the water supply of an institution.[16]

1.5 Consequences of Exposure to CBW

The victims of a CBW attack will develop clinical syndromes that may respond to the appropriate emergency treatment followed by more prolonged therapy. A patient who survives exposure to CBW agents will develop the characteristic clinical signs and symptoms that ascribed to a particular type of CBW agent.

These patients should undergo the clinical examination that includes laboratory procedures that will enable the identification of the responsible

Table 1.1
CBW Agents Available to Terrorists

- Vesicants
  - sulfur mustard
  - lewisite
  - nitrogen mustards
- Nerve agents
  - tabun
  - sarin
  - soman
  - VX
- Chemical asphyxiants
  - cyanogen chloride
  - hydrogen cyanide
- Respiratory irritants
  - chlorine
  - phosgene
  - diphosgene
- Bio-weapons
  - anthrax
  - smallpox
  - botulism
  - plague
  - brucellosis
  - tularemia
  - hemorrhagic fevers
  - encephalitides
  - Q fever

Those above are regarded as having a high priority as bio-weapons.

- Biological toxins
  - ricin
  - aflatoxin
  - treothecenes
- Fecal matter

CBW agent. The more specific examination using imaging techniques will be valuable in cases that survive the initial exposure and this will diagnose in many cases the presence of complications resulting from exposure to CBW agents.

1.6 Clinical Syndromes Following Exposure to Biological Agents

A. Respiratory syndromes

These syndromes can be caused by the various biological agents. In each of these syndromes the respiratory symptoms are the prominent aspect of the victim's clinical state and will be the ultimate cause of death. Clearly the associated clinical symptoms such as the effects on the eyes, the skin and on the cardiovascular, renal, hepatic and neurological systems may be secondary manifestations and complications that cause serious disabilities and in fatal circumstances may be a contributory factor in the causation of death.

1. Inhalation anthrax

Infection from the weaponized anthrax bacillus can follow the inhalation of the spores. In the alveoli and smaller bronchi the spores germinate to the gram negative bacillus and infection of the lung ensues. There is an incubation period of 1–3 days. Symptoms of the prodromal stage described by Bogucki and Weir[17] include fever, chills, general malaise, headache, and profuse diaphoresis.

There is a nonproductive cough, dyspnoea, chest discomfort and pleuritic pain. Chest x-rays at this stage reveal a mediastinitis and pleural effusions. There is an enlargement of the paratracheal glands (lymph nodes).

In the fulminant stage the pulmonary distress becomes more severe. A pneumonial process can be present in both lungs and may lead to adult distress respiratory syndrome (ADRS), septic shock, cardiorespiratory failure and death.[18,19]

Differential diagnosis. Laboratory diagnosis of the presence of the gram-neg anthrax bacillus will confirm the diagnosis. Samples of blood, sputum or lymph node aspirates will show the presence of the typical gram-neg. bacillus. Staining with Wright or Giemsa will distinguish the anthrax bacillus from other gram negative bacillus by its typical bipolar appearance. Blood culture specimens will also be positive for anthrax bacillus.[21–23] Acute virus respiratory diseases may resemble inhalation anthrax in the early stages. The characteristic x-ray appearance of the widened mediastinum will differentiate anthrax from other respiratory diseases.

The presence of the associated symptoms caused by anthrax will assist in the diagnosis. In many cases cutaneous anthrax lesions will be present. In many cases gastrointestinal symptoms will be present. In the early stages, inhalation anthrax can be differentiated from influenza. Rhinorrhoea, present in influenza, is not present in anthrax nasal congestion.[20]

2. Plague (*Yersina pestis*)

The weaponized gram negative bacillus or coccobacillus constitutes a major threat because of its contagiousness. Pneumonic symptoms are the prominent features of the effect of the weaponized bacillus. The weaponized bacillus in aerosol format can be readily distributed over a wide area. Exposed individuals can inhale the airborne bacillus and this will infect the respiratory system. The incubation period is 1–6 days. Fever, cough producing a bloody thin but rarely purulent sputum, hemoptysis and cyanosis will be prominent. Chest pain, dyspnea, myalgia and malaise will be early symptoms. Plague can be fulminating and lead rapidly to pulmonary consolidation with the clinical signs of pneumonia. In some cases these signs may be absent. ARDS will also develop. Septic shock will lead to death. Death can occur 24–26 hours after symptoms such as nausea, vomiting, diarrhoea and abdominal pain. In areas where there are enlarged lymph nodes the suspicion of bubonic plague will arise. Radiographic examination of the chest can show areas of lung infiltration.

Disseminated intravascular-coagulation will complicate the clinical features. Bubonic plague as a clinical entity, the most frequent finding in epidemic plague outbreaks, is not an intended result of the use of weaponized *Yersina pestis*. This bacillus can be weaponized primarily to infect the lungs. In the setting of a bioterrorist attack on previously healthy patients, the bacillus will cause a rapidly developing pneumonia with hemoptysis.

Laboratory tests carried out on sputum, blood, lymph node aspiration and cerebrospinal fluid will demonstrate *Yersina pestis* bacilli. The tests used (i.e., Gram, Wright and Giemsa stains) will show the typical bipolar gram negative bacilli or coccobacilli.[24–26]

Differential diagnosis. The differential diagnosis includes Hanta, viral lung infections, community acquired pneumonia and influenza-like pneumonia.

3. Tularemia

The weaponized form of *Francisella tularensis* is in the form of an aerosol. This is the most efficient mode of infection. This organism is a facilitative intracellular gram negative coccobacillus. Inhalation causes inhalational or pneumonic tularemia. The incubation period is 3–5 days followed by an abrupt onset.

The symptoms will include the following:

- high fever with chills and rigors
- temperature-pulse dissociation
- headache
- myalgia
- angina like chest tightness
- nonproductive cough, sometimes sputum
- occasional gastrointestinal symptoms
- radiology. early stage: penvascular cuffing; later stages: there will be small discrete pulmonary lesions and widespread bronchopneumonia.

Pulmonary symptoms may intensify leading to a fulminant disease. At this stage radiology reveals wide areas of diffuse infiltrates and areas of consolidation. The illness will progress rapidly to ARDS, pulmonary failure and cardiorespiratory arrest and death.

The diagnosis is confirmed by the laboratory examination of blood culture, sputum and pharyngal and gastric washings. Microscopy after gram, Wright and Giemsa stain reveals a gram negative coccobacillus. Fluorescent antibody techniques are indicated.[27]

Differential diagnosis. Tularemic pneumonia must be differentiated from the following:

- mycoplasma pneumonia
- chlamydia pneumonia
- *C. psittoci* (psittocosis)
- *Legionella pneumophilo* (legionellosis, Legionnaire's disease)
- *Coxiella burnelti* (Q fever)
- *Histoplasma capsulatum* (histoplasmosis)

4. Brucellosis (*Brucella melitensis*)[28,29]

Weaponized Brucella bacilli in an aerosol form can be inhaled in the respiratory tract where flu-like symptoms such as sore throat, tonsillitis and dry cough develop. In most cases the symptoms are mild. The death rate in untreated cases is less than 2 percent.

Brucellosis can be complicated by endocarditis. Although rare the endocarditis can be fatal. The physical examination of the chest wall reveals symptoms and signs consistent with an influenza-type disease.

Brucellosis contracted from the inhalation of the aerolized bacillus will also cause bone and joint involvement.

Laboratory tests may show anemia and thrombocytopenia.

Blood and bone marrow can be cultured but the colony rate is slow and must be incubated for twenty-one days.

Gram, Wright and Giemsa stains are used. The organism is a small gram negative coccobacillus.

Serum can be tested by the ELISA or agglutination tests.

The differential diagnosis includes all the influenza-like illnesses.

5. Q Fever (*Coxiella burnetti*)[30]

This can be a weaponized rickettsial organism that can be inhaled causing acute illness. The illness is generally self limited. It has significant morbidity but a low mortality.

Respiratory tract symptoms are prominent and the illness presents as a flu like syndrome. The incubation is from 3–30 days. Q fever may present in various clinical ways but as a potential bioterrorist agent it cannot easily be differentiated from viral illnesses such as atypical pneumonia.

The clinical symptoms are the following:

- fever
- extreme fatigue
- severe headache
- chills and sweating
- nausea and vomiting
- diarrhea
- cough and physical signs of pneumonia
- non specific rash in 4–18 percent of patients

Laboratory investigations include the following tests:

- full blood count especially platelet counts
- isolation of the organism *C. Burnetti*
- serology:
  - complement fixation
  - immunofluorescence
  - enzyme-linked immunosorbent assay (ELISA)

Differential diagnosis. Q fever must be differentiated from other flu-like syndromes as listed in respect of other microorganisms elsewhere in this chapter.

B. Pulmonary syndromes

1. Ricin

Ricin is derived from the castor bean. It can be produced in liquid or crystalline forms. Inhalation of ricin by experimental animals caused necrosis of the upper and lower respiratory epithelium after a latent period of eight hours. Symptoms such as tracheitis, bronchitis, bronchiolitis and interstitial pneumonia with perivascular arial alveolar edema are dose-dependent and death occurs 36–72 hours after the inhalation exposure.[31]

In humans the inhalation of ricin produces the following symptoms after 4–8 hours:

- fever
- chest tightness
- cough
- dyspnea

- nausea
- arthralgia

Inhaled ricin causes a high-permeability pulmonary edema, adult respiratory distress syndrome and respiratory failure. This leads to deterioration and death from cardiorespiratory failure. There are other routes of ricin exposure: ingestion of ricin by humans causes necrosis of internal organs.[32]

Via intramuscular injection of ricin local necrosis of muscle and regional lymph nodes will be caused.

Ricin intoxication causes severe dehydration, tachycardia, oliguria, hypotension, lethargy and shock results.

The autopsy report on Georgi Markov,[33] who was allegedly assassinated with an injection of ricin, recorded change in the liver. Death results from the combination of all the factors mentioned above and from cardiorespiratory failure.

The diagnosis of ricin as the cause of death depends on the pathological findings of widespread necrotic and hemorrhagic changes in organs such as liver, kidney, intestinal tract and respiratory tract.

2. Staphylococcal enterotoxin B

The weaponized form of this toxin is prepared as an aerosol.

The inhalation causes a respiratory tract disease. Symptoms include

- fever,
- headache,
- myalgia,
- nonproductive cough,
- retrosternal chest pain and, in severe cases, dyspnoea.

The use of these toxins as weapons by terrorists is not of importance if the population is not exposed to massive quantities of the material. When massive quantities are used, fatal results may follow respiratory failure and adult respiratory distress syndrome (ARDS).

Confirmation of the diagnosis depends on examination of clinical samples that include serum, respiratory secretions and urine.

In addition, antibody tests will confirm the diagnosis in acute and convalescent. Sera ELISA tests can also confirm the diagnosis.[34,35]

3. Clostridium perfringens epsilon toxins

Perfringens epsilon (E) toxin is one of a group of four major lethal toxins. It is known to increase capillary permeability.[36] It is capable of causing acute toxemia. The weaponized form of this toxin has potential for mass distribution as an aerosol.

Inhalation of this toxin will cause early irritation of pulmonary epithelium cells. Severe pulmonary edema may result. The toxin readily spreads in the circulation and can cause severe renal cardiac and central nervous system damage.

The clinical symptoms caused by the damage to the respiratory tract, including the lungs, will resemble other respiratory syndromes and lead to respiratory failure and ARDS.[37]

C. Fevers and rashes

All these viruses have either already been weaponized or are potential viruses for weaponization.

1. Smallpox (a DNA virus *Orthopoxvirus*)

The smallpox virus has already undergone weaponization.[60,61] Clinical symptoms include:[62]

- incubation period 7–17 days
- high fever, malaise, prostration, headache, backache
- maculopapular rash on oral, pharyngeal mucosa, face, forearms, trunk and legs
- vesicular rash, later pustular 1–2 days
- pustules round tense deep
- crusts after 8–9 days
- encephalitis occasionally
- death in second week of illness secondary to toxemia

Approximately 10 percent of cases smallpox occur in a fatal hemorrhagic form. The symptoms of the hemorrhagic form are

- shorter incubation period
- high fever
- abdominal pain
- headache
- petechiae and hemorrhages in skin or mucous membranes
- death occurs 5–6 days after the rash

In malignant (usually fatal) forms, the incubation period shorter as in hemorrhagic form; there are confluent soft flat velvety vesicular lesions; and, in the event of survival, lesions peel away leaving no scabs.

Variola minor is a lesser virulent form of the disease. This occurs in people with partial immunity from earlier vaccination.

Differential diagnosis. Cases of smallpox (Variolar major) must be differentiated from varicella chicken pox. This can done on the basis of symptoms.

- In smallpox all lesions on the skin progress at the same rate.
- Varicella (chicken pox) lesions progress in clusters and four stages of lesions can be present at the same time.
- Varicella lesions concentrate on the trunk and less on the limbs and not on the palms and soles.
- Smallpox is distributed centrifugally.[63]

Laboratory tests that confirm the diagnosis of smallpox can be performed on specimens taken from the vesicles, pustules or from the scabs. Care must be taken during the collection of specimens. Collection should be made by someone who has been vaccinated against smallpox.

Specimens can be collected on cotton swabs or the collection of scabs with a forceps. The specimen is then placed in a vacutainer tube enclosed in a second watertight container. The specimens should be sent to institutes with high containment facilities for diagnosis. Biological assays such as PCR, and restriction fragment length polymorphism can be done in such highly specialized laboratories.

The definitive identification of the virus depends on growing the virus in cell culture or on chorioallantoic egg membrane.

The orthopoxvirus can then be identified on electronmicroscopic examination. During the second half of the incubation period antibodies to the virus can be quantified by hemagglutination inhibition, complement fixation, neutralization and gel precipitation techniques.

Histological examination of biopsy specimens taken from the intraepidermal vesicles in the skin and mucous membranes are the most dominant features of smallpox.[64]

The histological examination of the earlier stages of the rash shows

- hyperemia, swelling of capillary endothelium and perivascular infiltrates of lymphocytes and histiocytes in the upper dermis;
- rupture of the membranes between the degenerating epithelial cells leads to multiloculated vesicles;
- ballooning of cells in the lower levels of the stratum spinosum and some degenerating cells fuse into giant cells with 2–4 nuclei; and
- Guarnieri's bodies (i.e., eosinophilic intracytoplasmic inclusion bodies) present in the ballooned epithelial cells.

Secondary infection in the pustular stage may cause a number of complications, including[65]

- keratitis and secondary bacteriological inflammation of the eyes leading to blindness;
- laryngitis, bronchitis and bronchopneumonia (inflammation of the respiratory tree);
- encephalitis (inflammation of the brain);
- osteomyelitis (inflammation in the long bones of the skeleton); and
- orchitis (inflammation of the testicle).

2. Hemorrhagic fever virus syndromes[66,67]

There are a number of hemorrhagic fever viruses that have undergone weaponization. This process can convert a virus that is naturally limited in its distribution and capacity to cause disease, into a virus that can be spread intentionally in areas where the populations have never faced this type of health challenge.

Virus disease such as Ebola hemorrhagic fever, Manbury hemorrhagic fever, Lassa fever, New World hemorrhagic fever, Rift Valley fever, yellow fever, Omsk fever and Kyasanur forest fever were originally described in limited geographical zones. In nature these diseases are vector borne. These vectors may be mosquitoes, rodents or ticks. The viruses are readily transferred from these vectors to human hosts and from human to human. These are the epidemiological characteristics of the virus in nature. When these viruses are weaponized and aerosolized, their contagious capacity and their pathological properties may be enhanced:

- high morbidity and mortality
- potential for person-to-person transfer
- low infective dose with large outbreaks.
- effective vaccines not available or in limited supply.

Any one of the hemorrhagic fever viruses is a potential or a current weaponized aerosolized CBW agent. The agent has a very high capacity for causing a high morbidity and mortality.

- pathogenesis; the hemorrhagic symptoms are caused by vascular instability and decreased vascular integrity in all forms of VHF
- Blood pressure is decreased.
- Shock may supervene.
- cutaneous flushing and conjunctival effusion
- Hemorrhage is inconstant.
- Disseminated intravascular coagulation occurs occasionally.
- Specific organs can be effected depending on the type of virus; e.g.:
  - filovirus VHF. The kidneys will be affected in Ebola and Marbury virus infections.
  - Hanta virus VHF. The lungs will be affected causing a severe pulmonary syndrome
  - yellow fever virus VHF. The liver will be severely affected causing liver necrosis and jaundice in severe cases

Circulatory disturbances with increased injury to vascular integrity will be an important pathological feature in all cases of VHF.

Platelet function will be affected due to a decrease in platelet totals in the blood.

The following are the prodromal symptoms that are common to all the VHF syndromes.

- There is an incubation period of a few days.
- Fever, myalgia and increasing prostration herald the onset of the illness.
- Dizziness, photophobia, hyperesthesia are frequent symptoms.
- Abdominal and chest pain will be present.
- Gastrointestinal symptoms such as anorexia vomiting will vary in intensity. Other gastrointestinal symptoms will be present.

The examination of the ill patient will elicit symptoms and signs of the established disease.

- The patient is acutely ill.
- Conjunctival suffusion will be present.
- There will be tenderness on palpation of the muscles and the abdominal wall.
- Hypotension and tachycardia will be present.
- There may be petechiae in the axillae and on other areas of the body.
- The skin over the head and thorax will be reddened and suffused.
- Periorbital edema will be present.
- ASR. (aminotransferase) levels will be elevated.
- There will be hemoconcentration due to vascular leaks.

In the seriously ill patient more severe symptoms will develop:

- shock
- multifocal bleeding
- CNS symptoms—encephalopathy
- coma and convulsions may develop

Symptoms due to the responsible virus will be superimposed on the VHF clinical diagnosis

a. Lassa fever. Characteristic symptoms include:

- bleeding in 15–30 percent of cases
- maculopapular rash in light skinned patients
- effusions are common
- male dominant pericarditis

- blood counts normal or slightly elevated
- platelet counts normal or less
- deafness in 20 percent cases
- high level of viremia or high AST levels predict fatal outcome.

b. Rift Valley fever manifests in one of four syndromes:

- febrile myalgia
- high fever. with liver involvement
- retinal vasculitis with edema, hemorrhages and infarction
- viral encephalitis

c. Hanta virus pulmonary syndrome. In the cardiopulmonary phase there is

- lowered blood pressure
- tachycardia, tachypnea and hypoxemia
- early radiographic pulmonary edema
- decompensation may lead to hypoxemia and respiratory failure
- cough may develop late in the illness
- late radiography shows severe edema in central as well as peripheral lung areas
- plural effusions
- thrombocytopenia
- disseminated intravascular coagulation
- severe kidney involvement.

The laboratory diagnosis can be made by using the following:

- IgM testing of serum
- IgC ELISA usually indicative of viral infection
- RT PCR (polimerase chain reaction) usually positive in first 7–9 days of the illness

Differential diagnosis. The differential diagnosis includes abdominal conditions. Meningococemia pyelonephritis, rickettsial disease, plague, sepsis, tularemia, influenza and relapsing fever.

d. Yellow fever virus. The clinical syndrome will include prominent hepatic necrosis. There is a phase of uremia. In a later phase jaundice, hemorrhages, black vomit, anuria and terminal delirium develop. Renal failure occurs with a rise in blood urea levels. There are marked liver function test aberrations.

e. Ebola and Marburg viruses. Symptoms are[68]

- continued fever with diarrhea
- chest pain with cough
- maculopapular rash in first seven days.
- desquamation of lesions
- bleeding from skin and mucosal sites found in most cases; some fatal cases may not bleed
- edema of face, neck, scrotum
- hepatomegaly
- secondary bacterial infection may occur
- late hepatitis, uvectis, orchitis

Laboratory findings are[69]

- leukopenia
- platelet count below 50,000
- disseminate intravascular coagulation
- serum levels of alanine and aspartate aminotransferase rise progressively
- jaundice
- pancreatitis may be suspected if the serum amylase increases
- proteinuria
- shock and decreased renal function

The definitive diagnosis of the Ebola or Marburg virus depends on detecting a high concentration of the virus in the blood. The ELISA tests detect the antigen.

Virus isolation is an effective diagnostic tool.

RT-PCR tests are sensitive to the presence of the virus antigen.

IgM and IgC antibodies are detected by ELISA and by fluorescent antibody tests.

Skin biopsies in autopsy diagnosis in both virus diseases are useful.

D. Neurological syndromes

1. Botulism

The toxins produced by the *Cl. botulinum* has been weaponized and is available in an aerosolized form.[82–85] The toxin can be inhaled, ingested or infect open wounds.[86]

The toxin binds irreversibly to the peripheral cholinergic synapses causing blockage of acetylcholine release, resulting in paralysis.

Symptoms start 12–24 hours after exposure.

- clinical symptoms descending flaccid paralysis
- dysphagia
- dysarthria
- diplopia
- ptosis

The differential diagnosis of the acute paralysis includes the following:

- Guillain-Barré syndrome. Acute severe fulminant polyradionucleoneuropathy
- Lambert-Eaton syndrome (i.e., myasthenic syndrome)
- tick paralysis
- myasthenia gravis

Laboratory diagnosis:

- Serum feces gastric specimens for toxin assays
- Vomitus for toxin assays

2. Mycotoxins (fungi)

a. Aflatoxin. This toxin, derived from the fungi *Aspergillus flavus* and *Aspergillus parasiticus*, has been weaponized (notably Iraq, 1991). The striking pathological result of exposure to this toxin is in its causation of hepatocellular cancer in humans. However as a weaponized agent, aflatoxin can cause acute aflatoxicosis, vomiting, abdominal pain, hepatitis leading to death.[87]

b. Trichothecens. These toxins are produced by the *fusarium* and *stachybotris* species. Acute toxicosis from inhalation of stachybotris mycotoxin is characterized by sore throat, blood nasal discharge, cough, high-grade fever and chest tightness.

Ingested, these toxins cause necrotic ulcers in nose, mouth, throat, stomach, intestines.

1.7 Clinical Syndromes Following Exposure to Chemical Agents

A. Pulmonary syndromes

The differential diagnosis of the particular etiological agent causing the pulmonary syndromes can be difficult. Associated pathological effects on other parts of the body typical of those caused by a particular chemical agent will facilitate the diagnosis of the particular chemical agent that caused the pulmonary syndrome.

Factors that influence the site and nature of the pathological damage caused to the respiratory system include

- the concentration of the chemical agent in the atmosphere,
- the inherent toxicity of the agent,
- the duration of exposure to the agent, and
- the water solubility of the agent.

1. Ammonia

This agent is readily available for use as a terror weapon. It can inflict major damage to the respiratory system.

A water-soluble chemical, it reacts with water to form ammonium hydroxide. This can cause widespread chemical burns to the eyes, the mucosal surfaces of the mouth and the upper and lower airways. Lung parenchymal damage is readily caused leading to respiratory failure.

Inhalation of excessive amounts of ammonia can lead to poisoning. The exposure of the lung parenchyme to ammonia causes a chemical pneumonitis and to chronic bronchitis. Symptoms can also indicate damage to the esophageal-gastrointestinal tract.

Severe symptoms such as hypotension, shock, metabolic acidosis, hemopoietic, renal and hepatic dysfunction and disseminated intravascular coagulation may precede death.[38,39]

2. Phosgene

This is a "lung choke" agent. This gas causes severe injury to the lung parenchyma. Used in the first world war as a chemical warfare agent, it is now used in many industrial chemical processes and is readily available and cheap.[40]

The use of phosgene as a terror weapon is a possibility that must be considered.

The pulmonary syndrome that results from exposure to phosgene has the following symptoms.

- Mild phosgene exposure produces cough, chest tightness, dyspnoea.
- Moderate exposure produces lacrimation, severe cough, sputum, dyspnoea.
- Severe exposure produces pulmonary edema.

These symptoms follow an asymptomatic period of up to 24–72 hours. A chronic state may last months to years. The symptoms of that state are exceptional dyspnoea and reduced exercise tolerance.

- Exposure to phosgene may aggravate pre-existing obstructive pulmonary disease.
- The acute very severe exposure to phosgene of the gastrointestinal tract, hemorrhage and hepatic, splenic and renal necrosis.
- The acute very severe exposure to phosgene leads to a high-permeability pulmonary edematous ARDS that may be fatal. The LCt50 of phosgene is 3,200 mg·min/m^3.

3. Chlorine

Like phosgene, chlorine is a "lung choke" agent. Inhalation of chlorine is the exclusive mode of exposure. It has a World War I record.

The agent does not need to be weaponized; it is a weapon.[41]

Chlorine spreads rapidly throughout the lung and effects mainly the central airways, damaging the mucous membranes. The pulmonary symptoms are the prominent features of this syndrome:

- cough and an increasing choking sensation
- chest tightness, more masked in people with hyperactive airways
- nasal irritation and ocular irritation will be the first indication of chlorine exposure
- hoarseness and aphemia
- exceptional dyspnoea
- inspiratory cough
- moderate exposure leads to pulmonary edema in twenty-four hours
- severe exposure leads to pulmonary edema in 30–60 minutes.

Sudden death from laryngospasm may follow.[42]

4. Chemical asphyxiants ("blood agents")

These are hydrogen cyanide (HC) and cyanogen choride (CK).[43,44] They are available now and used in many industrial processes.

The only occasion that HC was used as a chemical warfare agent was during the first world war. The cyanide compounds are very volatile. Their use as a CW outdoors is limited. In confined spaces these compounds are very toxic and inhalation can be fatal.

The cyanide compounds affect the use of oxygen in the tissues.

The LCt50 for hydrogen cyanide is 500–2,500 mg·min/m^3.

The LCt50 for cyanogen chloride is 1.1 g mm/m^3.

The LD50 for intravenous hydrogen cyanide is 1 mg/kg.

The LD50 for liquid dermal exposure 100 mg/kg.

The pulmonary syndromes that result from inhalation of hydrogen cyanide or cyanogen chloride are mainly caused by the development of hypoxia. The pulmonary stage in severe exposure to inhalation is relatively short and leads to deterioration of general body function. Symptoms include:

- immediate pulmonary symptoms
- hypertension followed by hypotension tachycardia
- loss of consciousness, apnoea, secondary cardiac arrest; death can occur within minutes;

Late symptoms following severe exposure include CNS, depression, coma, apnea and death.

Patients exposed to lower concentration of cyanide compounds or to dermal exposure will develop symptoms more slowly and they will be less serious. They may include[45,46]

- a smell of bitter almonds;
- hyperventilation, headache, dyspnoea, respiratory depression, pulmonary edema;
- in the central nervous system: anxiety, personality changes, agitation, seizures;
- flushing, diaphoresis, weakness;
- irritation of nasal, oral, respiratory mucosa.

Clearly only those patients who survive exposure to low concentrations of cyanide compounds will present themselves for clinical examination.

Diagnosis. This depends on the clinical history and the physical examination. Whole blood cyanide level assays confirm the diagnosis.[47]

5. Vesicants or blistering agents

Vesicants such as sulfur mustard (SM), nitrogen mustard (NM), Lewisite and phosgene cause serious and possibly fatal clinical states in people exposed to these chemical agents. SM has a smell of garlic. Inhalation of these vesicants cause the most serious of the clinical states. Damage to the respiratory tract results, leading to respiratory pathology that can be immediately fatal.

Other symptoms can result from exposure to the vesicants by direct contact with the eyes or skin or via the esophageal gastrointestinal tract by ingestion causing serious discomfort and disability and absorption of vesicants causing respiratory and cardiovascular pathology.

a. Sulfur mustard (SM). The respiratory symptoms appear early after exposure to SM.[48,49] The early symptoms are the following.

- irritation or burning of the nares
- epistaxis
- sinus pain
- irritation of nasopharynx
- tracheobronchitis several hours after exposure.

Later symptoms may result from pathological changes in the whole length of the respiratory tract especially after moderate to high dose exposure.

- bronchospasm
- bronchial obstruction
- hemorrhagic pulmonary edema
- respiratory failure
- secondary bacterial pneumonia

Symptoms that are caused by these pathological changes:

- severe cough
- dyspnoea
- hemorrhagic pulmonary edema

Death from SM is caused by respiratory failure with superimposed bacterial infection. Deaths from SM exposure are uncommon; in military experiences, the reported rate was less than 5 percent casualties.

The LD50 of sulfur mustard is 100 mg/kg. This is approximately 1–1.5 teaspoons of liquid. Exposure to vapor causing airway injury causes damage to the mucosa of the respiratory tract starting with the upper airways and reaches the lower airways. As the concentration of the vapor increases the extent of mucosal epithelial necrosis varies from mild to severe.

A pseudomembrane made up of inflammatory exudate forms in the respiratory tract from the larynx to the lower elements of the bronchial tract. Bronchoscopy reveals the presence and extent of the pseudomembrane and the presence of complications caused by necrosis of the bronchial wall leads to scarring and narrowing of the bronchial lumen leading to obstruction. Bronchopneumonia and bronchiectasis are frequent complications.

Repeated bougienage of tracheal and main bronchial stenosis may be needed.

In these circumstances bronchoscopic procedures will be both diagnostic and therapeutic.[50]

B. Eye lesions

The eye symptoms due to SM exposure, while not liable to be fatal can be very painful and the pathological changes caused by SM can cause limited vision and blindness.

Of 7,000 SM victims in the first world war, the eyes were the most frequently damaged organ (86 percent). There is a latent period between exposure and the appearance of symptoms:

- 2–8 hours after contact feeling of sand grains in the eye
- painful sensation with tearing
- eyelids and conjunctiva swell to point of closure
- hypersensitivity to light and lid cramp and practical loss of vision.
- corneal damage
- preliminary opacity ore common than necroses
- ulceration
- conjunctivitis
- blepharospasm
- iritis and mucous discharge

These symptoms appear in the acute stage. At a later period there is a keratitis and keratopathy that may occur 8–40 years after exposure and lead to a vision loss.

The none effect dose of SM on the eyes is 12 mg·min/m^3. The incapacitating dose is subjective depending on the individual 200 mg·min/m^3.

If the ulceration of the cornea is severe this may lead to perforation and subsequent vision loss.[51]

C. Skin lesions[52]

Although the skin lesions resulting from SM exposure are the most prominent they are not of themselves fatal. The skin lesions can be disfiguring and painful and in rarer cases lead to malignant change.

Approximately 20 percent of SM is absorbed by the skin. SM rapidly breaks down in the extra cellular water of the body. The compounds quickly bind to intracellular enzymes and nuclei acids causing irreversible cell damage.

SM is an alkylating agent and reacts readily with DNA, RNA and proteins. The effects of the alkylation of the biological molecules in the cell lead to severe disorganization of their biological functions. SM is a cell poison and is toxic to mitotic cells. Cytostasis (cell inactivity), mutation and slow cell death may result. The skin epithelium is a target because of the proliferating basal cell layer. The poisoning of the basal cell layer of the skin is the factor that directly leads to the separation of the basal layer of the skin leading to the formation of the blisters or bullae. The effects of SM are moisture, temperature and concentration dependent.

The pathological effects of SM on the skin:

- separation of the epidermis from the underlying dermis
- edema from vascular permeability
- inflammatory changes
- vascular leakage of fluid and accumulation under the separated epidermis
- bullae
- blisters

The symptoms caused by skin exposure to SM:

- skin rashes 4–16 hours after exposure
- skin swollen and reddened 24 hours
- development of mild to moderate erythema
- within twenty-four hours, erythematous areas begin to develop into blisters or bullae.[53] These bullae can be extensive and reach to the dermis.

Rupture of the blisters and bullae lead to denudation of the skin. The exposed skin is open to infections. Infected ulcers and boils are frequent.

Nikolsky's sign is elicited by scratching the skin surrounding the bullae or the denuded area of skin that closely resembles a "burn" or bullae or blisters appear because the intra-epidermal blisters are formed because of the effect of SM on the basal cells of the epidermis.

The healing of the blisters and bullae that are not secondarily infected will take about a week. The necrotic tissue of the blister or bulla sloughs off after a week and a granulating process starts at the border.

If the exposure of SM to the skin has been excessive a deep bulla may develop in 6–8 hours. There is necrosis which reaches the subcutis.

Ulcers develop that become infected and heal slowly. The ulcers may take months to heal and leave deep marginal pigmentation. The denudation of the skin may take 6–8 days (mean). The average time for healing was nineteen days.[54]

D. Neurological syndromes[70–73]

This group includes a number of organophosphate compounds:

- tabun LD50 1.9 mg/70 kg LCt50 400 mg·min/m^3
- sarin LD50 1.7 mg/70 kg LCt50 100 mg·min/m^3
- soman LD50 350 mg/70 kg LCt50 50 mg·min/m^3
- VX LD50 10 mg/70 kg LCt50 10 mg·min/m^3

These substances are acetylcholinesterase inhibitors. The four substances mentioned above are members of a wider group of organophosphate compounds.[74] Included in this group are organophosphate insecticide analogues such as

- parathion,
- malathion,
- dieldrin, and
- methylparathion.

These are the most frequently used organophosphate insecticides in agriculture. They are lethal if humans are exposed to even small quantities.. The other organophosphates such as taban, sarin, soman and VX have been used as chemical warfare nerve agents and also as terrorist agents.

The syndromes that follow exposure to the organophosphate compounds consist of symptoms that result from the combination of three processes that occur simultaneously.

1. Muscarinic

These effects are caused by interference with cholinergic synaptic functions at the neuroeffector junction. This is due to the over stimulation of the synaptic end-plate by the accumulation of acetylcholine.

- miosis
- hypersecretion of salivary, sweat, lachrimal and bronchial glands
- broncho constriction
- nausea
- vomiting
- cramp-like abdominal pain
- urinary and fecal incontinence
- bradycardia

2. Nicotinic

These effects result from over stimulation by accumulated acetylcholine at skeletal myonuclear junctions and autonomic ganglia.

These effects include:

- fasciculation
- skeletal muscle twitching
- weakness
- flaccid paralysis
- obscure parasympathetic effects
- hypertension due to adrenal stimulation

3. Central nervous system effects

The nerve agent can be inhaled once it has become aerosolized. Tabun, sarin and soman are readily volatile and the danger they present is mainly from inhalation of aerosolized particles.

VX is much less volatile and remains in liquid form. This agent is more readily absorbed through the skin. As long as the agents tabun, sarin and soman remain liquid they will also be absorbed through the skin.

Acetylcholine is a neurotransmitter in the parasympathetic nervous system and in the muscles. The brain's ascending activating system is also cholinergic, controlling consciousness, and it transmits control from the midbrain to the cerebral cortex. Acetylcholine is stored in the synaptic vesicles in the neurons. On depolarization it is released into the synaptic cleft and reaches the specific molecule in the sarcolemma of the distal neurons and transmits the signal to the distal neurons.

The enzyme acetylcholinesterase is found in the synaptic cleft and breaks down the acetylcholine to choline and water. The choline is transported back to the axon to be reconstituted as acetylcholine. Thus the synapse is prepared for the next signal transmission. The nerve agent (anticholinesterase) disrupts this cycle by combining with the acetylcholinesterase and prevents it from clearing acetylcholine from the synaptic cleft.

Toxic levels of acetylcholine accumulation in the synaptic cleft and paralyzes the cholinergic synaptic transmission.

Cholinergic synapses are found in the central nervous system, at the termination of somatic nerves, in ganglion synapses of the autonomous nerves, at parasympathetic nerve endings and at some sympathetic nerve endings such as those in the sweat glands.

In "ageing" the organophosphate compound and the enzyme cannot be separated.

While the anticholinesterase action of the organophosphate compounds can be prevented or reversed by the antidotes such as atropine sulfate, pralidoxime, pyridoxamine and physostigmine, once the processes of "ageing" have occurred, these antidotes are not effective.

E. Diagnosis of nerve agent poisoning

The symptoms depend on the vapor concentrations to which the victim was exposed.

1. General symptoms

- low vapor concentration inhalation
  - miosis and visual disturbances (dim vision)
  - rhinorrhea
  - dyspnoea

  These symptoms may appear within a few seconds to minutes.

- inhalation of high vapor concentrations
  - loss of consciousness within a few minutes

- seizures
- flaccid paralysis
- miosis
- copious secretions
- involuntary micturition or defecation
- death

- skin exposure to liquid nerve agents
  - small droplet on skin no effects for eighteen hours
  - clinical effects 2–3 hours after thorough decontamination
  - percutaneous absorption depends on site and temperature
  - muscular fasciculation and sweating at contact site
  - larger droplets cause gastrointestinal effect
  - malaise and weakness
  - droplets with lethal doses cause loss of consciousness, seizures, flaccid paralysis, apnoea
  - sudden onset after thirty minutes.

2. Specific system symptoms

- nervous system symptoms
  - seizure activity which may develop into status epilepticus
  - subtle CNS changes persist for some weeks after exposure
  - complete recovery if severe anoxia has not caused residual brain damage
  - psychological symptoms (e.g., depression, insomnia, irritability, nervousness, impairment of attention)
  - EEC changes present

- pulmonary symptoms
  - copious bronchial glands secretion
  - broncospasm
  - weakness and paralysis of respiratory muscles

- cardiovascular symptoms
  - increase vagal nerve effect on heart rate
  - slowing down of heart rate (bradycardia)

  - cardiac function abnormalities
  - idioventricular dysrhythmia
  - multiform ventricular extrasystoles
  - Corsades de Tors point
  - ventricular fibrillation
  - complete heart-block

- miosis (frequently the signal symptom of nerve agent exposure)
  - appears rapidly if eye exposed to splash of nerve agent
  - may get unilateral miosis
  - deep aching pain
  - constricted pupil or visual disturbance
  - dim vision from constricted pupil or inhibition of cholinergic fibres of the retina or central nervous system.

3. Differential diagnosis[75]

- *Cl. botulinum*
- paralytic fish poisoning
- ciguatera bacterial fish infection
- totrodotoxin (TTX fungal) poisoning
- myasthenia gravis (in chronic nerve agent poisoning)

4. Laboratory diagnosis

- Reduction of anticholinesterase activity plasma, reduction of red cell cholinesterase to less than 50 percent of normal,[76] activity in red cells less than 50 percent of normal. These low percentages confirm the diagnosis of nerve agent exposure or organophosphate insecticide exposure .
- Blood plasma cholinesterase values below 20 i.u. (normal is 100 i.u.)[77]
- Red blood cell cholinesterase inhibition test is the best diagnostic test. Severe symptoms occur when 70 percent inhibition is recorded.[78,79]

The test is not specific for this type of poisoning. Other causes include acute hepatitis, cirrhosis advanced carcinoma, first trimester of pregnancy, myocardial infarction and pulmonary embolism.

5. Conventional injuries and nerve agent intoxication

The combination of these two clinical aspects in the same casualty aggravates the prognosis in respect of each of these states.

Berkenstadt and others[80] stressed the pathological interactions between these two types of injury, a neck or a chest injury there is an inability to wear a mask.

The absorption of nerve agents by the body causes muscarinic, nicotincic and central nerve system pathology that intensifies the hypovolemic shock and other symptoms caused by the conventional wounds.

6. Symptoms

The synergistic effect of trauma and nerve agent intoxication was discussed by Abraham et al.[81] They stress the serious consequences of this joint pathology. The nerve agent reduces the respiratory and cardiovascular ability of the body to compensate for the shock and hypovolemia caused by the trauma.

The trauma to the body with tissue lacerations facilitates the entry of the nerve agent into the body. There are essential diagnostic steps that must be followed.

- The anamnesis must be meticulous.
- Symptoms and signs of both the nerve agent and the trauma must be recorded.
- Severe muscle weakness should be noted.
- Assess adequacy of the antidotes given before admission to the emergency ward.

F. Gastrointestinal symptoms

Exposure to SM causes unspecific general symptoms:

- nausea
- vomiting
- abdominal pains

- headache
- fatigue
- apathy
- diarrhea
- weight loss
- tachycardia

SM either through ingestion or penetration through the skin into the tissues of the body can produce these symptoms parallel to the development of the skin and eye lesions.

SM also depresses the bone marrow leading to effects on the leucopoietic cells. There is release of lymphocytes into the system with the depletion of the spleen and lymph nodes; while the hemopoietic cells are resistant, leukopoeinia appears in the blood stream; in severe cases, agranulocytosis occurs.[55]

Differential diagnosis . The diagnosis of the pulmonary syndrome due to exposure to SM is based on the pulmonary symptoms as well as the totality of symptoms affecting the eyes, the skin and the gastrointestinal tract.

This pulmonary syndrome has to be differentiated from the syndromes resulting from the exposure to other vesciants such as nitrogen, mustard, Lewisite and the irritating chemical effects of chlorine gas and phosgene.

The laboratory confirmation of SM was reported by Drasch and others.[56]

1. Lewisite (chlorovinyldichloroarsine)

This vesicant causes immediate symptoms due to the absence of the need for cyclization. Sulfur mustard requires cyclization which necessitates a delay of some hours before action starts. Lewisite inhibits SH (percentage saturation of hemoglobin) group-containing enzymes and disrupts energy pathways, resulting in the depletion of adenosine triphosphate and cell death.

The antidote BAL (2,3-dimercaptopropanol) effectively stops the action of lewisite. The knowledge that there is an effective antidote to lewisite may reduce the possibility that lewisite may be used as a terrorist weapon.

The pulmonary syndromes caused by lewisite are similar to those of SM. The development of pulmonary symptoms is more rapid and early respiratory obstruction from the formation of the pseudo membrane in the respiratory tract may necessitate early intubation and removal of the obstructions. Other complications such as bronchopneumonia and bronchiectosis can occur, but with earlier development than in cases of SM poisoning.

The other regions of the body such as the eyes, skin, alimentary tract will be more rapidly and more seriously affected.

Permanent blindness from corneal scarring can occur if lewisite is not removed rapidly from the eye.

Lewisite shock caused by intravascular volume depletion secondary to capillary leaking can be fatal. This may also lead to hepatic necrosis and renal failure from hypoperfusion.[57,58]

2. Nitrogen mustard (NM)

This vesicant has been used as a chemical war agent (e.g., in the first world war, 1914–18).

Since that date the antineoplastic properties of NM have been employed to treat many forms of cancer. NM is not regarded as a chemical war agent at present. It is readily available in hospital pharmacies. NM is less potent than SM but the consequences of exposure are similar.[59]

1.8 Autopsies and Special Pathological Findings

When the victim does not survive the exposure in the immediate post-exposure time frame, or does not respond to the more prolonged therapy, the cause of death necessitates a full autopsy. The autopsy must include a detailed description of the external appearance of the body. In this chapter only those special pathological findings relating to the individual CBW agents will be described.

A full internal examination must include histopathology, microbiology and toxicology. The following samples are to be taken for laboratory examination: blood, urine, stomach contents, eye fluids, and cerebrospinal fluids.

Specimens must be taken from organs such as liver, kidney, heart, lung and brain.

The routine autopsy examination procedures are included in standard forensic pathology textbooks.

A. Infections of the respiratory tract

1. Inhalation anthrax

There is a widened mediastinum due to bilateral enlargement of hilar glands. There are bilateral pleural effusions. There is an hemorrhagic destructive pneumonia. Ulceration of the airways is marked with alveolar distension by edema fluid. Many gram positive bacilli are found.

2. Pneumonic plague

This presents as a spreading hemorrhagic bronchopneumonia. There are enlarged hilar glands. Inguinal glands and other glands such as cervical or pelvic may be enlarged in some cases.

3. Francisella pneumonia

Ulcerative bronchitis with a fibrinous pneumonia is present.

4. Smallpox

Apart from the diagnostic skin rash, there are secondary complications:

- keratitis
- laryngitis
- bronchitis
- bronchopneumonia
- encephalitis
- osteomyelitis
- orchitis

5. Tularemia

Pneumonia causes a bronchopneumonia. This starts as a pneumonitis that rapidly develops into the pneumonic stage. Complications such as meningitis, endocarditis, pericarditis, osteomyelitis occur. The pneumonia can be accompanied by endotoxic shock. This shock may be the terminal factor causing death. The autopsy will confirm this.

B. The effects of chemical agents on the respiratory tract

1. Vesicants

All vesicants produce the same pathological changes in the respiratory tract. They differ in the degree of toxicity and in the extent of damage they can cause.

Severe pseudomembranes inflammation of the trachea, bronchial tubes and broncho-pneumonic complications such as tracheal or main bronchus obstruction by the pseudomembrane by causing suffocation may be the cause of death.

The inflammatory changes associated with the pseudomembrane may lead to bronchiectasis in patients who develop long-term symptoms.

The other associated changes in the body will be typical blisters and bullae and blisters on the skin and pathological changes in the eyes. There may be a membranous film inside the ascending colon, cloudy swelling of the myocardium, liver and kidneys and enlargement of the spleen may be present.

2. Microscopic examination of SM

Specimens of tissues removed from lesion either by biopsy from the patient or taken from the body at autopsy reveal the following findings:

- Skin lesions in erythematous stage show inter and intracellular edema and nuclear pyknosis of the epidermis. Perivascular lymphocyte infiltration is present in the dermis.
- Bullous lesions are subepidermal and infiltrated with leukocytes and lymphocytes.
- Ulcerating lesions of the epidermis are necrotic with severe inflammatory cell response.
- The pigmented lesions show hyperactivity of the melanocytes with increased melanin in the dermis.

The microscopic examination of autopsy lung tissue shows pseudomebranous layers of fibrin and inflammatory cells that block the excretory ducts of the mucous glands. Blockage of mucous ducts is followed by necrosis.

The substances such as chlorine, phosgene, ammonia produce widespread epithelial damage and death from pulmonary edema, if these substances are released in high concentrations.

Bronchial and bronchiolar irritation causes inflammation leading to bronchiectasis.

3. Chemical asphyxiants: Cyanide compounds

The hypostasis postmortem lividity will be brick red or deeply cyanotic there may be black vomit around the lips. The body will have a bitter almond like smell. The stomach lining may be eroded with a black surface, or be streaked with dark red lines. Erosions and hemorrhages from the walls may lead to dark blood in the stomach.

Esophagus may show mild erosive damage.

Toxicology will reveal the cyanide and determine the amount in the body.[88]

C. The effects of nerve agents

The autopsy macroscopic findings are nonspecific and in themselves do not establish the diagnosis of death caused by the various nerve agents. There is deep cyanosis, pulmonary edema may be marked. Other signs of an acute cardiorespiratory failure is present. The miosis which is an early clinical sign in the living does not persist more than a few hours after death.

The excessive accumulation of sweat on the skin is also valid in the living patient. After death the sweat on the skin is only present for a short period of time.

Microscopic examination of brain and other tissues

In experimental treatment of animals with nerve agents hypoxic changes are found in the frontal cortex, entorhinal center, amygdala, caudate nucleus and the hippocampus. These changes are also seen in humans who die after status epilepticus from other causes.

Heart hemorrhage, myofiber necrosis and myocarditis are present.[89]

Toxicology will provide a clear diagnosis of nerve agent exposure in blood examination to determine the presence of the nerve agent.

Determination of the red blood cell acetylcholinesterase inhibition and the serum cholinesterase inhibition percentages, or both, will confirm the diagnosis. In acute parathion poisoning the percentage inhibition will be 30–50 percent of normal.

Appendix
Foiled Osmium Tetroxide Attack Reported (April 6, 2004)

After preparation of this chapter had been completed, breaking news was reported of a planned CBW attack in London that was foiled by U.K. and U.S. intelligence agents. The chemical believed to be involved is osmium tetroxide, a corrosive substance used by scientists to stain materials and as a catalyst.

The suspects were allegedly sympathetic to al-Qa'eda, which has produced training manuals containing plans for use of choking agents as a method of attack. Although this plot did not progress beyond planning stages, the potential use of osmium tetroxide has raised new fears about al-Qa'eda's pursuit of dual-use chemicals as terrorist weapons and has generated a debate about the potential lethality of this type of chemical, when combined with a conventional explosive.

Until news broke of this attempted attack, osmium tetroxide had not been regarded as a likely terror weapon due its relatively high cost and the extreme difficulty which would be encountered in weaponizing the chemical. It is dangerous to touch or inhale and must be handled with extreme care. In the laboratory it is only handled inside a fume cupboard.

Osmium tetroxide is readily available and there are no restrictions on its purchase. At the time of writing this addendum, scientists are expressing divided opinions on its possible effectiveness as a weapon.

While many experts warned of extreme dangers, *Times on Line* quoted Professor Alastair Hay, an expert on chemical weaponry, as saying that osmium tetroxide is not nearly as dangerous as experts are suggesting. He added that if it had any role in an explosive device, it would be as a catalyst rather than creating a major chemical hazard through release of the osmium and the contamination problem which would result from that and, that as a chemical hazard, osmium is only a minor irritant. After an explosion, it would have much the same effect as dust and smoke in irritating the lungs.

The yellow crystalline solid is volatile turning from solid to gas at room temperature. The vapors corrode skin and eyes and the fumes damage the lungs when inhaled.

If inhaled the fumes cause a burning sensation and may produce cough, headache, wheezing, shortness of breath and visual disturbances. These symptoms may not manifest immediately and may be delayed.

Contact with the skin causes burns, painful irritation blisters. The tetroxide reduces to black dioxide on contact with the skin, leaving a black stain.

Effects in the eyes include redness, pain, blurred vision and, in severe cases, loss of vision and deep burns.

Ingestion of the chemical leads to abdominal cramps, a burning sensation, and shock.

Bibliography

Abraham R.B., B. Rudick and A.A. Weinbraum. "Practical guidelines for acute care of victims of bioterrorism: Conventional injuries and concomitant nerve agent intoxication." *Anesthesiology V.* 97(4):989–1004 (2003).

Abrutyn, G. "Botulism." In E. Braunwald et al., eds. *Harrison's Principles of Internal Medicine*, 15th ed. (NY: McGraw-Hill, 2001).

Atlas, R.M. "The threat of bio terrorism returns the fear of smallpox." *Curr. Opin. Microbiol.* 1:719–727 (1998).

Barajes, K., A. Stewart and C.R. Combs. "The army chemical/biological SMART-CB Team: The nurse's role." *Crit. Care Nurs. Clin. N. Am.* 15:257–264 (2003).

Baze, W.B. "Soman induced morphological changes: An overview in non human primates." *Journal of Applied Toxicology* 13(3):173–177 (1993).

Berkenstadt, H., B. Marganitt and J. Atsmon. "Combined chemical and conventional injuries: Pathophysiological, diagnostic and therapeutic aspects." *Isr. J. Med. Sci.* 27:623–626 (1991).

Bogucki, S. and S. Weir. "Pulmonary manifestations of intentionally released chemical and biological agents." *Clin. Chest. Med.* 23:777–794 (2002).

Borio L. et al. "Hemorrhagic fever virus as a biological weapon." *JAMA* 287 (18):2391–2405 (2002).

Bozeman W., D. Dilbero and J.L. Schauben. "Biological and chemical weapons of mass destruction." *Emerg. Med. Clin. N. Am.* 20:975–993 (2002).

Campbell, G.L. and D.T. Dennis. "Plague and other Yersina infections." In E. Braunwald et al., eds. *Harrison's Principles of Internal Medicine*, 15th ed. (NY: McGraw-Hill, 2001).

Cohen, A. et al. "History of biological warfare." *Harefuah* 141:7–12 (2002).

Drasch, G., B. Kretchmer and K.L. Von Mayer. "Concentration of mustard gas bis (2-chlorethyl) sulphide in the tissues of a victim of vesicant exposure." *Journal of Forensic Science* 21:1788–1793 (1987).

Eisenmenger, W. et al. "Clinical and morphological findings on mustard gas bis (2-chlorethyl) sulphide poisoning." *J.F.S.C.A.* 36.(6):1688–1698 (1991).

Etzel, R.A. *JAMA* 287(4):425–426 (2002).

Freitag, L. et al. "The role of bronchoscopy in pulmonary complications due to mustard gas inhalation." *Chest* 100:1436–1441 (1991).

Greenfield, R.A. et al. "Microbiological, biological, chemical weapons of warfare and terrorism." *Am. J. Med. Sci.* 393(6):326–334 (2002).

Gunderson, C.H., C.R. Lehman and F.R. Sidell. "Nerve agents." *Neurology* 42:946–950 (1992).

Jortani, S.A., J.W. Snyder and J.R. Valdes. "The role of the clinical laboratory in managing chemical and biological victims." *Clin. Chem.* 46:(12)1883–1893 (2000).

Kasper, D.L. and Zalesnik, D.F. "Gas gangrene, antibiotic associated with colitis and other clostridial infections." In E. Braunwald et al., eds. *Harrison's Principles of Internal Medicine*, 15th ed. (NY: McGraw-Hill, 2001).

Knight, B. "Agrochemical poisoning." *Forensic Pathology* 1996:559.

Korpeter, M. et al. 2001USA N - RHDS Medical management of biological casualties 2001 in Greenfield, R.D., Brown, B.R. and Hutchins. J.B. *Am. J. Med. Sc.* 26(6):326–340 (2002).

Lee, E.C. "Clinical manifestations of sarin nerve gas exposure." *JAMA* 290 (5):659–662 (2003).

Linden, C.H. and M.J. Burns. "Illness due to poisons, drug overdosage and envenomation." In E. Braunwald et al., eds. *Harrison's Principles of Internal Medicine*, 15th ed. (NY: McGraw-Hill, 2001).

Madkov, M. and D. Kaspers. "Brucellosis." In E. Braunwald et al., eds. *Harrison's Principles of Internal Medicine*, 15th ed. (NY: McGraw-Hill, 2001).

Mason, J.K. and B.N. Purdue. *The Pathology of Trauma* (London: Arnold, 2000), p.378.

McCarthy, M. "Anthrax attack in U.S.A." *The Lancet. Infectious Disease* 1: 288–289 (2001).

Moore, D.W. and J.R. Keeler. "Mustard gas poisoning, pathophysiology and nursing implications." *Crit. Nurs.* 1993:62–67.

Morita, H. et al. "Sarin poisoning in Matsumoto Japan." *Lancet* 346:290–293 (1995).

Noah, D.L, K. Huebner and J.F. Wackele. "The history and threat of biological warfare and terrorism." *Emerg. Med. Clin. N. Am.* (20):255–271 (2002).

Norris, L.R. and P.S. Auerbach. "Disorders caused by reptile bites and marine animal exposures." In E. Braunwald et al., eds. *Harrison's Principles of Internal Medicine*, 15th ed. (NY: McGraw-Hill, 2001).

O'Tool, T. "Smallpox: An attack scenario." *Emerg. Infect.* Dis. 5:540–546 (1999).

Okumura, T. et al. "Report on 640 Victims of the Tokyo Subway Sarin attack." *Ann. Emerg. Med.* (28)129–135 (1991).

Patt, H. and R.D. Feigin. "Diagnosis and management of suspected cases of bioterrorism: A pediatric perspective." *Pediatrics* 109(4):1685–692 (2002).

Peters, C.J. "Infections caused by arthropods and rodent-borne viruses." In E. Braunwald et al., eds. *Harrison's Principles of Internal Medicine*, 15th ed. (NY: McGraw-Hill, 2001).

———. "Filoviridea, Marburg and Ebola viruses." In E. Braunwald et al., eds. *Harrison's Principles of Internal Medicine* (NY: McGraw-Hill, 2001).

Rubin, E. and J.L. Farber., eds. *Pathology* (Philadelphia: Lippincott, 1988) pp. 333–354..

Robbins, S.L. and R.S. Cotran. *Infectious Diseases: Pathological Basis of Disease*, 6th ed. (Philadelphia: W.B. Saunders, 1979), p. 374.

Robinson-Dunn, B. "The microbioloby laboratory's role in response to bioterrorism." *Arch. Pathol. Lab. Med.* 126:291–294 (2002).

Sausville, E.N. and D.L. Long. "Principles of cancer therapy." In E. Braunwald et al., eds. *Harrison's Principles of Internal Medicine*, 15th ed. (NY: McGraw-Hill, 2001).

Sidell, F.R. "Chemical warfare agents II: Nerve agents." *Emerg. Med.* 865–871 (1992).

Simpson, K.G., ed. *Taylor's Principles and Practice of Medical Jurisprudence* (London: Churchill Livingstone, 1965).

Trundle, D. and G. Marcial. "Detection of cholinesterase inhibition: The significance of cholinesterase measurements." *Ann. of Clin. and Lab. Science* 18(3):345–352 (1998).

Watson, A.P. and G.D. Griffin. "Toxicity of vesicant agents scheduled for destruction by the chemical stockpile disposal program." *Environmental Health Perspectives* 98:259–280 (1992).

Wormser, U. "Toxicology of mustard gas." *TIPS* 12:164–167 (1991).

Yergler, M. "Nerve gas attack: Emergency mass casualty." *AJAN* 102(7):57–60 (2002).

Zilinskas, R.A. "Iraq's biological weapons." *JAMA* 278(5):418–424 (1997).

Endnotes

1. K.G. Simpson., ed. *Taylor's Principles and Practice of Medical Jurisprudence*. (London: Churchill Livingstone, 1965).

2. J.K. Masson and B.N. Purdue, eds. *The Pathology of Trauma*, 3rd ed. (London: Arnold, 2000).

3. H. Patt and R.D. Feigin. "2002 Diagnosis and management of suspected cases of bioterrorism." *Pediatrics* 109(4) (2002).

4. Masson, note 2, p.378.

5. H. Morita et al. "Sarin poisoning in Matsumoto Japan." *Lancet* 346:290–3 (1995).

6. S.A. Jortani, J.W. Snyder and J.R. Valde. "The role of the clinical laboratory in managing chemical and biological victims." *Clin. Chem.* 46:(12)1883–1893 (2000).

7. C.E. Lee. "Clinical manifestations of sarin nerve gas exposure." *JAMA* 290(5):659–662 (2003).

8. Barajes, K. et al. "The army chemical/biological SMART C.B. team: The nurse's role." *Crit. Care Nurs. Clin. Nam.* 15:257–264 (2003).

9. http://www.cdc.gov/ncidod/EID/vol8no10/02-0353.htm.

10. Barajes, note 8.

11. A. Cohen et al. "History of biological warfare." *Harefuah* 141:7–12 (2002).

12. Cohen, note 11.

13. At the time of writing osmium tetroxide was not considered a possible warfare agent. See Addendum.

14. A. Greenfield et al. "Microbiological, biological, chemical weapons of warfare and terrorism." *Am. J. Med. Sci.* 393(6):326–334 (2002).

15. W. Bozeman, D. Dilbero and J.L. Schauben. "Biological and chemical weapons of mass destruction." *Emerg. Med. Clin. N. Am.* 20:975–993 (2002).

16. Cohen, note 11.

17. S. Bogucki and S. Weir. "Pulmonary manifestations of intentionally released chemical and biological agents." *Clin. Chest Med.* 23:777–794 (2002).

18. H. Patt and R.D. Feigin. "Diagnosis and management of suspected cases of bioterrorism: A pediatric perspective." *Pediatrics* 109(4):1685–692 (2002).

19. M. McCarthy. "Anthrax attack in U.S.A." *Lancet: Infectious Diseases* 1: 288–289 (2001).

20. Jortani, note 5.

21. Jortani, note 5.

22. Bogucki, note 17.

23. McCarthy, note 19.

24. Patt, note 18.

25. G.L. Campbell and D.T. Dennis. "Plague and other yensina infections." In E. Braunwald et al., eds. *Harrison's Principles of Internal Medicine*, 15th ed. (NY: McGraw-Hill, 2001).

26. Bogucki, note 17.

27. Bogucki, note 17.

28. M. Madkov and D. Kaspers. "Brucellosis." In E. Braunwald et al., eds. *Harrison's Principles of Internal Medicine*, 15th ed. (NY: McGraw-Hill, 2001).

29. Patt, note 18.

30. Patt, note 18.

31. M. Kortepeter et al. *USAMRIID's Medical Management of Biological Casualties Handbook* (Fort Detrick, MD: U.S. Army Medical Research Institute of Infectious Diseases, 2001); R.A. Greenfield et al. "Microbiological, biological, and chemical weapons of warfare and terrorism." *Am. J. Med. Sci.* 323(6):326–40 (2002).

32. Korpeter, note 31.

33. Cohen, note 11.

34. Greenfield, note 31.

35. Patt, note 3.

36. D.L. Kasper and D.F. Zalesnik. "Gas gangrene, antibiotic associated with colitis and other clostridial infections." In E. Braunwald et al., eds. *Harrison's Principles of Internal Medicine*, 15th ed. (NY: McGraw-Hill, 2001).

37. Kasper, note 36.

38. Bogucki, note 17.

39. C.H. Linden and M.J. Burns. "Illness due to poisons, drug overdosage and envenomation." In E. Braunwald et al., eds. *Harrison's Principles of Internal Medicine*, 15th ed. (NY: McGraw-Hill, 2001).

40. Bogucki, note 17.

41. Bogucki, note 17.

42. Bogucki, note 17.

43. Bogucki, note 17.

44. Greenfield, note 34.

45. Bogucki, note 17; Greenfield, note 34.

46. Linden, note 39.

47. Linden, note 39.

48. U. Wormser. "Toxicology of mustard gas." *TIPS* 12:164–167 (1991); M. Yergler. "Nerve gas attack: Emergency mass casualty." *AJAN* 102(7)57–60 (2002).

49. D.W. Moore and J.R. Keeler. "Mustard gas poisoning, pathophysiology and nursing implications." *Crit. Nurs.* 1993:62–67.

50. L. Freitag et al. "The role of bronchoscopy in pulmonary complications due to mustard gas inhalation." *Chest* 100:1436–1441 (1991).

51. W. Eisenmenger et al. "Clinical and morphological findings on mustard gas bis (2-chlorethyl) sulphide poisoning." *J.F.S.C.A.* 36.(6):1688–1698 (1991).

52. A.P. Watson and G.D. Griffin. "Toxicity of vesicant agents scheduled for destruction by the chemical stockpile disposal program." *Environmental Health Perspectives* 98:259–280 (1992).

53. Eisenmenger, note 51.

54. Eisenmenger, note 51.

55. Eisenmenger, note 51.

56. G. Drasch, B. Kretchmer and K.L. Von Mayer. "Concentration of mustard gas bis (2-chlorethyl) sulphide in the tissues of a victim of vesicant exposure." *Journal of Forensic Science* 21:1788–1793 (1987).

57. Greenfield, note 31.

58. Watson, note 52.

59. E.N. Sausville and D.L. Long. "Principles of cancer therapy." In E. Braunwald et al., eds. *Harrison's Principles of Internal Medicine*, 15th ed. (NY: McGraw-Hill, 2001).

60. T. O'Tool. "Smallpox: An attack scenario." *Emerg. Infect.* Dis. 5:540–546 (1999).

61. R.M. Atlas. "The threat of bio terrorism returns the fear of smallpox." *Curr. Opin. Microbiol.* (1)719–727 (1998).

62. S.L. Robbins and R.S. Cotran. *Infectious Diseases: Pathological Basis of Disease*, 6th ed. (Philadelphia: W.B. Saunders, 1979), p. 374.

63. Patt , note 3.

64. Robbins, note 62

65. Robbins, note 62

66. L. Borio et al. "Hemorrhagic fever virus as a biological weapon." *JAMA* 287 (18):2391–2405 (2002).

67. C.J. Peters. "Infections caused by arthropods and rodent-borne viruses." In E. Braunwald et al., eds. *Harrison's Principles of Internal Medicine*, 15th ed. (NY: McGraw-Hill, 2001).

68. Peters, note 67.

69. Borio, note 66.

70. F.R. Sidell. "Chemical warfare agents II: Nerve agents." *Emerg. Med.* 865–871 (1992).

71. C.H. Gunderson, C.R. Lehman and F.R. Sidell. "Nerve agents." *Neurology* 42:946–950 (1992).

72. Lee, note 7.

73. Greenfield, note 31.

74. Bozeman, note 15.

75. L.R. Norris and P.S. Auerbach. "Disorders caused by reptile bites and marine animal exposures." In E. Braunwald et al., eds. *Harrison's Principles of Internal Medicine*, 15th ed. (NY: McGraw-Hill, 2001).

76. C.H. Linden and M.J. Burns. "Illness due to poisons, drug overdosage and envenomation." In E. Braunwald et al., eds. *Harrison's Principles of Internal Medicine*, 15th ed. (NY: McGraw-Hill, 2001).

77. T. Okumura et al. "Report on 640 Victims of the Tokyo Subway Sarin attack." *Ann. Emerg. Med.* (28)129–135 (1995).

78. M. Yergler. "Nerve gas attack: Emergency mass casualty." *AJAN* 102(7):57–60 (2002).

79. D. Trundle and G. Marcial. "Detection of cholinesterase inhibition: The significance of cholinesterase measurements." *Ann. of Clin. and Lab. Science* 18(3):345–352 (1998).

80. H. Berkenstadt, B. Marganitt and J. Atsmon. "Combined chemical and conventional injuries: Pathophysiological, diagnostic and therapeutic aspects." *Isr. J. Med. Sci.* 27:623–626 (1991).

81. R.B. Abraham, B. Rudick and A.A. Weinbraum. "Practical guidelines for acute care of victims of bioterrorism: Conventional injuries and concomitant nerve agent intoxication." *Anesthesiology V.* 97(4):989–1004 (2003).

82. Sidell, note 70.

83. Gunderson, note 71.

84. Greenfield, note 31.

85. Lee, note 7.

86. R.A. Zilinskas. "Iraq's biological weapons." *JAMA* 278(5):418–424 (1997)

87. R.A. Etzel. "Mycotoxins." *JAMA* 287(4):425–426 (2002).

88. B. Knight. "Agrochemical poisoning." *Forensic Pathology* 1996:559.

89. W.B. Baze. "Soman induced morphological changes: An overview in non human primates." *Journal of Applied Toxicology* 13(3):173–177 (1993).

Chapter 2

Infectious Agents of Bioterrorism

Lindsey R. Baden, M.D.

Synopsis

2.1 Introduction

September 11, 2001 and its aftermath brought forth the need for law enforcement and public health authorities to plan and work together to counter future threats. The need to understand the potential means by which terror maybe inflicted on the civilian population is essential to developing reasonable defense strategies. Prior episodes of domestic bioterrorism have been largely unappreciated until recently.[1,2] Agents of bioterrorism are especially concerning given the potential for person-to-person transmission, and the diversity of biological agents which may be used by a terrorist organization. The Centers for Disease Control (CDC) and others have developed a list of priority threats. These agents have been divided into three categories: Category A agents are easily disseminated, may be transmitted from person to person, result in high mortality rates, may cause social disruption and require special public health preparedness. Category B agents are those which are moderately easy to disseminate, result in low mortality rates, and require specific enhancements of diagnostics. Category C agents include emerging pathogens that could be engineered for mass dissemination in the future. The biologic agents in these categories are presented in Table 2.1.[3] This chapter will focus on the agents of greatest concern, those in Category A.

2.2 Anthrax

Anthrax is a ubiquitous, global disease of animals caused by the gram-positive organism, *Bacillus anthracis*. As this organism is colorless, odorless, and relatively easy to manufacture it is a likely candidate to be developed and deployed by terrorist organizations.[4] The events in Sverdlovsk in 1979,[5,6] in which anthrax was accidentally released from a Russian bioweapons facility, and the anthrax attacks in 2001 using the U.S. Postal System,[7–9] highlight this concern. The challenges of optimizing aerosol dissemination limited the extent of illness associated with these episodes.

There are several aspects of the biology of *B. anthracis,* which make it an attractive agent for bioterrorism. First, it is relatively easy to grow in culture, thus making large-scale manufacture simple. Second, it has two important forms—active bacterial replication, which causes disease and is susceptible to antimicrobial therapy, and the spore form, which is relatively inert and extremely difficult to eradicate (thus potentially contaminating an environment for decades). When the spore form is in an environment rich in nutrients then it can activate and begin replication thus causing disease. Third, the organism has certain virulence factors (lethal factor and edema factor), which cause accelerated severe disease. In addition it can be engineered to have antimicrobial resistance determinates, thus decreasing the ability to be treated effectively. Fourth, this is an ubiquitous disease of animals with approximately 2,000 human cases occur-

Table 2.1
Potential Biologic Agents of Bioterrorism

Category A	Category B	Category C
Anthrax	Brucellosis	Nipah virus
Botulism	Food safety threats	Hantavirus
Plague	Glanders	Multi-drug resistant *Mycobacteria ttuberculosis*
Smallpox	Melioidosis	Tickborne hemorrhagic fever viruses
Tularemia	Psittacosis	
Viral hemorrhagic fevers	Q fever	
	Typhus fever	
	Viral encephalitis	
	Water safety threats	

Adapted from the CDC guidelines (www.bt.cdc.gov/agent/agentlist-category.asp, accessed June 2004) ring annually worldwide (predominantly cutaneous), thus potentially obscuring (at least initially) a terrorist event or raising the specter of a terrorist event when natural disease occurs.

Anthrax causes three important types of human illness: cutaneous, gastrointestinal, and pulmonary. The site of human infection depends on how one comes into contact with the organism: touching, ingestion, and respiration, respectively. Cutaneous disease is associated with a pustule, which ulcerates and develops into a black scab (eschar). This is associated with systemic toxicity, such as fever and malaise, and is rarely fatal if identified and treated early. Gastrointestinal illness is extremely rare and is caused by the ingestion of contaminated food, presents with hemorrhagic intestinal illness with mesenteric lymph node enlargement and bloody diarrhea and is associated with a high mortality. Respiratory infection is associated with enlargement and necrosis of the mediastinal lymph nodes and is often rapidly fatal. Of these three syndromes respiratory disease is the most worrisome as it may be difficult to distinguish from the "common cold," is a rapidly progressive illness, and has the potential to be delivered by aerosol.[10] In the 2001 U.S. attacks there were eleven cases of inhalation disease of whom five died,[4] while in the Sverdlovsk episode a 70–80 percent mortality has been reported.[5,6]

When an outbreak of anthrax has been diagnosed early treatment is essential to diminish the subsequent morbidity and morality. As observed in the Sverdlovsk episode, mortality was high in individuals who developed clinical illness within thirty days of exposure, however, cases of illness still occurred between one and two months past the release of the spores from the bioweapons facility. Thus treatment and post exposure prophylaxis (PEP) should be continued for sixty days, see Table 2.2 for recommendations.[4,11,12] An anthrax vaccine (six-dose series), which appears to induce modest protection is available and appears safe,[13-15] however, due to limited supply, use is restricted to those at highest risk (military, high risk groups, and potentially for PEP). Research is underway to better delineate the safety and efficacy profile of vaccination for anthrax.

An important consideration in managing an anthrax attack is that there is no data to suggest person-to-person spread. Risk of infection is greatest if exposed to the primary aerosol and quite low subsequently.[16] However, the challenge of decontaminating an environment of anthrax is extremely difficult and costly, thus magnifying the effects of terror and

Table 2.2
Treatment and Post Exposure Prophylaxis for Agents of Bioterror

Agent	Regimen		Post Exposure Prophylaxis	
	1st	2nd	1st	2nd
Anthrax	Ciprofloxacin x60d	Doxycycline x60d	Ciprofloxacin x60d	Doxycycline x60d Amoxcilin x60d
Plague	Streptomycin x10d Gentamicin x10d	Doxycycline x14–21d Ciprofloxacin x10d Chloramphenicol x10d	Doxycycline x7d Ciprofloxacin x7d	Chloramphenicol x7d
Tularemia	Streptomycin x10d Gentamicin x10d	Doxycycline x14–21d Ciprofloxacin x10d Chloramphenicol x 14–21d	Doxycycline x14d Ciprofloxacin x 14d	
Botulinum Toxin	Anti-Toxin			
Small Pox	Cidofovir VIG		Vaccination**	
Viral hemorrhagic fever*	Ribavirin x6d			

- d= days, VIG=variola immune globulin
- Dose adjust for children.
- Consult a physician as soon as possible.
- *VHF which are potentially susceptible to ribavirn include Arenaviruses and Rift Valley Fever virus.
- ** Vaccination is effective if given within four days of exposure.

social disruption when investigating a possible anthrax release. Enhanced collaboration between public health and law enforcement authorities will be required to ensure safety and optimize preservation and identification of critical pieces of evidence.[17–20]

2.3 Smallpox

Smallpox is caused by the variola virus and was globally eradicated in 1977.[21] Smallpox vaccination ceased in the United States in 1972 except for the military and a few laboratory personnel. Currently only two laboratories, one in the U.S. and the other in Russia, are know to possess wild type variola, however, there is significant concern that "others" may also possess the virus. Given that vaccination for smallpox has ceased for over twenty-five years, a large population of variola-naive individuals and those with waning immunity to variola exist. This is probably the single most important reason why variola is a leading concern as a weapon of bioterror. Other aspects of variola which enhance the concern that it maybe used by terrorist organizations include: (1) highly contagious, thus person-to-person spread could facilitate rapid dissemination; (2) nearly 100 percent of infected individuals become ill and there is approximately a 30-percent mortality (which is likely higher in immunosuppressed individuals such as those with HIV/AIDS, cancer or status post organ transplantation); (3) limited treatment option for those with clinical illness (see Table 2.2); and (4) easily transported either in a vial or by an infected individual prior to developing clinical illness.[22]

Certain aspects of the biology of smallpox are pivotal to understanding the emerging strategy to defend against an attack. Infection results from inhalation of infectious particles. The incubation period provided is approximately twelve days, see Table 2.3. Illness is characterized by fever, malaise and the development of a characteristic vesicular or pustular rash. This must be carefully distinguished from chickenpox, which is most easily done by carefully assessing the rash; in smallpox the rash is uniform in nature while chickenpox has crops of lesions in different stages of evolution. Smallpox is most contagious during the first week of illness. Vaccination for smallpox within two to three days of exposure typically prevents illness and within four to five days prevents death.[23]

One strategy to obviate the threat of a smallpox attack would be to vaccinate the entire population with vaccinia (smallpox vaccine). Current U.S. stockpile of vaccinia would allow vaccination of the entire U.S. population.[23-28] As vaccinia is a live viral vaccine. Rare but well-described complications exists, including; progressive vaccinia, severe generalized vaccinia, ocular vaccinia, eczema vaccinatum, and death. These rare complications are more likely to occur in individual with a suppressed immune system (such as that caused by HIV/AIDS, cancer, and use of corticosteriods) and those with skin disease (such as eczema).[23,24,29] In addition, secondary transmission of the vaccine virus can occur to close contacts, such as family members, thus broadening those at risk of complications from vaccination. Given these risks it is difficult to justify universal vaccination for smallpox when the last known case of wild-type infection was in 1977. Developing a safer smallpox vaccine is an area of active investigation.

The current strategy to defend against the smallpox threat is based on the following observations: (1) nearly 100 percent of smallpox-infected individuals are symptomatic with a characteristic rash; (2) an infected individual is most infectious with the onset of the rash, not before; and (3) vaccination within two to three days of exposure typically prevents disease. Thus if a case of smallpox infection is diagnosed then immediate vaccination of all contacts, and as needed, all contacts of contacts should control the outbreak, which was the strategy used to successfully eradicate the disease twenty-five years ago. This strategy is predicated on early disease detection[30] and rapid mobilization of public health resources.[23–25]

2.4 Plague

Plague has been associated with at least three global pandemics. The second pandemic also known as the Black Death occurred in Europe in the fourteenth and fifteenth centuries and was associated with 20–30 million deaths, or one third of the European population.[31] Person-to-person transmission along with other factors contributed to the significant morbidity and mortality associated with the Black Death and the specter of this organism being used as an agent of bioterror.

Plague is caused by the gram-negative bacterium *Yersinia pestis.* There are three major syndromes associated with infection: bubonic (enlarged regional lymph nodes), septicemia (blood stream infection), and pneumonic (infection of the lungs.) Plague is a naturally occurring infection typically spread between rats by fleas. Human infection is incidental, with approximately 1,700 human cases annually worldwide. The overwhelming majority of these cases are the bubonic form. In the U.S. over the last fifty years approximately 400 cases of the plague were reported with 84 percent bubonic and only 2 percent pneumonic, with an associated fatality rate of 14 percent and 57 percent respectively.[32] Symptoms of bubonic plague typically develop two to eight days after being bitten by an infected flea while symptoms in primary pneumonic plague typically occur more quickly, over two to four days[33] (see Table 2.3). Delay in diagnosis and the initiation of appropriate antimicrobial therapy will likely contribute to increased mortality.

Warning signs of a bioterror incident would include: occurrence of plague infection in communities without prior episodes, in individuals without proper risk factors, and in an area without associated rodent deaths.[31] In addition, the likely method of dissemination would be via an aerosol thus primary pneumonic disease would be the likely form of illness. The importance of distinguished pneumonic plague from other respiratory illnesses as early as possible would be essential to contain the outbreak and minimize the potential morbidity and mortality. Use of a mask has been effective in prior epidemics of plague to diminish transmission and would be an essential part of a containment strategy. Suspect

Table 2.3
Treatment and Post-Exposure Prophylaxis

Agent	Typical IP	P-t-P Tx	Risk Factors for Natural Infection	Estimated #US cases/yr	Environmental Decontamination Complicated
Anthrax	2-6d	N	association w/ animals	5	Y
Plague	2-8d	Y	association w/ rodents	20	N
Tularmia	3-5d	N	association w/ animals	150-200	N
Botulinum toxin	12-72 hour	N	contaminated foods or colonized wounds	200	N
Smallpox	7-17 d	Y	none	none	N
Viral hemorrhagic fevers	4-21d	Y/N*	geographic restrictions, exposure to arthropods or rodents	none	N

* Person to person transmission documented for filoviruses and arcnaviruses
IP= incubation period, P-t-P= person to person transmission, d = days, Y= yes, N= no

or confirmed cases of pneumonic plague would require at least thirty-six hours of effective antimicrobial therapy before they were no longer potentially contagious. As plague does not have a spore form and is sensitive to heat and sunlight, environment decontamination would unlikely be required as it would be for anthrax. Treatment and post-exposure prophylaxis are presented in Table 2.2. A vaccine against plague was discontinued in 1999, but is an area of active research.

2.5 Tularemia

Tularemia is a global disease affecting widely diverse animal hosts and is caused by the gram-negative bacterium *Francisella tularensis.* Human disease is incidental and not necessary for the perpetuation of this organism in nature. As *F. tularensis* requires a small inoculation, as few as ten organisms to cause disease, and is relatively easy to manufacture and disseminate, and has the ability to cause severe human infection, it has been considered a candidate for development as a biological weapon. In the 1930–40s in Japan and later in the Soviet Union substantial effort in this vein occurred.[34, 35] In addition to optimizing production and dissemination capabilities, an effort toward bioengineering antimicrobial resistant organism has occurred.

Human illness caused by *F. tularensis* includes the following syndromes: ulceroglandular, oropharyngeal, pneumonic, and septic. Ulceroglandular disease is associated with an ulcer occurring at the site of inoculation, typically after handling an infected carcass or being bitten by an infected arthropod, followed by the development of regional adenopathy and systemic symptoms such as high fever (see Figure 2.1). Oropharyngeal tularemia occurs after ingesting the organism via contaminated food or drink. Pharyngeal ulceration with exudate and cervical adenopathy then follow. Pneumonic disease is rare and occurs as a result of inhaling contaminated aerosols (primary disease) or by secondary spread from bacteremia (secondary disease). Fatality rates as high as 30–50 percent have been reported with primary pneumonic infection. Approximately, 150–200 human cases of tularemia are reported in the U.S. per year, predominately of the ulceroglandular or glandular variety, and are associated with a low case fatality rate (approximately 1.4 percent).[34–37] Most cases occur during summer months when the vector (arthropods) is most active.

The most likely bioterror scenario with tularemia would be an aerosol deployment, thus leading to greater dissemination and the more severe pneumonic disease. Illness would likely develop over the next three to five days, initially as a nondescript respiratory process. Treatment and

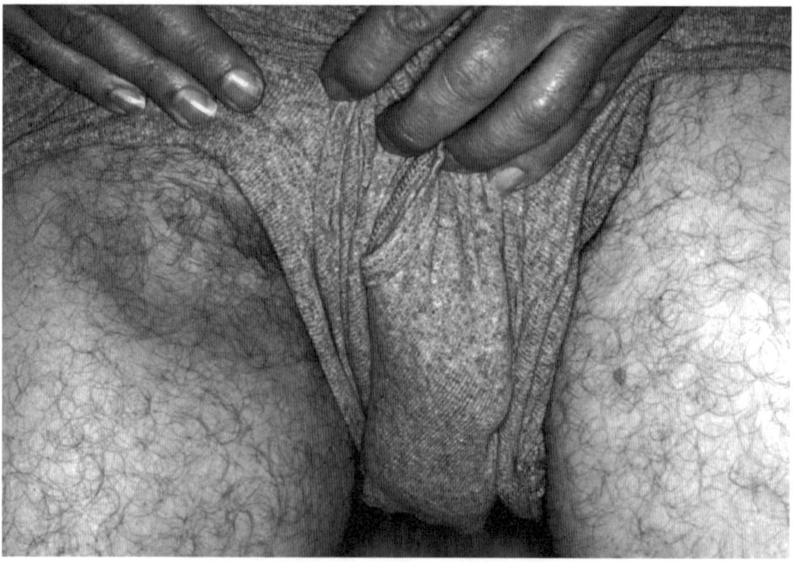

Figure 2.1 *Severe right inguinal adenopathy in a fifty-year-old male with naturally acquired tularemia*

post-exposure prophylaxis are outlined in Table 2.2. As tularemia is not spread by person-to-person contact no special infection control procedures are warranted. However, any procedure, which may lead to the development of aerosol from infected tissue, such as bone cutting, should be performed with caution. A vaccination for tularemia is currently under review by the FDA, thus its optimal use at this time is unknown. As tularemia does not have a spore form and the organism is sensitive to environmental conditions, decontamination of a contaminated area is relatively straight forward, using bleach- or alcohol-based cleansers. Municipal water supplies are unlikely to be vulnerable to attack given current chlorination practices.[34]

2.6 Botulinum Toxin

Botulism is a disease associated with profound muscle weakness due to blockage of acetylcholine release at the neuromuscular junction. This disease is not caused by direct bacterial invasion but rather by the secretion of an exotoxin from the gram-positive organism *Clostridium botulinum.* There are seven distinct types of toxin in nature, denoted A-G. Given the ease of manufacture, transport, and potency (most poisonous substance known approximately 0.1 gram would be fatal), this agent has been developed by several groups for use as a bioweapon including the U.S., Iraq, Iran, North Korea, Syria, and the Soviet Union.[38] In addition, the Aun Shinrikyo group were attempting to develop this toxin as a weapon of terror at the time they released sarin gas in Tokyo.

In the U.S. there are approximately 200 human cases of natural occurring botulism per year.[39,40] These cases are typically associated with the consumption of contaminated foods or colonization of a wound by *C. botulinum.* Once an ingestion of preformed toxin or absorption of toxin from a colonizing organism occurs, clinical illness associated with a descending, flaccid paralysis occurs over the next twelve to seventy-two hours. Difficulty with breathing and vision are characteristic features. Mechanical ventilation may be required as respiratory insufficiency is the most severe complication which may last for several months, until nerve regeneration occurs. An important characteristic of botulism is the lack of sensory or higher cognitive impairment. The difficulty of diagnosing botulism is highlighted by a Canadian outbreak, which infected twenty-eight travelers over one two months with a myriad of clinical illnesses being diagnosed, such as multiple sclerosis, stroke, and Guillane-Barré syndrome, before the point source outbreak was identified.[33]

The majority of food borne outbreaks of botulism in the U.S. are associated with toxins A, B, E, and F. Treatment of botulism is largely supportive in nature along with antitoxin (against toxins A, B, and E). An investigational heptavalent antitoxin is available if non-A, B, E toxin were released. A vaccine for botulism is under development, however, mass vaccination must be weighed carefully against the potential loss of botulism toxin's ability to treat a variety of medical conditions associated with muscular spasm, such as strabismus, cervical torticollis, and blepharospasm, due to the development of antitoxin immunity. Botulism is not spread from person to person and cannot penetrate intact skin, thus no special precautions are required when treating affected patients. The toxin is predicted to decay at approximately 17 percent per minute thus within two days little residual environmental contamination would be present after a malicious release.[38]

2.7 Hemorrhagic Fever Viruses

The hemorrhagic fever viruses (HFV) are a diverse group of viral pathogens, which cause significant human disease associated with fever and bleeding. The family of viruses of concern include: Filoviruses (e.g. Ebola and Marburg), Arenaviridae (e.g., Lassa, Junin, Machupo, Guanarito, Sabia), Bunyaviruses (e.g., Rift Valley fever), and Flaviviruses (e.g., yellow fever, Omsk hemorrhagic fever, and Kyasanur Forest disease). These viruses are considered potential candidates for use as bioweapons due to several factors: high morbidity or morality, potential for person-to-person transmission, limited treatment options, and feasibility of large-scale production.[41] The consequence of an outbreak of a HFV would depend on which virus was used. For example, Ebola, Marburg and Arenavirus have the potential for person-to-person transmission as demonstrated in a variety of reported naturally occurring outbreaks[42]. Associated mortality is high for Ebola (50–80 percent), Marburg (23–70 percent), Arenaviruses (15–30 percent) and Yellow Fever (20 percent). Limited treatment options are available only for Arenaviruses and Rift Valley fever with ribavirin, see Table 2.2. A preventative vaccine is only available for yellow fever.[41] There are currently only two laboratories in the U.S. with the capability to conduct viral isolation for this group of pathogens at the CDC and USAMRIID (BSL-4 capability). Thus initial diagnosis of an outbreak would likely be by serology. Optimal infection control practices would depend on the virus involved, but initial containment efforts (pending viral identification) should include aerosol precautions.

2.8 Laboratory Preparedness

The breadth of pathogens and toxins, which could be used in a bioterror event, is formidable. A cornerstone of biodefense is to develop the infrastructure that would allow early, rapid, accurate diagnosis, thus facilitating a determination if an event represents natural disease as opposed to a malicious release. Proper disease containment and treatment is essential if significant illness and social disruption are to be avoided. The CDC, in conjunction with the local health authorities, is in the process of enhancing local and national laboratory capacity to address these concerns by creating a Laboratory Response Network (LRN) for bioterrorism, which consists of over 100 laboratories with at least one in each state.[30] It is essential that law enforcement agencies develop the proper collaborations with the scientific community to be optimally positioned to investigate potential malicious use of biologic agents.[43–48] A secondary benefit of these diagnostic enhancements will be the improved diagnosis of naturally occurring disease thus facilitating treatment.[49] Activities which bring together law enforcement and public health officials are an important means of developing strategies to deal with potential incidents and also uniquely assist in developing a network of individuals with varying expertise who can confer as needed.[44,48]

2.9 Conclusion

Infectious diseases cause significant human mortality as the pandemics of influenza, plague, and HIV and the recent outbreaks of SARS, West Nile virus, and monkeypox highlight. The ease of access to various organisms, the ability to manufacture, and the potential for person-to-person transmission make biologic agents a major concern as a weapon of terrorists. The potential for causing panic and social disruption is evident from the recent anthrax attack via the postal system. A critical aspect of preparing and responding to a bioterror attack is building the infrastructure and expertise necessary to diagnose a malicious release from naturally occurring disease.[1,2,40] The difficulties of this are highlighted by many recent investigations. More research into optimal diagnostics, therapeutics, and vaccines are urgently needed. Enhanced cooperation between public health and law enforcement authorities will be essential.[17]

Endnotes

1. T.J. Torok et al. "A large community outbreak of salmonellosis caused by intentional contamination of restaurant salad bars." *JAMA* 278:389–95 (1997).

2. S.A. Kolavic et al. "An outbreak of Shigella dysenteriae type 2 among laboratory workers due to intentional food contamination." *JAMA* 278:396–8 (1997).

3. www.bt.cdc.gov/agent/agentlist-category.asp.

4. T.V. Inglesby et al. "Anthrax as a biological weapon, 2002: Updated recommendations for management." *JAMA* 287:2236–52 (2002).

5. M. Meselson et al. "The Sverdlovsk anthrax outbreak of 1979." *Science* 266: 1202–8 (1994).

6. R. Brookmeyer et al. "The statistical analysis of truncated data: Application to the Sverdlovsk anthrax outbreak." *Biostatistics* 2:233–47 (2001).

7. J.A. Jernigan et al. "Bioterrorism-related inhalational anthrax: The first 10 cases reported in the United States." *Emerg. Infect. Dis.* 7:933–44 (2001).

8. L.M. Bush et al. "Index case of fatal inhalational anthrax due to bioterrorism in the United States." *N. Engl. J. Med.* 345:1607–10 (2001).

9. T.A. Mayer et al. "Clinical presentation of inhalational anthrax following bioterrorism exposure: Report of 2 surviving patients." *JAMA* 286: 2549–53 (2001).

10. CDC. "Update: Investigation of anthrax associated with intentional exposure and interim public health guidelines." *MMWR* 50:889–893 (2001).

11. D.M. Bell, P.E. Kozarsky and D.S. Stephens. "Clinical issues in the prophylaxis, diagnosis, and treatment of anthrax." *Emerg. Infect. Dis.* 8:222–5 (2002).

12. C.W. Shepard et al. "Antimicrobial postexposure prophylaxis for anthrax: Adverse events and adherence."*Emerg. Infect. Dis.* 8:1124–32 (2002).

13. "Use of anthrax vaccine in the United States." *MMWR Recomm. Rep.* 49:1–20 (2002).

14. P.R. Pittman. "Anthrax vaccine: Short-term safety experience in humans." *Vaccine* 20:972–8 (2001).

15. A.R. Wiesen and C.T. Littell. "Relationship between prepregnancy anthrax vaccination and pregnancy and birth outcomes among U.S. Army women." *JAMA* 287:1556–60 (2002).

16. K.P. Fennelly et al. "Airborne infection with *Bacillus anthracis*: From mills to mail." *Emerg. Infect. Dis.* 10:996–1001 (2004).

17. J.C. Butler et al. "Collaboration between public health and law enforcement: New paradigms and partnerships for bioterrorism planning and response." *Emerg. Infect. Dis.* 8:1152–6 (2002).

18. "Diagnosis and management of foodborne illnesses: A primer for physicians." *MMWR Recomm. Rep.* 50:1–69 (2001).

19. E.P. Richards. "Collaboration between public health and law enforcement: the constitutional challenge." *Emerg. Infect. Dis.* 8:1157–9 (2002).

20. J.L. Gerberding, J.M. Hughes and J.P. Koplan. "Bioterrorism preparedness and response: Clinicians and public health agencies as essential partners." *JAMA* 287:898–900 (2002).

21. F. Fenner. "A successful eradication campaign: Global eradication of smallpox." *Rev. Infect. Dis.* 4:916–30 (1982).

22. D.A. Henderson et al., Working Group on Civilian Biodefense. "Smallpox as a biological weapon: Medical and public health management." *JAMA* 281:2127–37 (1999).

23. V.A. Fulginiti et al. "Smallpox vaccination: a review, part I: Background, vaccination technique, normal vaccination and revaccination, and expected normal reactions." *Clin. Infect. Dis.* 37:241–50 (2003).

24. V.A. Fulginiti et al. "Smallpox vaccination: a review, part II: Adverse events." *Clin. Infect. Dis.* 37:251–71 (2003).

25. M. Wharton et al. "ecommendations for using smallpox vaccine in a pre-event vaccination program. Supplemental recommendations of the Advisory

Committee on Immunization Practices (ACIP) and the Healthcare Infection Control Practices Advisory Committee (HICPAC)." *MMWR Recomm. Rep.* 52:1–16 (2003).

26. S.E. Frey et al. "Clinical responses to undiluted and diluted smallpox vaccine." *N. Engl. J. Med* 346:1265–74 (2002).

27. S.E. Frey et al. "Dose-related effects of smallpox vaccine." *N. Engl. J. Med.* 346:1275–80 (2002).

28. K.A. Sepkowitz. "How contagious is vaccinia?" *N. Engl. J. Med.* 348:439–46.

29. J.S. Halsell et al. "Myopericarditis following smallpox vaccination among vaccinia-naive U.S. military personnel." *JAMA* 289:3283–9 (2003).

30. J.M. Hughes and J.L Gerberding. "Anthrax bioterrorism: Lessons learned and future directions." *Emerg. Infect. Dis.* 8:1013–4 (2002).

31. T.V. Inglesby et al., Working Group on Civilian Biodefense. "Plague as a biological weapon: medical and public health management." *JAMA* 283:2281–90 (2000).

32. "Fatal human plague: Arizona and Colorado, 1996." *MMWR Recomm. Rep.* 46:617–20 (1997).

33. M. Ratsitorahina et al. "Epidemiological and diagnostic aspects of the outbreak of pneumonic plague in Madagascar." *Lancet* 355:111–3 (2000).

34. D.T. Dennis et al. "Tularemia as a biological weapon: Medical and public health management." *JAMA* 285:2763–73 (2001).

35. S. Harris. "Japanese biological warfare research on humans: A case study of microbiology and ethics." *Ann. N.Y. Acad. Sci.* 666:21–52 (1992).

36. J.M. Boyce. "Recent trends in the epidemiology of tularemia in the United States." *J. Infect. Dis.* 131:197–9 (1975).

37. S.M. Teutsch et al. "Pneumonic tularemia on Martha's Vineyard." *N. Engl. J. Med.* 301:826–8 (1979).

38. S.S. Arnon et al. "Botulinum toxin as a biological weapon: Medical and public health management. *JAMA* 285:1059–70 (2001).

39. R.L. Shapiro, C. Hatheway and D.L. Swerdlow. "Botulism in the United States: A clinical and epidemiologic review." *Ann. Intern. Med.* 129:221–8 (1998).

40. M.E. St. Louis et al. "Botulism from chopped garlic: Delayed recognition of a major outbreak." *Ann. Intern. Med.* 108:363–8 (1988).

41. L. Borio et al. "Hemorrhagic fever viruses as biological weapons: Medical and public health management." *JAMA* 287:2391–405 (2002).

42. S.F. Dowell et al., Commission de Lutte contre les Epidemies a Kikwit. "Transmission of Ebola hemorrhagic fever: A study of risk factors in family members, Kikwit, Democratic Republic of the Congo, 1995. *J. Infect. Dis.* 179 Suppl 1:S87–91 (1999).

43. J.Y. Richmond and S.L. Nesby-O'Dell, CDC. "Laboratory security and emergency response guidance for laboratories working with select agents." *MMWR Recomm. Rep.* 2002; 51:1–6 (2002).

44. K.D. Nolte et al. "Medical examiners, coroners, and biologic terrorism: A guidebook for surveillance and case management." *MMWR Recomm. Rep.* 53:1–27 (2004).

45. www.cdc.gov/programs/bio.htm.

46. B. Robinson-Dunn. "The microbiology laboratory's role in response to bioterrorism." *Arch. Pathol. Lab. Med.* 126:291–4 (2002).

47. Weilbocher J ME. *J. Lab. Clin. Med.* 24:34–8 (1938).

48. CDC. "Responding to detection of aerosolized *Bacillus anthracis* by autonomous detection systems in the workplace." *MMWR Recomm. Rep.* 53:1–11 (2004).

49. M. Dworetzky. "Smallpox, October 1945." *N. Engl. J. Med.* 346:1329 (2002).

Chapter 3

Smallpox

Louis C. Tripoli, M.D., John G. Bartlett, M.D. and William Stanhope, PA

Synopsis

3.1 History

Smallpox is an ancient scourge. While no one knows for certain how and when it arose, there are many interesting clues. Understanding the biology of variola leads to some logical deductions as to its origin.

Since it has no animal reservoir, and since infection confers either death or lifelong immunity after a relatively brief infection, the virus can only survive where there is sufficient density of people and entry of naive individuals into the infected population. These conditions did not exist in Europe, for example, until the Roman Empire, but they existed in Asia and northern Africa much earlier, and this is where the story of variola's contribution to human misery begins. But first, let us digress for a few words on terminology.

A. Terminology

1. "Variola"

In the sixth century A.D., Bishop Marius of Avenches (modern Switzerland), used the Latin word *variola* to describe an epidemic illness that was prevalent in southern Europe at the time (Hopkins 1983, 25). The word literally means "pustule," from the Latin *varius* (spotted). Constantinus Africanus (1020–1087), a Dark Ages know-it-all, was the first to use the word variola to describe the disease we call smallpox.

2. "Smallpox"

Smallpox as a word did not arise in the English language until the return of Columbus's crews from the new world. They carried a new disease with them, syphilis, which, because it caused an exanthem, it was called the "great pox." Before that, the term "pox" referred to variola as well as a number of other eruptions. The term "great pox" is actually translated from the French *la grosse vérole*, as the soldiers of Charles VIII seem to have acquired it in Italy during the siege of Naples in 1494, and ultimately, the term reached England. (Of interest, to this day the German language still uses only the term *Pocken* to denote the English smallpox.) In earlier editions of Osler's books from the late nineteenth century, the convention was to write the term as "small-pox," but around 1914, the word lost its hyphen.

B. Ancient history

Population density rose concurrent with the introduction of large-scale agriculture, perhaps around 10,000 B.C. The Ebers Papyrus, written between 3730 and 1555 B.C., contains descriptions of an illness that may have been smallpox (Hopkins 1983, 15).

The earliest visual evidence of smallpox is believed to be the vesicular skin lesions seen on three Egyptian mummies from the Eighteenth and Twentieth Dynasties (1570 to 1085 B.C.) (Hopkins 1983, 14). The mummy of the Pharaoh Ramses V, who died in Egypt in 1157 B.C., still exhibits a rash that is distributed like smallpox and looks like smallpox to experienced eyes.

Cuneiform tablets indicate that the Hittites contracted smallpox from Egyptian captives during their wars with Egypt between 1380 and 46 B.C. (Hopkins 1983, 16). Thereafter, smallpox changed human history. The outcome of history was decided largely by warfare, and the outcomes of wars were clearly affected by smallpox. In many cases, the population that had grown accustomed to the infection had a strategic advantage of those who did not. Invariably, one side would give it to the other, but there is little evidence to show that smallpox was used as a strategic weapon until the French and Indian Wars, which will be mentioned later.

Here are some examples of the strategic influence of smallpox in ancient history:

- In 430 B.C., smallpox destroyed one-fourth of the Athenian army and left Athens vulnerable to Sparta.
- In 395 B.C., Carthage had to lift its siege of Sicily because its army was ravaged by smallpox.
- In the second century A.D., Galen wrote that smallpox caused a major epidemic in Rome, at its peak claiming up to 2,000 lives daily. The disease ultimately claimed the life of the Emperor Marcus Aurelius. According to modern estimates, this outbreak claimed 3.5 to 7 million lives and weakened the empire (Littman 1973).

C. European history

St. Nicaise became the patron saint of smallpox victims. He was the Bishop of Rheims and was martyred by the Huns who invaded France in 451. He had recovered from smallpox the year before his death.

Chilperic I, King of the Francs from 561 to 584, had ten children by three marriages, but only one child, Clotaire, survived his father. At least two of his sons, Dogobert and Clodobert, died of smallpox, but the king recovered. After the death of their sons, the Queen persuaded Chilperic to acts of charity for his subjects because she saw their deaths as warning from God about building up riches on the earth.

Guntram, another Merovingian King and brother of Chilperic, was married to Queen Austrigilde. She contracted smallpox but looked at it differently from her sister-in-law. Her physicians were to be held accountable for any bad outcome, and she instructed her husband to have them executed if she died. She did, and they were—a form of medieval medical liability.

Since European history is the history of its rulers from the Middle Ages until the nineteenth century, smallpox played a crucial role in shaping European history as it became increasingly prevalent. There are dozens of examples of rulers dying from smallpox in the sixteenth, seventeenth, and eighteenth centuries that became history-altering events. These are some of the most important events according to Hopkins (Hopkins 1983):

- Queen Elizabeth I is still one of the world's celebrated smallpox victims. She survived, but was bald and marked for life as a result, clearly shaping her *Weltausschauung*.
- In the seventeenth century, smallpox killed the Duke of Mantua and his male heirs, sparking the War of Mantuan Succession.
- When Ferdinand IV, emperor-elect of the Holy Roman Empire, died of smallpox in 1654, the crown went to his brother Leopold I, who stopped the Turkish advances into the Empire.
- The English royal Stuarts seem to have been particularly susceptible to death from smallpox, and their line of succession was affected by it.
- Smallpox so affected the Habsburgs that the line of Austrian succession was shifted four times by smallpox deaths.

- The French royal line was also shifted several times by smallpox in the eighteenth century.

D. North American history

Smallpox arrived in the New World in 1507, in the Caribbean. It devastated the native populations so extensively that it is largely credited with making the conquest of the Americas possible or at least easier (Best 2004). Whole tribes were exterminated. The disappearance of the Lucayan Indians is chiefly ascribed to smallpox (Dixon 1962, 192). After reaching Mexico in 1520, it has been estimated that 31 million people died in a short time (Dixon 1962, 192). It exterminated innumerable people in South America. In the early seventeenth century, as colonists and traders arrived in North America, the New England Indian tribes were virtually wiped out by smallpox and other diseases (Jones 2004, 21). In 1634, an outbreak of smallpox in New England had a recorded case-fatality rate of 90 percent (Jones 2004, 3).

Perhaps the most chilling example of smallpox in human history is its intentional use as an offensive strategic weapon in the French and Indian War (1754–1763). The English forces are credited with giving blankets to the Indians that had been used and contaminated by smallpox victims. A letter from Lord Jeffrey Amherst to Colonel Henry Bouquet, dated July 16, 1763, contains a long post script in which Amherst approves Bouquet's plan to use smallpox against the Indians:

> P.S.:
> You will do well to try to Innoculate the Indians by means of Blanketts, as well as to try every other method that can serve to extirpate this execrable Race. I should be very glad you Scheme for hunting them down by dogs could take effect.

From the historical record, it appears that the plan succeeded in helping to defeat the Indian forces.

In March, 1775, as a smallpox epidemic raged in Boston, which was occupied by British troops, the Continental Army chose not to enter Boston for fear of a biological attack that was rumored as being planned by the British. A year later, Washington still had not entered the city. The following passage appears in records of George Washington's General Orders of March 14, 1776:

> The General was informed Yesterday evening, by a person just out of Boston, that our Enemies in that place, had laid several Schemes for communicating the infection of the small-pox, to the Continental Army, when they get into the town (Fenn 2001).

Following the Louisiana Purchase and westward expansion, smallpox further devastated Native American populations, along with measles, tuberculosis, and other diseases. Fur traders brought smallpox into the lands along the Missouri River, and in June 1838 the Madan, Assinboine, and Blackfeet were decimated by it. This example shows what can happen if smallpox is introduced into populations with no natural immunity (Jones 2004, 1).

E. Variolation

Inhalation of the virus results in more severe disease than does inoculation into the skin. In fact, the practice of introducing variola into the skin, variolation, was a common method of inducing immunity prior to the introduction of vaccination by Jenner in 1796. In the early eighteenth century, Europe became increasingly aware of the practices in Asia, Greece, and North Africa using material from smallpox pustules to induce immunity in uninfected persons. The Chinese were reported to use dried scabs for nasal inhalation in order to induce immunity. Other practices involved introduction of infected material into the skin.

One of the prominent and famous personalities credited with the successful introduction of variolation into England was Lady Mary Whortley Monatgue, herself a smallpox survivor with cosmetic sequelae. Her life was one of unusual boldness for a woman at the time. She came from a lowly birth and married into the English aristocracy. Her husband was a diplomat who was posted to Constantinople, where Lady Montague and Charles Maitland, a surgeon, observed the practice and adopted it. The first record of variolation in England was that of Charles Maitland's successful inoculation of Lady Montague's four-year-old daughter on their return to England. While much of the credit for the successful adoption of variolation in England rightly belongs to her, Charles Maitland, and the president of the Royal Society and physician to the king, Sir Hans Sloane, also deserve credit.

Variolation was opposed by religious leaders, particularly Calvinists, because it was seen as interference with God's will. It was also opposed on medical grounds because it carried some danger to the inoculee and to those around him. Two developments came together to dispel fear. England had started to accumulate death records in the late sixteenth century, and analysis of this robust database became possible with the maturation of the study of probability and its growth into the study of statistics. In an address to the Royal Society in January 1723, physician James Jurin used statistics to show that the risk of dying from natural smallpox was one in every five or six victims, whereas the risk of dying from variolation, as practiced at that time, was one in ninety-one (Hopkins 1983, 50).

As opposed to oft-repeated estimates of the danger of this process, the rate of fatality from this procedure was probably far less than the 2-percent rate that is often seen in modern discussions of the subject. (The American figure of 2 percent probably derives from the report of Mather and Boylston in 1721, in which 2 pecent of 287 people who underwent variolation died; they compared that risk to the 14.9-percent case-fatality rate from natural infection in their experience (Rudolph 1965; Blake 1959)) The major disadvantage of the procedure was not to the patient but to those around him: it was known to cause outbreaks of smallpox among the non-immune (Klebs 1914). In fact, purposeful inoculation of infectious products was a method of immunization among the Chinese for centuries and even was a cause of outbreaks in China in the twentieth century (Yutu 1988).

A family of English physicians, the Suttons, was influential in creating a franchise approach to variolation, setting up variolation centers as one of the first examples of a medical business enterprise. The Suttons were able to make the process so much more efficient (the Sutton method), that they inoculated many people in Europe and made a handsome living from it. It appears as well that the mortality rate from the process dropped as the Suttons and others realized that even a small inoculum passed from one person to another (variola inoculata) was sufficient to provide lasting immunity. Watson, a Suttonite, published his case series in 1768 (see Table 3.1).

Table 3.1

Date	No. Of Cases	Inoculum Properties and Quality	Medications	Number of Pustules				Course	
				Total	Average	Max.	Min.	With Exanthem	Without exanthem
Oct. 19, 1767	10	**A.** Watery (serum) from variola vera	Jalap. Calomel before and after inoculation	72	9	25	3	Only 1 patient has headache (Variolois)	2 only local inflammation. Re-inoculation after 12 days negative.
	10	Same	Inf. Sennae Syr. Rosae as above	66	8	30	2	No complaints of ill health (Variolois)	2 only local. Re-inoculation wounds disappear after 1-2 days.
	11	Same	None, only purgatives at end	288	32	200	7	5 Headache 2 Slight Fever	1 (fever) localized large areola. 1 (no fever) re-inoculation after 14 days negative.
Nov. 1, 1767	8	**B.** Thin pus from variola inoculata	Calomel as above, without other ingredients or purgatives	576	72	440	7	6 Headache 1 Worms (Variolois)	
	8	Same	Inf. Sennae as above	215	29	64	3	1 Headache (Variolois)	
	7	Same	None, Gatti Method	125	18	60	2	2 Headache. 20 days after inoculation the exanthem is gone.	
Nov. 24, 1767	15	**C.** Thick pus from variola inoculata (Exanthem)	None, diet 19 days before operation	727	55	260	2	7 Headache and nausea. Localized inflammation persisted until the course of the exanthem had run. All pustules larger and riper than above.	2 only local inflammation. Re-inoculation after 14 days. Not visible after 3 days.
	5	Same	None, diet only 3 days before operation	293	73	168	4		
	62	From above cases, with pustules		2362	38	440	2	Trivial sickness. Together fewer pustules than in the usual case of smallpox.	All cases appear as if protected. All mingled with the other patients without contracting infection
	12	From above cases, without pustules		0	0				
	74								

Source: A.C. Klebs. *Die Variolation im achtzehnten Jahrhundert; ein historischer Beitrag zur Immunitätsforschung* (Gießen: Verlag von Alfred Töpelmann, 1914).

Variolation in continental Europe was slower to take hold because of two traditions, religion and the French medical establishment, both of which opposed variolation but for different reasons. One of the great progenitors of European continental variolation was Angelo Gatti, who popularized the process and made it more efficient. However, the practice took hold later in the eighteenth century and was ultimately replaced in practice by vaccination, which will be described in a separate section.

In the Western hemisphere, variolation was practiced among the African slaves. The Americans picked up the practice and popularized it a about the same time that it was gaining acceptance in England.

Cotton Mather, a famous cleric in Boston, who also practiced an early form of public health management, learned the practice from his slaves in 1712 and used the pulpit to instruct others on the practice. According to one account, his servant said, ". . . take the Juice of the Small Pox, and Cut the Skin and put in a drop: then by 'nd by a little Sick, then a few Small Pox; and no body dye of it; no body have Small Pox any more" (Lienhard 1997).

Boston ignored Mather for another nine years. On April 22, 1721, the British ship HMS Seahorse arrived in Boston Harbor from Barbados, carrying smallpox. The city was ripe for an epidemic. One physician, Boylston, began doing inoculations. That unleashed a firestorm. People questioned whether we should trust the "groundless Contrivances of Men" instead of the "all-wise providence of God Almighty" (Lienhard 1997). Another threw a bomb through Mather's window. It didn't go off, so the note was preserved. It said, "Cotton Mather, you Dog, Dam you, I'l inoculate you with this; with a pox to you" (Best 2004). Despite these challenges, the practice of variolation took hold in New England and probably saved many lives. However, the lesson did not hold for long, and the city was open for another epidemic during the Revolutionary War. Even though vaccination became widespread in the nineteenth century, Boston would not see its last epidemic end until 1903.

The advent of vaccination in 1796 and its popularization made the systematic elimination of smallpox outbreaks possible for the first time. Popular resistance to vaccination, as well as lack of systematic public health policy, led to situations in which the population became susceptible to outbreaks as the memory of the last one faded.

F. Historical vignettes from North America

1. Montreal, 1885

Sir William Osler wrote,

> The disease smoulders here and there in different localities, and when conditions are favorable, becomes epidemic. Perhaps the most remarkable instance in modern times of the rapid extension of the disease occurred in Montreal in 1885. Small-pox had been prevalent in that city between 1870 and 1875, when it died out, in part owing to the exhaustion of suitable material and in part owing to the introduction of animal vaccination. The health reports show that the city was free from the disease until 1885. During these years, vaccination, to which many of the French Canadians are opposed, was much neglected, so that a large unprotected population grew up in the city. On February 28th a Pullman-car conductor, who had travelled from Chicago, where the disease had been slightly prevalent, was admitted into the Hotel-Dieu, the Civic Small-pox Hospital being at the time closed. Isolation was not carried out, and on the 1st of April, a surgeon in the hospital died of small-pox. Following her decease, with the negligence absolutely criminal, the authorities of the hospital dismissed all patients presenting no symptoms of contagion, who could go home. The disease spread like fire in dry grass, and within 9 months there died in the city, of smallpox, 3,164 persons (Osler 1892).

2. Milwaukee, 1894

The smallpox epidemic in Milwaukee in 1894 led to widespread rioting and revolts against the health department. The policies of the health department under its director Walter Kempster were generally responsible for the disaster, in which 1,079 people suffered from smallpox, and 244 died. There was widespread resistance to vaccination and to isolation policies, in which the rich victims were allowed to remain quarantined in their homes, and the poor were required to be isolated in the smallpox hospital (Leavitt 2003). Milwaukee serves the modern public health professional as an example of what *not* to do in a crisis.

3. Boston, 1901

The Boston outbreak of 1901 started with problems similar to those that Milwaukee had experienced in 1894. By 1903, when it ended, there were 1,596 reported cases and 270 deaths (Albert 2002). Very firm tactics had to be used to overcome initial resistance. In both Milwaukee and Boston, there was considerable resistance to vaccination among the immigrant groups especially, who were traditionally suspicious of authorities, particularly those in uniform. In Boston, several bills were introduced into the sate legislature aimed at limiting the state's ability to require vaccination. The turning point finally came when one of the most vocal anti-vaccinationists, Dr. Pfeiffer, was exposed to smallpox and contracted the disease. He recovered, but this event led to the discrediting of the anti-vaccine faction, and their bills were defeated (Albert 2001).

Patients were quarantined in one of two city-operated isolation hospitals: the Southampton Street Hospital or a hastily-improvised hospital on Gallop's in Boston Harbor. (The island is now abandoned, but it can be seen on the approach to the airport from almost any commercial flight today). Excellent records survive from the Southampton Street Hospital that give us an insight into an oft-asked question today: what was the effect of prior vaccination on the natural history? The caveat to this analysis is that most of the young adult men were sent to Gallop's Island, leaving women, children, and older men at Southampton. The twenty-one-day case-fatality rate among those patients at Southampton Street was 27 percent for the unvaccinated and 11 percent for the vaccinated. Those vaccinated were further divided into unsuccessful vaccination, case-fatality rate, 23 percent; successful vaccination, 9 percent; and recent primary vaccination, 0 percent (Albert 2002).

4. New York City, 1947

In 1947, New York City had its last outbreak of smallpox. New York had not seen smallpox for quite a while and vaccination had been neglected. The initial case was brought in to New York City by a man who was on his way from Mexico to Maine. He spent some time walking around the streets of New York before he went to Bellevue hospital. There, his rash was not recognized by the hospital physicians. He was ultimately transferred Willard Parker Hospital, and he died. The initial presentation went unrecognized, and it wasn't until two more cases arose after death of the index patient, that smallpox was suspected.

After the initial delay, the city got it right, and, under Health Commissioner Israel Weinstein, undertook a mass of vaccination campaign as well as a careful case tracing epidemiological investigation to track down all of the potential contacts of the index case.

The vaccination campaign was well thought out and went well with a great deal of publicity. People stood in lines that wound around the city streets waiting for their turn to be vaccinated. The mayor of New York, Mayor O'Dwyer, locked representatives of drug companies inside City Hall and told them that they were going to produce more vaccine and make it available to the city at a reasonable price, or they were not leaving the building. He succeeded (Leavitt 2003).

The city's handling of this event serves as a model for later crises. There were valuable lessons from the successful containment of the New York exposure that should not be neglected by the modern reader:

- Communicate skillfully and often with the press and with government entities.
- Ask for help from other agencies.
- Treat people and victims with even-handedness.
- Take charge.

Fifty-four years later, the performance of another mayor of New York would underscore the importance of these lessons.

3.2 Smallpox as a Virus

The agent of smallpox was not definitively identified until 1947 (Nagler 1948). Before the eighteenth century, there were several competing beliefs. The minority opinion, the "animalcular" theory, held that tiny organisms, "animalcules" caused the disease. The two dominant theories were the "seed" theory and the "miasmic" theory. In the "seed" theory, everyone was born with smallpox as a genetic condition that would eventually be released. The unintended advantage of this theory is that it allowed an opportunity for preventive inoculation (variolation) to be undertaken, which was otherwise opposed by mostly Calvinist theologians of the time as interfering with God's will. In the "miasmic" theory, certain types of atmospheric conditions were thought to give rise to the infection. This theory arose in part by observations about the seasonal variation of smallpox epidemics. Modern observations have confirmed that the virus is better transmitted in cool, dry climate. Another theory, the "corpuscular" theory, held that smallpox was a poison that was introduced into the body in an unknown fashion. The main difference between this idea and the animalcular one is that the poison was not capable of reproduction; however it could be conveyed from one person to another. Of course, many believed that the disease was simply punishment from God (or, in the pre-Christian era, the gods).

In 1764, the Italian physician Angelo Gatti reasoned that smallpox was caused by a microorganism. Gatti hypothesized that smallpox came from foreign bodies that could be transmitted by direct contact either through the air or by ingestion. He specifically used the word "virus" to describe this foreign body and further hypothesized that it was able to multiply in the victim (Klebs 1914). The notion that smallpox was a specific disease with a specific cause took hold, and ultimately led to better accuracy of differential diagnosis when compared to other diseases like the measles or chickenpox.

In the early twentieth century, the prevailing hypothesis was that smallpox was caused by an intracellular parasite, which could be seen on stained specimens as Guarnieri bodies, after the observations of Giuseppe Guarnieri in 1893 (Councilman 1904b).

In the twentieth century, a new variant of variola emerged, variola minor. The genetic code was not available during the eradication campaign, but it was clearly a different species. Modern techniques have allowed us to look into the genetic code of the variola virus (Nitsche 2004), and to determine its genetic relatedness to other orthopoxviruses.

A. The eradication of smallpox and its potential re-emergence

One of the two greatest achievements of modern medicine was the eradication of smallpox. The other was the discovery of antibiotics in the form of penicillin by Fleming. Of note, the eradication of smallpox was perhaps the only time in history that a species was intentionally made extinct to benefit another. Inexplicably, this achievement has not yet been awarded the Nobel Prize, though it has saved more lives and relieved more human suffering than almost any other medical advance. In its heyday, smallpox claimed over 2 million lives a year. The one person who stands out as the architect of the eradication campaign is D.A. Henderson, at that time working for the WHO and Johns Hopkins University; at the time of this writing the resident scholar at the University of Pittsburgh Center for

Biosecurity (http://www.upmc-biosecurity.org/). His strategy for containing and eradicating the disease stands as one of the greatest achievements of mankind, and is chronicled elsewhere. It is also noteworthy in the twenty-first century to point out that the eradication of smallpox was achieved with an investment of $100 million, thus making this arguably one of the most cost-effective interventions in the history of medicine.

In fact, variola major was eradicated prior to variola minor. The last case of variola major in nature was that of a young girl in Bangladesh, Rahima Banu, diagnosed on October 16, 1975. The last case of variola minor that occurred naturally—and the last smallpox case in the world, was that of Ali Maow Maalin on October 26, 1977, in Somalia. (He is reported to have cried on learning of a laboratory outbreak in 1978 that deprived him of being the last known case (Preston 2002).)

Smallpox made its final appearance in the United States in 1949, in Hidalgo County, Texas. In 1971, with no cases having been reported in the United States in the previous twenty-two years but with six to eight deaths per year due to complications of vaccination, the U.S. Public Health Service formally recommended the discontinuation of routine vaccination, and vaccination of children was stopped in 1972. Most people born before that year were vaccinated. The U.S. military continued to provide vaccination until the early 1980s, and in fact many servicemen were vaccinated multiple times.

The World Health Organization officially certified that smallpox had been eradicated on December 9, 1979, two years after the last case in Somalia. In 1980, the World Health Assembly recommended that all countries cease routine vaccination.

Learning from the accidental release of variola in 1978, WHO recommended destruction of all stocks of smallpox except for two official repositories: the Centers for Disease Control and Prevention (CDC) in Atlanta, Georgia, and the Institute of Viral Preparations in Moscow, Russia. These two stocks were slated for destruction in the year 2000, but the former Soviet Union decided to divert their stocks for the development of offensive biological weapons. Later, viral stocks were moved to the Russian State Research Center of Virology and Biotechnology in Koltsovo (Alibek 1999). The United States decided not to destroy its stocks out of fear that the potential to study the virus to develop countermeasures would be lost. If it were not for these events, this publication might be superfluous to the modern healthcare provider, but the Soviets produced virulent strains of smallpox in mass quantities, and the stocks as well as the scientists who made them are unaccounted for to this day. The accidental release of Anthrax in the former Soviet Union as well as a possible outbreak of smallpox in Aralsk, Kazakhstan (Zelicoff 2003), have provided further evidence of the offensive biological weapons programs under development.

The world's population is vulnerable to infection by smallpox because of the cessation of vaccination. Even those who have been previously vaccinated may only have partial protection. There is evidence from multiple sources that vaccination in the distant past (greater than five years) may protect against mortality but not provide complete immunity (Eichner 2003). Recognizing the potential threat of the re-emergence of smallpox, recommendations exist as to how to deal with a potential outbreak (Henderson 1999a). Those who are tasked with constructing the worst possible scenarios for biodefense have fertile ground for speculation (Inglesby 2000).

One particular passage serves an ample illustration: "A clandestine aerosol release of smallpox, even if it infected only 50 to 100 persons to produce the first generation of cases, would rapidly spread in a now highly susceptible population, expanding by a factor of 10 to 20 times or more with each generation of cases" (Henderson 1999a, 2132). A smallpox outbreak in modern times—with greater population density, greater mobility, more people with medically-altered immune systems, and virtually no immunity among the majority of the population—would be a true challenge.

Smallpox in its natural form is at least an understood entity to a certain extent, but the methods used to eradicate it were practiced by those who also made it into a weapon. It is likely and even probable that genetic engineering has created more virulent and biologically diverse strains of smallpox. Experiments to combine the genes of hemorrhagic fever viruses with those of variola were probably carried out by the Soviets (Preston 2002). Researchers have been able to make the mousepox virus 100-percent virulent in experimental infections in mice by inserting the interleukin-4 gene into the genetic sequence of the virus (Jackson 2001). The technology necessary to perform this feat of molecular biology is well within the grasp of the average microbiologist and could be predicted

(Mullbacher 2001). In fact, the experiment has been reproduced in a microbiology laboratory in St. Louis (Hesman 2003) .These discoveries and other suspected bioengineering programs combine to create considerable fear of the potential for a genetically-engineered virus to be released on the human race, one with the potential for devastating consequences that would make even our ancestors shudder.

B. Biodefense implications

In May, 2000, the U.S. Department of Justice conducted a simulation of a biological attack on a major city. The name of the exercise was TOPOFF, derived from top officials, because it was designed to test the leadership of those in charge. The theoretical agent was *Yersinia pestis*, or plague. The experiment was complex and had many conceptual leaps of faith, and will not be exhaustively examined here. While the agent was not smallpox, the public health lesson was universal: the systems are not in place to deal with a large-scale outbreak of a serious infectious disease, whether natural or intentional (Inglesby 2001). The analysis of this exercise (or, the unauthorized biography of it) by Inglesby, Grossman and O'Toole is a masterpiece of observation and is a must-read for anyone involved in public health, medicine or health law.[1]

C. Clinical manifestations

Much has been written about smallpox in the twenty-first century primarily by authors that have never seen a case of human smallpox. We have therefore decided to concentrate on the observations of those who performed first-hand observations, such as Osler, Dixon, Rao, Fenner, and Henderson. Many of the references that we will draw from are no longer in print and are therefore difficult to find. For this reason, we will attempt to summarize and in some cases repeat their findings. Our objective is not to create new knowledge, but to preserve what has been observed in the past in the hope that it will not be needed in the future.

Pox viruses are the largest and most complex viruses that infect humans (Bray 2004). They probably descended from organisms that infected early forms of life because they have widespread distribution in both vertebrates and invertebrates. They may have evolved with us. There are many varieties of insect pox, some that infect caterpillars. Once infected, the caterpillars become virus producing machines and ultimately die, leaving virus is on the vegetation so that other caterpillars ingest it and become themselves infected.

Variola is a DNA virus and belongs to the genus orthopoxvirus, the member to cause skin lesions in mammals. Some orthopoxviruses are quite fastidious and infect only one species, such as smallpox. An alternate hypothesis of smallpox evolution is implied by its genetic similarity to other pox viruses. Smallpox may have jumped from another species to humans (cross-species transfer) and became established as a human disease in endemic form in large cities. Epidemics occurred when travelers brought the agent to other populations (Bray 2004).

This cross-species transfer was not accompanied by successful adaptation of the smallpox virus to its new host. Variola does not have any animal factor or reservoir and it causes a brief infection that requires close contact for transmission. Infection with variola also causes immunity. Orthopoxviruses also have high replicative fidelity that, among other factors, enables inoculation with the related vaccina virus to protect against variola (Bray 2004).

D. Typical clinical course

Smallpox follows a fairly regular predictable course in the majority of the infections. Up to the twentieth century, there was only one form of variola, but it had several manifestations. The ordinary, pustular type was by far the most common, occurring in about 90 percent of patients. Several other variants occurred in the remaining patients. More benign variants were modified smallpox and variola sine eruptione. Dreaded and much more virulent variants were the hemorrhagic and flat forms. Ordinary smallpox was further subdivided into discrete, semiconfluent, and confluent rashes. In the twentieth century, a new form of smallpox emerged, called variola minor. It had distinctly different clinical manifestations and will be discussed separately.[2]

Then overall fatality rate of variola major is 25–30 percent, but some forms are much more likely to lead to a fatal outcome than others.

1. Acquisition

The virus is generally acquired by inhaling infectious particles, droplet nuclei or aerosols expelled from the oropharynx of infected persons and by direct contact. The critical mass of virus that needs to be inhaled is unknown. (Henderson 1999) The size of the smallpox virion is within the range of particles that can easily be deposited into the alveoli, but most often, the transmission is from droplet nuclei. These particles have a shorter range than suspended nuclei, so most of the time transmission is from "face contact"—three feet or less. However, there have been cases in which infection has been acquired at considerable distance. In England in 1962, four cases of smallpox were documented to have occurred in persons whose only likely source contact was travel to within 10,000, 4,000, 4,000, and 3,000 feet respectively of a smallpox hospital (Bradley 1962). In 1978, one year after the last case of naturally-occurring smallpox, a laboratory accident in Birmingham, England caused the release of enough smallpox to infect a woman on a different floor of the building. (The woman died, and the researcher who inadvertently released the virus committed suicide as a result (Preston 2002).) In a natural outbreak in a German hospital in 1970, there were several cases in which infection took place at some distance from the index patient, carried by air currents and the ventilation system of the hospital (Wehrle 1970).

Many sources have reported that contaminated clothing or bed linens can also spread the virus (as in the example of its intentional use as a bioweapon in the eighteenth century). Dixon goes on the point out several other ways in which smallpox can be transmitted (Dixon 1962, 300–301):

- **The smallpox corpse**. There are many documented cases of contagion from the dead bodies of victims, even after minimal exposure.
- **Clothing and bedding**. Dixon gives several examples of how infection has been carried from victim to a third party by clothing. Outbreaks among laundry workers and their families are well documented, and he provides other examples of healthcare workers and tradesmen transferring the infection from hospital to others.
- **Flies**. There is some evidence to suggest that flies might carry infected material short distances, in areas where flies are found in abundance.
- **Cotton**. While evidence for the survival in cotton is not very convincing, there have been examples in which viable virus was recovered from scabs preserved in cotton at room temperature up to eighteen months after the scab was shed.

- **Animals** have often been blamed for outbreaks, but there is no evidence to support this conclusion, and Dixon dismisses animals as being vectors.

2. Incubation period

After inhalation, the virions are taken up by alveolar macrophages and transported to the lymph nodes, where they multiply. During this time, there is a paucity of symptoms. If there is a known exposure, the person exposed does not need to be quarantined, but should take a nocturnal temperature for seventeen days. At the first sign of fever or illness, the exposed person should be placed in droplet isolation (quarantine), preferably at home.

Once acquired, the smallpox incubation period lasts twelve to fourteen days with a range of seven to seventeen days.[3] Viral proliferation but not viremia is taking place. This phase is believed to be largely asymptomatic.

3. Prodrome

After two weeks of incubation, the prodromal phase starts. The virus infects white blood cells and solid organs. Symptoms appear as the host mobilizes its resources to fight the infection. This is a nonspecific flu-like illness, but some of the manifestations tend to give clues toward smallpox: intense pain in the back, hips, or groin, and headache. Nausea and vomiting are characteristic in this phase, but gastrointestinal function is remarkably normal in most cases for the rest of the illness.

A Sanskrit text from India circa 1500 B.C., the Susruta Samhita, provides this description: "Before [smallpox] appears, fever occurs, with pain over the body, but particularly in the back . . . severe pain is felt in the large and small joints, with cough, shaking, listlessness, and languor; the palate, lips, and tongue are dry with thirst and no appetite" (Hopkins 1983, 16). Severe abdominal pain or delirium may also occur, complicating efforts at diagnosis.

This prodromal phase lasts three to five days and is not associated with the risk of contagion. In general, virus particles are not expelled into the air until the patient develops an enanthem. While the enanthem may precede the exanthem by approximately one day, it is a general axiom that patients are not infective until the rash appears (Henderson 1999). Because of the prodromal illness, smallpox was usually not spread as rapidly or as widely as chickenpox or measles, because those with smallpox were sick at home as a result of the prodrome.

However, William Osler points out that early petechial rashes could be found in about 10–16 percent of patients during this phase of the disease (13 percent in his case series in Montreal in 1885). Osler provided a good description of the early rashes as petechial, as sometimes "measly" or easily confused with measles (Osler 1892). Since very few people alive today have seen smallpox in Caucasians, this observation may have been lost to modern physicians.

> In this stage of invasion the so-called initial rashes may occur, of which two forms can be distinguished—the diffuse, scarlatinal, and the macular or measly form; either of which may be associated with petechiae and occupy a variable extent of the surface . . . The scarlatinal rash may come out as early as the second day and be as diffuse and vivid as in a true scarlatina. The measly rash may also be diffuse and identical in character with that of measles. Urticaria is also occasionally seen. (Osler 1892, 50)

Fenner and Henderson provide an example in their book, *Smallpox and Its Eradication*, now out of print. However, they argue that this fleeting rash may be an "allergic" phenomenon and may be limited to people who have been previously vaccinated. It appears behind the knees, in the axillae, and groin (Fenner 1988).

Contaminated clothing, sheets, blankets, and other items can also transmit the infection. It is well known through history that disinfection of contaminated items was necessary to prevent spread of infection, even before the viral theory emerged.

According to Rao, the symptoms of the prodrome consist of the following (Rao 1972):

- fever, 100 percent
- headache, usually severe 90 percent
- backache, 90 percent
- chills, 60 percent
- vomiting, 50 percent

- pharyngitis, 15 percent
- delirium, 15 percent (mostly in adults)
- abdominal colic, 13 percent
- diarrhea, 10 percent
- convulsions, 7 percent (mostly in children)

Other common symptoms include nausea, anorexia and malaise. Males may manifest groin or testicular pain.

On the second or third day (rarely the fourth day), the fever breaks and the patient feels better, and the macular rash appears.

4. The rash

The phase of the disease following the prodrome is the eruptive phase. The eruption proceeds through several stages, each one taking several days before the next stage appears. The entire sequence takes about two weeks, but the distal portion of the eruptive phase is the most variable.

The clinical manifestations of the disease are largely manifestations of oropharyngeal and dermal invasion and proliferation. While organ manifestations are not uncommon, orthopoxviruses of mammals all tend to be dermatropic. Variola makes and secretes a substance similar to epidermal growth factor, which stimulates the proliferation of skin cells and provides more substrate on which the viruses can grow and multiply. It also appears that the viral machinery works best at temperatures lower than human body temperature (Bray 2004).

The earliest eruption is in the mouth and oropharynx, but it is often overlooked. Macules quickly yield to shallow ulcers on the soft palate, pharynx, and mouth (Dixon 1962). This is followed rapidly or sometimes simultaneously with a macular eruption on the face and forearms that quickly becomes papular while spreading to the trunk and legs (Fenner 1988, 1460). In ordinary smallpox, the pustular rash follows, but other variants may occur.

E. Clinical types of variola major

While other classification schemes exist, perhaps the most familiar is the one devised by Rao and further refined by Fenner and Henderson. The system is as follows.

1. **Ordinary type**. Raised pustular skin lesions. Three subtypes:
   a. **confluent**. Confluent rash on face and forearms.
   b. **semiconfluent**. Confluent rash on face; discrete elsewhere.
   c. **discrete**. Areas of normal skin between pustules, even on face.
2. **Modified type**. Like ordinary type but with an accelerated course.
3. **Variola sine eruptione**. Fever without rash caused by variola infection.
4. **Flat type**. Pustules remain flat; usually confluent or semiconfluent. Usually fatal.
5. **Hemorrhagic type**. Widespread hemorrhages in skin and mucous membranes. Two subtypes:
   a. **early**, with purpuric rash. Always fatal.
   b. **late**, with hemorrhages into base of pustule. Usually fatal.

Adapted from (Rao 1972) and (Fenner 1988, 4).

It is striking to note the case-fatality rates according to these clinical types based on Rao's careful observations of hospitalized patients in Madras. These statistics were modified by Fenner and Henderson to yield the statistics in Table 3.2. One notes the value of vaccination. In the twenty-first century, many ask the question whether previous vaccination confers any benefit. These figures give some consolation, but the effect of vaccination seems to wane over time.

1. Ordinary type

a. Eruptive phase. The first rash is the enanthem, present in the mouth, pharynx and tongue. It starts as small red macules and evolves into ulcerated lesions. Some patients complain of sore throat. The enanthem progresses rapidly and may spread extensively or be almost absent. Fenner and Henderson point out that the saliva would be heavily laden with virus if the enanthem was severe, a significant mode of transmission.

The skin rash (exanthem) starts on the second to fourth day after the onset of fever, first as macules on the face and forehead (herald spots). The rash quickly spreads to the proximal extremities and the trunk, and then the distal extremities, so that within twenty-four hours, it is extensive. The macules quickly give way to papules, but the evolution in any one bodily area tends to be synchronous. There may, for example, be pap-

Table 3.2

	Unvaccinated		Vaccinated	
	% of total cases	Case-fatality rate	% of total cases	Case-fatality rate
Ordinary Type	88.8%	30.2%	70.0%	3.2%
• Confluent	• 22.8%	62.0%	• 4.6%	26.3%
• Semiconfluent	• 23.9%	37.0%	• 7.0%	8.4%
• Discrete	• 42.1%	9.3%	• 58.4%	0.7%
Modified Type	2.1%	0	25.3%	0
Flat Type	6.7%	96.5%	1.3%	66.7%
Hemorrhagic Type	2.4%	96.4%	3.4%	93.9%
• Early	• 0.7%	100%	• 1.4%	100%
• Late	• 1.7%	96.8%	• 2.0%	89.8%
Total		35.5%		6.3%

ules on the face and macules on the extremities at the same time. Each stage of the rash lasts about a day before moving on to the next stage until the rash results in scabs. The progression is from macule to papule to vesicle to pustule. After that, the scab forms, dries, falls off, and leaves a shallow scar that may progress to permanent scarring if deep enough in the skin.

The face, palms, and soles bear the greatest burden of lesions, and the scabs are the most persistent on the palms and soles because of the thickness of the skin.

Evolution of skin lesions (ordinary type smallpox):

Day 1. Erythematous macules.

Day 2. By the second day, the initially flat or macular lesions become papules, but are histologically actually vesicles.

Days 4–5. Clinically, the papules give way to obvious vesicles, which start with clear fluid and then become more pustular within 24–48 hours.

Day 7. All the skin lesions have evolved to the pustular stage and continue to grow in size. At some point in the vesicular phase, the lesions become umbilicated, but once they reach the large pustular stage they lose the umbilication and as the pustules start to mature, they harden and feel very much like small hard beads or buckshot under the skin.

Day 14. By this time, the fluid within the pustules diminishes, and ultimately a scab forms, which separates leaving an area that has become depigmented.

Because of its thickened upper skin layers, the palms and soles of the feet tend to have vesicles formed underneath the skin, which can be seen, but generally are not as raised. Because of this, it may take some time for the skin of the palms and soles to separate and sometimes full casts of the hands and feet could be recovered from the patients.

b. Distribution of the rash. The rash of smallpox is often described as centrifugal, as opposed to that of chickenpox, which is called centripetal. In this respect, the smallpox rash is most dense on the face and extremities; and on the extremities, it is denser distally than proximally. It tends to aggregate on extensor rather than on flexor surfaces and on convexities rather than on concavities. Rickett's sign, named after the physician who described many detailed cases, is a skin sign used in the differential diagnosis of smallpox. Rickett's sign is positive if the apex of the axilla is relatively free of pustules compared to the folds of the axilla (Fenner 1988).

On the trunk, there tends to be more and denser lesions on the back than on the front. On the abdomen, the upper half is usually more affected than the lower, which is also true of the face.

c. Fever. As noted previously, the fever usually falls by the second or third day after the onset of the disease when the rash first appears. However, the fever usually returns by the seventh or eighth day and continues to remain high through the course of the illness until scabs form over the lesions. Sometimes secondary skin infection occurs, and in that case, the fever persists.

The above descriptions are generally applied to the ordinary type of smallpox. Variations smallpox according to the Classification System of

Rao will now be described. It should be pointed out that approximately 88–90 percent of cases observed by Rao were of the ordinary type.

2. Confluent smallpox, ordinary type

This term refers to cases in which there was no evidence of normal tissue occurring between the pustules. If this confluence occurs only on the face, it is known as semi-confluent. In Rao's series, the case fatality rate of confluent ordinary smallpox was 62 percent in the patients who were unvaccinated and, in the semi-confluent type, was fatal in 37 percent.

3. Modified type smallpox

It is somewhat difficult to keep the concept of modified smallpox straight from variola minor, as well as from variola major occurring in patients who had previously been vaccinated. The WHO Scientific Group on smallpox eradication from 1968 defined modified smallpox as an eruption that occurs mostly in vaccinated patients in which crusting is complete within ten days. The skin lesions tend to evolve more quickly, are more superficial and may not show the characteristic uniformity of the more typical smallpox eruption. Ultimately in 1972, the WHO expert committee on smallpox eradication qualified this description by relating modified smallpox specifically to smallpox in vaccinated persons.

4. Variola sine eruptione

This is a febrile illness that occurs among vaccinated people with no rash. Usually, there is a high fever with headache and backache. Within forty-eight hours, the fever subsides. Viral isolation experiments, conducted before the advent of modern DNA analysis, indicated the presence of smallpox in the oropharyngeal secretions of patients with this illness.

5. Flat-type smallpox

This type of smallpox was given this appellation because of the fact that the lesions did not become raised or form the characteristic papules or pustules. It was unusual—occurring in only 6.7 percent of unvaccinated people in Rao's series, and the majority of cases occurred in children (72 percent). This form carried a very high fatality rate. The enanthem was quite severe, which usually occurred on the mouth and tongue, but could sometimes be found in other mucous membranes such as the rectal area.

The lesions on the skin mature slowly and, although they start out as discrete lesions, do not take on the characteristics of raised lesions but rather seem to be inside or under the skin, actually starting with a small depression in the skin. Many times these lesions are accompanied by some hemorrhage, although not as extensive as in the hemorrhagic type of smallpox. In contrast to the "shotty" feel of the ordinary smallpox, the skin in this eruption feels soft and velvety (Fenner 1988).

The skin may become quite friable. Sometimes, the skin is diffusely affected rather than in the typical smallpox distribution. In this particular form of smallpox, the enanthem extends even into the lungs causing pneumonia or adult respiratory distress syndrome (ARDS, as we define it today), or both. In addition, the gastrointestinal tract is characteristically affected and an acute gastric dilatation was noticed 24–48 hours before death in many subjects. Dilatation of the stomach and change in color of the lesions from red to grey portend a very poor prognosis. In some cases, the rectal mucous membranes completely sloughed. Fenner and Henderson hypothesized that flat smallpox occurred in people with deficient cellular immunity (Fenner and Henderson 1988, 32).

6. Hemorrhagic type

The hemorrhagic syndromes carry an especially poor prognosis, and it appears that the early and late forms should be classified as two physiologically and pathologically distinct syndromes with similar clinical manifestations and outcomes. These manifestations are particularly striking in the reports that describe them, with the skin turning dark purple to black. Hemorrhage occurs from the mucous membranes, lungs, and urinary tract. The conjunctivae accumulate dark blood, giving a frightful appearance to the victim. There is an erythematous rash that is common in the early stages of hemorrhagic smallpox and this may be difficult to distinguish from the prodromal rash of ordinary smallpox.

In earlier writings, hemorrhagic smallpox was called "purpura variolosa" and "variola pustulosa hemorrhagica." Rao probably started the convention to call them early and late hemorrhagic type smallpox. When the hemorrhage enters the skin and the mucous membranes early in the disease, this is called the early hemorrhagic phase. It appears to be a vigorous form of disseminated intravascular coagulopathy, though modern studies on the blood of victims have never been performed. This type of smallpox leads invariably to death and can be quite dramatic, with extensive hemorrhage from the mouth, gums, nose, stomach, lungs, urinary tract, and female genital tract.

This type of smallpox is exceptionally rare but, perhaps because of how dramatic it is, it has been written about extensively. It is interesting to hypothesize that it is caused by some sort of immune phenomenon because it tended to occur in generally healthy adults and is as common in vaccinated subjects as it is in unvaccinated subjects. In the early hemorrhagic type of smallpox, the rash starts on the second day with a generalized erythema quickly giving rise to petechiae (pinpoint skin hemorrhages) and areas of ecchymoses (bruising). In addition, the patients develop high fever and continue to have severe headache and backache. In this respect, the illness may easily be confused with meningococcal meningitis. Authors in the early twentieth century described a characteristic expression of the face and fetid odor of the breath. (Ricketts 1908) Usually the patients die on the sixth day of the fever and usually remain conscious until the end. It appeared that lung congestion with or without congestive heart failure was common in these patients. Pregnant women were especially susceptible to this subtype.

7. Late hemorrhagic type smallpox

Occasional descriptions survive from even as far back as the fifteenth and sixteenth century about victims who seem to be getting better and resolving the fever and rash only suddenly to develop the hemorrhagic form. In this type, hemorrhage appears as the lesions mature from papules into pustules, but instead of pustules, the lesions develop hemorrhagic characteristics, starting at the base of the lesions. Patients continue to remain febrile or septic throughout the whole course of the illness. The majority of cases of late hemorrhagic smallpox were fatal, death occurring between the eighth and tenth day (Fenner 1988, 38). However, as opposed the early type, the fatality rate was not 100 percent. Fenner and Henderson postulate "haemorrhagic type small pox was primarily due to defects and the response to infection by individual patients" (Fenner 1988, 38). They go on to say, ". . . these cases were characterized by high and sustained viraemia, severe depletion of platelets, and a poorly developed humoral immune response."

F. Laboratory findings

In general, in the patients with smallpox the white blood cell count is variable, the number of neutrophils falls, and the number of lymphocytes rises during the infection. However, as the patients developed the pustular stage, granulocytes become more numerous in the blood, thrombocytopenia is common in the hemorrhagic form, again suggesting disseminated intravascular coagulation.

G. Organ complications

Pneumonia was a common complication of pustular smallpox, being reported in many autopsy series. One typical report is that of Councilman, Magrath, and Brinckerhoff in the 1904 Boston outbreak. They reported forty-five cases of bronchopneumonia or lobar pneumonia out of fifty-four autopsy studies (83 percent) (Councilman 1904a). Other series reported pneumonia in at least half of fatal cases of pustular smallpox. The question whether actual involvement of the lungs by smallpox virus occurs remains unresolved to this day. There are those who propose that the evidence indicates a viral pneumonia could occur in the patients with smallpox and others who advocate that the only form of pneumonia was secondary bacterial superinfection. Tantalizing but indirect evidence from animal experiments in 1929 demonstrated the presence of Guarnieri bodies in the lung tissue of rabbits infected with vaccinia virus that developed pneumonia (Armstrong 1929), but human autopsy studies demonstrating Guarnieri bodies are unavailable. In 1876, Ivanowski reported seeing material in pathologic specimens of lung tissue from smallpox victims who had died with pneumonia. This material was described in a way that makes it seem very similar to Guarnieri bodies (Ivanowski 1876). This short passage appears in a widely-read text on pathology from 1948: "In fatal cases, pneumonia is often present. Although it is difficult to follow the sequences, there is evidence that the pneumonia is primarily of the interstitial or viral type, which is obscured later by superimposed streptococcal and other bacterial infections" (Anderson 1948, 359). However, Dixon notes that a viral pneumonia syndrome attributable to variola was never demonstrated with conviction (Dixon 1962). The final outcome of this controversy is unknown. It has also been described that people had severe liquefaction of internal organs in cases of hemorrhagic smallpox, but again this is probably secondary to diffuse intravascular coagulation.

H. Complications

Common complications with smallpox infection include the following.

- **Cellulitis** of the skin
- **Conjunctivitis**
- **Corneal ulceration and keratitis**
- **Arthritis or osteomyelitis variolosa**. This occurs most commonly in the elbow and is primarily from viral infection of the metaphyses of growing bones.
- **Bronchitis and pneumonitis**, as mentioned above. This could be either bacterial bronchopneumonia or other manifestations.
- **Gastrointestinal**. The occurrence of gastrointestinal complications from smallpox was observed, but was not attributable to smallpox for certain by the time the disease no longer appeared in humans.
- **Genitourinary** system. Orchitis sometimes occurred and, sometimes, hematuria.
- **Encephalitis**. Occurred in about one in 500 cases in variola major (Rao 1972), and about one in 2,000 cases of variola minor (Fenner 1988).

Many patients developed the characteristic pockmarks or scarring of the skin, which were permanent; some became blind, and some had limb deformities.

I. Variola minor

In 1904, Korte' described a form of smallpox with a low (1 percent) case-fatality rate know in South Africa as kaffir-pox or *amaas*, a word of uncertain origin (Fenner 1988, 3). Chapin later described a similar disease that had been present in North and South America since as early in 1896, called "alastrim" from the Portuguese word *alastra*, a derivation of what English-speakers would call "tinder fire." Ultimately, alastrim came to be called "variola minor," causing the more classical form to be named "variola major." The disease spread from South Africa to Florida, then to North and South America and Europe.

In retrospect, variola minor was a form of smallpox believed to be a strain that arose in the twentieth century and had case fatality rates of less than 1 percent. In addition, the occurrence of the disease was accompanied by less intensity of symptoms. Apparently, experiencing a case of variola minor conferred immunity to variola major. Also, of note is that some authors notice the prodromal rashes in this form of smallpox very commonly in people of fair skin origin, but almost never in people of dark skin origin. The individual lesions appeared smaller than those of variola major and the evolution of the rash was quite a bit faster.

There were also outbreaks in which the case-fatality rate was somewhere between that of variola major (greater than 20 percent) and variola minor (less than 1 percent), leading some to hypothesize that there was an "intermedius" strain, but this was never definitively proven and remains unsettled to this day.

J. The effect of immunity

Little is written about the clinical manifestations of smallpox in those with immune suppression. Most of the observations about immunity in modern times are associated with vaccinia and its complications and are discussed separately. Buller induced HIV-like immunosuppression in mice, then infected them with mousepox virus (ectromelia). The lack of immunity resulted in a failure of the virus-specific cytotoxic-T-cell response, which was associated with an increased susceptibility to the lethal effects of the virus (Buller 1987). In 10 HIV-positive military personnel who were inadvertently vaccinated in the modern vaccination program, no adverse events occurred (Tasker 2004). Smallpox vaccination could theoretically result in serious complications for patients with organ transplantation (Dropulic 2003) and AIDS (Bartlett 2003) so, by extension, smallpox would probably be worse. It is important to emphasize that there is no contraindication to vaccination in the face of an outbreak of smallpox, because whatever the vaccination could cause probably pales in comparison to an attack of variola.

Fewer than 100 percent of those exposed to smallpox actually develop the illness, but the reasons are obscure. Natural immunity certainly plays a role, and there are reports from the past of people who appeared to be completely resistant to infection despite no known previous infection. In addition to cell-mediated immunity, there is some question about whether factors related to the skin may play a role in the ability to resist the spread of poxviruses. For example, people with atopic dermatitis are at increased risk for eczema vaccinatum following inoculation with vaccinia (the smallpox vaccine), a condition in which the rash spreads to areas that are or have been affected by atopic disease. People with atopic dermatitis lack endogenous antimicrobial peptides in the skin (Ong 2002). These naturally-occurring peptides (defensins) have broad antimicrobial properties and are present in the skin of all mammals (Zasloff 2002). Whether the distribution and concentration of such peptides is a factor in susceptibility is unknown.

Endnotes

1. Another simulation was performed using smallpox as the weapon. The name of the exercise was "Dark Winter," and an analysis was done by Inglesby, O'Toole, and Henderson, but was not available at the time we were composing this chapter.

2. In the context of bioterrorism, it is unlikely that variola minor would be used as an agent. However, we consider this virus strain in the context that it might serve other uses, such as induction of immunity.

3. While the rule of 7–17 days always held in natural smallpox outbreaks, there is fear that in a deliberate smallpox attack with a highly concentrated load of infectious particles, the incubation period may be far shorter, even as short as two days. (Patrick 2004)

References

"25th anniversary of the last case of naturally acquired smallpox." *JAMA* 288(20):2533 (2002).

Albert, M.R. et al. "The last smallpox epidemic in Boston and the vaccination controversy, 1901–1903." *N. Engl. J. Med.* 344(5):375–379 (2001).

———. "Smallpox manifestations and survival during the Boston epidemic of 1901 to 1903." *Ann. Intern. Med.* 137(12):993–1000 (2000).

Alibek, K. *Biohazard: The Chilling True Story of the Largest Covert Biological Weapons Program in the World, Told from the Inside by the Man Who Ran It* (NY Random House, 1999).

Anderson, W.A.D. *Pathology* (St. Louis: Mosby, 1948).

Armstrong, C. and R.D. Lillie. "Vaccine virus pneumonia in rabbits." *Pub. Health Rep.* 44:2635 (1929).

Barbera, J. et al. "Large-scale quarantine following biological terrorism in the United States: Scientific examination, logistic and legal limits, and possible consequences." *JAMA* 286(21): 2711–7 (2001).

Barquet, N. and P. Domingo. "Smallpox: The triumph over the most terrible of the ministers of death." *Ann. Intern. Med.* 127(8 Pt. 1):635–42 (1991).

Bartlett, J.G. "Smallpox vaccination and patients with human immunodeficiency virus infection or acquired immunodeficiency syndrome." *Clin. Infect. Dis.* 36(4):468–71 (2003).

Baxby, D. "Smallpox vaccination techniques; from knives and forks to needles and pins." *Vaccine* 20(16):2140–2149 (2004).

Behbehani, A.M. "Rhazes. The original portrayer of smallpox." *JAMA* 252(22): 3156–9 (1984).

Best, M. et al. "'Cotton Mather, you dog, dam you! I'll inoculate you with this; with a pox to you': Smallpox inoculation, Boston, 1721." *Qual. Saf. Health Care* 13(1):82–3 (2004).

Blake, J.B. *Public Health in the Town of Boston 1630–1822* (Cambridge, MA: Harvard University Press, 1959).

Boylston, A.W. "Clinical investigation of smallpox in 1767." *N. Engl. J. Med.* 346(17):1326–1328 (2002).

Bradley, W.H. "Smallpox in England and Wales 1962." *Proc. Roy. Soc. Med.* 56:335–338 (1962)

Bras, G. "The morbid anatomy of smallpox." *Arch. Path.* 54(149):303–351 (1952).

Bray, M. "New data in a 200-year investigation." *Clin. Infect. Dis.* 38(1): 90–1 (2004a).

Bray, M. and M. Buller. "Looking back at smallpox." *Clin. Infect. Dis.* 38(6):882–9 (2004b).

Brown, T.H. "The African connection: Cotton Mather and the Boston smallpox epidemic of 1721–1722." *JAMA* 260(15): 2247–9 (1988).

Buller, R.M. et al. "Abrogation of resistance to severe mousepox in C57BL/6 mice infected with LP-BM5 murine leukemia viruses." *J. Viro.* 61(2):383–7 (1987).

Councilman, W.T. et al. *The Pathological Aanatomy and Histology of Variola* (Boston: Harvard Medical School, 1904a).

———. "Studies on the pathology and the etiology of variola and vaccinia." *J. Med. Res.* 11:1–235 (1904b).

Demkowicz, W.E. et al. (1996). "Human cytotoxic T-cell memory: Long-lived responses to vaccinia virus." *J. Virol.* 70(4):2627–31 (1996).

Dhar, A.D. et al. "Tanapox infection in a college student." *N. Engl. J. Med.* 350(4):361–366 (2004).

Dixon, C.W. *Smallpox* (London: J. & A. Churchill, 1962).

Dropulic, L.K. et al. "Smallpox vaccination and the patient with an organ transplant." *Clin. Infect. Dis.* 36(6):786–8 (2003).

Dworetzky, M. "Smallpox, October 1945." *N. Engl. J. Med.* 346(17):1329 (2002).

Eichner, M. "Analysis of historical data suggests long-lasting protective effects of smallpox vaccination." *Am. J. Epidemiol.* 158(8):717–23 (2003).

Fenn, E.A. *Pox Americana: The Great Smallpox Epidemic of 1775–82* (NY: Hill and Wang, 2001).

Fenner, F. "Nature, nurture and my experience with smallpox eradication." *Med. J. Aust.* 171(11–12):638–41 (1999).

Fenner, F. et al. *Smallpox and Its Eradication* (Geneva: World Health Organization, 1988).

Fornaciari, G. "Renaissance mummies in Italy." *Med. Secoli.* 11(1) 85–105 (1999).

Frey, S.E. and R.B. Belshe. "Poxvirus zoonoses: Putting pocks into context." *N. Engl. J. Med.* 350(4):324–327 (2004).

Grundy, I. "Montagu's variolation." *Endeavour* 24(1):4–7 (2000).

Hampton, T. "New smallpox vaccine shows promise." *JAMA* 291(15): 1825 (2004).

Henderson, D.A. "Lessons from the eradication campaigns." *Vaccine* 17 Suppl 3: S53–5 (1999a).

Henderson, D.A. et al. "Smallpox as a biological weapon: Medical and public health management: Working Group on Civilian Biodefense." *JAMA* 281(22):2127–37 (1999b).

Hesman, T. "Vaccine-evading mouse virus raises big issue." *St. Louis Post-Dispatch*, 2003.

Holmes, G. et al. "The death of young King Edward VI." *N. Engl. J. Med.* 345(1): 60–2 (2001).

Hopkins, D.R. *The Greatest Killer: Smallpox in History* (Chicago: University of Chicago, 1983).

Inglesby, T.V. et al. "A plague on your city: Observations from TOPOFF." Clin. Infec.t Dis. 32(3):436–45 (2001).

Inglesby, T.V. et al. "Preventing the use of biological weapons: Improving response should prevention fail." *Clin. Infect. Dis.* 30(6):926–9 (2000).

Ivanowski, N. "Die parasitaeren Knoten in den Lungen bei Variola." *Virchow-Hirsch Jahresbericht* 11:52 (1876).

Jackson, R.J. et al. "Expression of mouse ynterleukin-4 by a recombinant ectromelia virus suppresses cytolytic lymphocyte responses and overcomes genetic resistance to mousepox." *J. Virol.* 75(3):1205–1210 (2001).

Jones, D.S. *Rationalizing Epidemics: Meanings and Uses of American Indian Mortality since 1600* (Cambridge, MA: Harvard University, 2004).

Joseph, D.G. "MSJAMA: Uses of *Jacobson v. Massachusetts* in the age of bioterror." *JAMA* 290(17):2331 (2003).

Kim, M. et al. "Biochemical and functional analysis of smallpox growth factor (SPGF) and anti-SPGF monoclonal antibodies." *J. Biol. Chem.* M400343200 (2004).

Klebs, A.C. *Die Variolation im achtzehnten Jahrhundert: Ein historischer Beitrag zur Immunitätsforschung* (Gießen: Verlag von Alfred Töpelmann, 1914).

Leavitt, J.W. "Public resistance or cooperation? A tale of smallpox in two cities." *Biosecur. Bioterror.* 1(3):185–92 (2003).

Lienhard, J.M. *Slaves and Smallpox: Engines of Our Ingenuity* (Houston: University of Houston, 2004).

Lillie, R.D. "Smallpox and vaccinia: The pathologic anatomy." *Arch. Path.* 10(241):241–291 (1930).

Lipkowitz, E. "MSJAMA: The physicians' dilemma in the 18th-century French smallpox debate." *JAMA* 290(17):2329–30 (2003).

Littman, R.J. and M.L. Littman. "Galen and the Antonine plague." *Amer. J. Philol.* 94:243–55 (1973).

McIntyre, J.W. and C.S. Houston. "Smallpox and its control in Canada." *Cmaj.* 161(12):1543–7 (1999).

Mullbacher, A. and M. Lobigs. "Creation of killer poxvirus could have been predicted." *J. Virol.* 75(18):8353–8355 (2001).

Nagler, F.P.O. and G. Rake "The use of the electorn microscope in diagnosis of variola, vaccinia, and varicella." *J. Bact.* 55:45–51 (1948).

Naleway, A.L. et al. "Eczematous skin disease and recall of past diagnoses: Implications for smallpox vaccination." *Ann. Intern. Med.* 139(1):1–7 (2003).

Nitsche, A. et al. "Detection of orthopoxvirus DNA by real-time PCR and identification of variola virus DNA by melting analysis." *J. Clin. Microbiol.* 42(3): 1207–1213 (2004).

Ong, P.Y. et al. "Endogenous antimicrobial peptides and skin infections in atopic dermatitis." *N. Engl. J. Med.* 347(15): 1151–1160 (2002).

Osler, W. *The Principles and Practice of Medicine* (NY: D. Appelton, 1892).

Patrick, W. (2004). Potential shortening of incubation period of smallpox infection by increasing infectious load. L.C. Tripoli. St. Louis, MO: Dinner meeting with Bill Patrick and Bill Stanhope. This observation was based on experiments in animals with other pathogens. Mr. Patrick, a microbiologist who worked in the offensive bioweapons program at USAMRIID before it was closed in 1969, made this observation based on work he had observed but not done himself.

Patterson, K.B. and T. Runge "Smallpox and the Native American." *Am. J. Med. Sci.* 323(4):216–22 (2002).

Pepose, J.S. et al. "Ocular complications of smallpox vaccination." *Am. J. Ophthalmol.* 136(2):343–52 (2003).

Popov, S. "Commentary on Dr. Alan P. Zelicoff's analysis (No. 6)." *Crit. Rev. Microbiol.* 29(2):175–6; discussion 183–90 (2003).

Preston, R. (2002). The Demon in the freezer: a true story. New York, Random House.

Rao, A.R. *Smallpox* (Bombay: Kothari Book Depot, 1972).

Reed, K.D. et al. "The detection of monkeypox in humans in the Western hemisphere." *N. Engl. J. Med.* 350(4):342–350 (2004).

Ricketts, T.F. *A Classification of Cases of Smallpox by the Numerical Severity of the Eruption* (London: McCorquodale, 1893).

——— *The Diagnosis of Smallpox* (London, Cassell, 1908).

Rudolph, R. and D.M. Musher. "Inoculation in the Boston smallpox epidemic of 1721." *Arch. Int. Med.* 115:692–696 (1965).

Sarynov, E. et al. (2003). "Report on measures taken to contain and eradicate the smallpox outbreak locale in the city of Aralsk (September/October, 1971)." *Crit. Rev. Microbiol.* 29(2):109–44; discussion 149–52 (2003)

Schoepp, R.J. et al. "Detection and identification of variola virus in fixed human tissue after prolonged archival storage." *Lab. Invest.* 84(1):41–8 92004).

Stone, A.F. and W.D. Stone. "Lady Mary Wortley Montagu: Medical and religious controversy following her introduction of smallpox inoculation." *J. Med. Biogr.* 10(4):232–6 (2002).

Tasker, S.A. et al. Unintended smallpox vaccination of HIV-1 infected individuals in the United States military." *Clin. Infect. Dis.* 38:1320–1322 (2004).

Taylor, H.A. and R.R. Faden. "Ethical considerations in the formation of smallpox vaccine policy." *Biosecur. Bioterror.* 1(1):47–52 (2003).

Tucker, J.B. and R.A. Zilinskas. "The 1971 smallpox outbreak in the Soviet city of Aralsk: Implications for variola virus as a bioterrorist threat: Introduction." *Crit. Rev. Microbiol.* 29(2):81–95 (2003).

Watson, W. *An Account of a Series of Experiments, Instituted with a View of Ascertaining the Most Successful Method of Inoculating the Small-Pox* (London, 1768).

Wehrle, P.F. et al. "An airborne outbreak of smallpox in a German hospital and its significance with respect to other recent outbreaks in Europe." *Bull. World Health Organ.* 43(5):669–79 (1970).

Young, D.C. "Smallpox vaccination in the shadow of Jenner." *Lancet* 363(9410): 738 (2004).

Yutu, J. et al. "Outbreaks of smallpox due to variolation in China, 1962–1965." *Am. J. Epidemiol.* 128(1):39-45 (1988).

Zasloff, M. "Antimicrobial peptides in health and disease." *N. Engl. J. Med.* 347(15):1199–1200 (2002).

Zaucha, G.M. et al. "The pathology of experimental aerosolized monkeypox virus infection in cynomolgus monkeys (*Macaca fascicularis*)." *Lab. Invest.* 81(12):1581–600 (2001).

Zelicoff, A.P. "An epidemiological analysis of the 1971 smallpox outbreak in Aralsk, Kazakhstan." *Crit. Rev. Microbiol.* 29(2):97–108 (2003).

Appendix A. Smallpox Prevention

Contact precautions

Smallpox spreads from person to person primarily through droplet nuclei and aerosols expressed from the respiratory tract of infected patients and inhaled by susceptible persons who are generally in close contact.[1,2] The greatest risk is to household members. The period of contagion is dated from the onset of the rash and is greatest for the next 7–10 days.[3,4] Secondary cases are usually restricted to close contacts, an average of two to five cases/primary source. The reason for this restricted spread is that most patients are confined to bed by the time of the onset of rash and the period of transmission. Variola virus is present in high concentrations in skin lesions, especially scabs, but this does not appear to be a major factor in transmission because the virus is tightly bound to the scab matrix and is a less important source of aerosolization. Thus, the major mechanism of transmission is aerosolization from the respiratory tract similar to the mechanism for chickenpox. Although aerosolization over distances beyond close patient contact is unusual, there have been outbreaks within hospitals that have implicated spread to adjacent rooms, wards and even floors of hospitals.[5] The standard practice for smallpox control during the period of epidemics was to isolate victims until scabs had separated from the skin.

Another potential source of smallpox was infected clothing and bedding, which accounted for some cases in laundry workers. The potential for spread by contaminated surfaces, carpets, letters and so forth is unlikely due to the fragility of the virus at room temperature and the limitation of aerosolization. In the context of bioterrorism, the assumption is an aerosol release of the virus with the first recognition of cases after an incubation period of 12–14 days and then 2–3 days for the appearance of the rash. In terms of the susceptibility, it is assumed that all people are susceptible with adequate exposure if they do not have immunity from vaccination (discussed below). These observations account for current recommendations regarding prevention strategies according to the consensus statement of the Johns Hopkins Working Group on Civilian Biodefense.[6]

When a diagnosis of smallpox is made there should be an attempt to isolate all suspected cases immediately. Household contacts and other face-to-face contacts should be placed under surveillance and should be vaccinated unless already vaccinated with a documented response. It is preferred that patients are isolated in the home rather than hospitals where the potential for spread could be far more substantial. The emphasis is on contacts defined as persons who live in the same household or have had face-to-face contact after the onset of fever. These contacts should have temperature measurements daily in the evening for the seventeen-day period after exposure. In the event of fever, these contacts should be isolated at home.

Post-exposure prophylaxis

Vaccination is a critical part of the post-exposure prevention strategy which should be used for those who are exposed by aerosol release and those who are household or close face-to-face contacts as defined above. Vaccination should be given as quickly as possible after exposure and is probably effective for up to four days post-exposure.[7] The benefit is for prevention and, for those who nevertheless acquired disease, a significant reduction in mortality.[8]

Vaccination

Sources

The original vaccination for smallpox was cowpox strains tested by Jenner in the late eighteenth century. The current vaccine is vaccinia, another orthopoxvirus of uncertain origin, but distinct from both smallpox and cowpox.[9] Current vaccines are derived from one of four vaccinia strains: the Lister strain with vaccine, the New York City Board of Health (NYBOH) strain, the Temple of Heaven strain used in China and the Patwadanger strain used in India. In the US, the standard has been the New York Board of Health strain with vaccine produced by Wyeth Pharmaceuticals as DryVax. This product was grown in the skin of calves, freeze-dried and packaged in 100-dose vials that are reconstituted. Before 1972, smallpox vaccination was routinely given to all children at age one year in the US and for military recruits going to foreign countries. Routine vaccination was discontinued in the U.S. in 1972 so that relatively few U.S. citizens have been vaccinated who were born before 1971, which accounts for about half of the U.S. population.[10] The exception are some military personnel, participants in vaccine trials, and participants in the three-phase vaccination plan of President Bush for 2003–04 which included approximately 580,000 military personnel and 37,000 volunteers participating as smallpox response teams.[11] The freeze-dried DryVax may be preserved almost indefinitely at –20° C and probably at 4° C as well. This product shows potency after storage over thirty years of 1.6×107 pfu/ml.[12] The NYBOH strain has been grown in Vero cells and is currently undergoing trials that appear to show equivalence with DryVax in terms of immunogenicity.

Efficacy

The efficacy of vaccination has historically been judged at 90.7–96.7 percent.[13,14] Neutralizing antibody develops approximately ten days post vaccination, which is 4–8 days prior to the antigenic response of naturally occurring smallpox; this presumably accounts for the benefit of vaccination in the early post-exposure period.[15] The duration of protection is debated due to variations in the duration of humoral response (as measured by neutralizing antibody, complement fixation and hemagglutination inhibition assays) and cell-mediated response.[16,17] Prior teaching suggested that protection lasted 5–10 years and revaccination was customary at 3–10 year intervals. The debate is based on differences noted in the antigenic response according to humoral or cell-mediated responses, rates of disease or severity of disease during epidemics following varying duration of prior vaccination and responses with re-vaccination.[16–19] The current opinion by most authorities is that the duration of protection against infection is more than the 5–10 years as previously thought but specifics about duration of long-term protection are not clear.

Vaccination strategies

Indications for smallpox vaccination has varied through the years. The procedure was abandoned in the U.S. as a routine childhood vaccination in 1972 and abandoned in the rest of the world in 1980 when WHO declared smallpox eradicated. On December 13, 2002 President Bush announced a three-phase smallpox vaccination plan which included a mandatory vaccination for selected members of the armed forces and personnel who served in high-risk parts of the world as a mandatory phase one program that was initiated on December 13, 2002. The second part of the phase one plan was a voluntary program with a target of 440,000 public health response and health care teams initiated in February 2003. This latter phase was suspended after about 39,000 were vaccinated due to concerns about workmen's compensation, questions about liability, questions about the possibility of an association with myocardial infarction and concerns myopericarditis as a newly described side effect. Phase two of the plan was to include approximately 10 million additional health care providers as well as first responders and phase three would be an offering to the general public for voluntary vaccination anticipated in late 2003 or 2004. The destiny of these plans is now unclear.

Indications and contraindications

In the event of a confirmed, imminent or likely exposure to smallpox virus, there are no absolute contraindications to vaccinia vaccine. However, when the vaccine is voluntary and there are no direct benefits to the vaccinee, vaccine policies need to be ultra conservative to assure safety; a number of contraindications apply:[20,21]

- pregnancy or intended pregnancy within four weeks
- immunodeficiency, including HIV infection, congenital or acquired immunodeficiency disorder, organ transplantation, generalized malignancy, leukemia, lymphoma, and autoimmune disease
- immunosuppressive therapy including corticosteroid therapy (at least 20 mg/day prednisone for at least fourteen days), radiotherapy, enzyme metabolite therapy, alkylating HM therapy, chemotherapy and other immunomodulatory medications
- eczema or atopic dermatitis that is active or by prior history
- skin diseases including burns, wounds, contact dermatitis, recent surgical incisions, chickenpox, shingles, herpes, psoriasis, Darier disease and severe acne
- conjunctival or corneal diseases
- allergy to components of DryVax including polymyxin B, streptomycin, chlortetracycline, neomycin, or phenol

These contraindications apply when the potential vaccinee has any of these conditions or has a close contact, usually a household contact, with one of these conditions. It is estimated that 25–37 percent of Americans would be excluded on the basis of these contraindications and that about half of these would be contraindications due to a condition in a household contact.[6,20]

Method

Someone versed in the unique methods and also protected by vaccination should administer the vaccine. In the event of an emergency, the vaccinator can be vaccinated and then begin vaccinations immediately. The methods are unique to this vaccine.[21] There is no skin preparation, a bifurcated needle is dipped into the vaccine's vial and there are then three rapid epidermal punctures (primary vaccination) or fifteen rapid epidermal punctures (revaccination). Each puncture should be of sufficient depth for a trace of blood at the vaccination site after 15–30 seconds. The lesion is covered with sterile gauze or a semiocclusive cover such as Opsite. The vaccinee is instructed to not touch, rub or scratch the site which contains viable vaccinia virus that can be transmitted to an unvaccinated contact. The vaccination site then evolves with a papule at 3–4 days, vesicle at 5–6 days, pustule at 8–9 days, crusting with scab formation at about 12 days and scab detachment leaving a scar at 17–21 days. A "take" is defined as the presence of a papule, vesicle, ulcer or crusted lesion surrounded by an area of induration. More than 95 percent with this reaction will have a serologic response.[22] Other reactions are deemed "equivocal"; immunity is uncertain and it is recommended that these patients be revaccinated. The recent experience with DryVax to 680 previously unvaccinated healthy adults age 18–32 years indicated a take rate of 97–99 percent.[23] With revaccination, the same criteria applied, but evolution takes place over a shorter period. Systemic symptoms are common including headache, nausea, fever, chills, malaise and myalgias that typically peak at days 8–10 postvaccination and resolve in 1–3 days. Fevers greater than 38.9° C and fever after day 16 are seen in only about 1 percent of vaccine recipients.[24] The recent military experience with vaccinations of 580,000 military recruits showed approximately 3 percent took sick call for an average of 1.5 days.

Adverse reactions

Adverse reactions to the vaccine are common and have been extensively studied with several by Lane et al. in the 1960s[25–27] and in the more recent experience, especially in the military.[24,27] The major complications are summarized in Table 3A.1 and below:

- **eczema vaccinatum**. This occurs in vaccinated persons and unvaccinated contacts who have active or inactive eczema. This is now recognized as a T-cell defect disorder, which presumably accounts for the association.[29] Clinical features are multiple cutaneous lesions that look like the primary site of inoculation, especially in areas of eczema, but also in uninvolved skin. Prompt VIG therapy appears to be effective.[27,30]

Table 3A.1
Complications of Smallpox Vaccination

Complication	10 state 1960s (1 million)[26]	National survey (1 million)[25]	Military program (1 million)[24,38,39]
Postvaccinial Encephalitis	8.6	2.4	2.0
Progressive vaccinia	1.7	10	0
Eczema vaccination	40	11	0
Myopericarditis	0	0	60
Contact vaccinia	20	–	20

- **progressive vaccinia**. This is a devastating complication, usually fatal, in patients who have impaired immune defenses, especially impaired CMI.[30] In these cases, the vaccine injection site shows progressive enlargement, often complicated by 10–20 large, painless skin ulcers that expand concentrically without inflammation.[33–35] This complication has been described in a patient with AIDS raising concern about this risk in the HIV-infected population;[35] nevertheless, the majority of patients with HIV infection who are vaccinated do not appear to have any complications, presumably because of adequate CD4 cell counts.[24,27] Standard treatment in the 1960s was VIG, but it is uncertain that this conferred benefit and, for patients with HIV infection, HAART is probably more logical.
- **postvaccinal encephalitis**. This is thought to be an autoimmune reaction that usually occurs after primary immunization with two forms: postvaccinal encephalitis and postvaccination encephalomyelitis. Clinical features include mental status changes, seizures and CSF with mononuclear cells and increased protein. Mortality rates are as high as 25 percent and 25 percent of survivors have neurologic deficits.[30,31] There is no effective therapy other than support.
- **contact vaccinia**. Contact vaccinia represents spread of vaccinia from the vaccination site to another person. In the 1960s this was usually a child with exposure to a family member who was vaccinated.[25,26,30,31,36] The major concern at the time was this complication in a vulnerable contact, especially one with eczema. The more recent

military experience indicated just twenty-six reported cases of contact vaccinia among 580,000 military vaccine recipients[37] and this generally involved "bed partners."

- **myopericarditis**. This is a previously under appreciated complication of smallpox vaccination that has been reported in at least thirty-seven military recruits.[38,39] Risk factors were white men, primary vaccinees with a median age of twenty-six years with the onset of chest pain and other signs of myopericarditis at 7–19 days postvaccination. There were no deaths. In the civilian vaccination program there were fifteen such cases, but most occurred with revaccination, most were female and the median age was forty-eight years.
- **myocardial ischemia**. The recent experience with the vaccination program in the U.S. showed nine cases of angina or myocardial infarction in civilians and fifteen in military personnel.[24,41] However, analysis of these populations indicates that this rate is actually lower than would be expected on the basis of chance.[40] Scrutiny of these data has led to the conclusion that coronary ischemia is unrelated to the vaccination.

Policy options for prevention

Several policies have been considered for control of smallpox in the event of bioterrorism.[41] The following list the major options under consideration:

- **ring vaccination**. The method is to identify cases and contacts with the strategy of isolation and vaccination limited to these groups. The advantage is the ability to limit vaccine use and its complications. The challenge is to be able to identify the contacts.
- **quarantine**. Suspected and confirmed cases are isolated. The utility of this method for preventing transmission is obvious, but it is dependent on the legality of quarantine, availability of adequate facilities to do it, and compliance whether voluntary or compulsory.
- **target vaccination**. Vaccination is restricted to a geographic area based on epidemiological evidence of risk of exposure. An advantage is the utility of this method as demonstrated during the global

eradication campaign. The disadvantage is that this has not been tested in a population of high risk.

- **mass vaccination**. The implication is vaccination of the entire population. This would effectively eliminate dissemination and it would eliminate smallpox as a potential agent of bioterrorism if done preemptively. The obvious disadvantages are the vaccine-related morbidity and mortality, and the cost and difficulty of implementing this strategy.

A review of these strategies indicated that none could be identified as a preferred method that would satisfy all varieties of release scenarios. Instead, it was suggested that the preferred tactic would be real time statistical analysis and modeling at the time of the event based on the initial data with substantial attention to infrastructure combined with historical information as summarized above.[41]

References (Prevention)

1. P.F. Wehrle et al. "An airborne outbreak of smallpox in a German hospital and its significance with respect to other recent outbreaks in Europe." *Bull. World Health Organ.* 43:669–679 (1979).

2. W. Anders and J. Sosch. "Die Pockenausbrucke 1961/61 in Nordrhein-Westfalen." *Bundesgesundheitsblatt.* 17:265–269 (1962).

3. T.M. Mack. "Smallpox in Europe, 1950–71." *J. Infect. Dis.* 125:161–169 (1972).

4. T.M. Mack, D.B. Thomas and M.M. Khan. "Epidemiology of smallpox in West Pakistan, II: Determinants of intravillage spread other than acquired immunity." *Am. J. Epidemiol.* 95:157–168 (1972).

5. P.F. Wehrle et al. "An airborne outbreak of smallpox in a German hospital and its significance with respect to other recent outbreaks in Europe." *Bull. World Health Organ.* 43:669–679 (1970).

6. D.A. Henderson et al. "Smallpox as a biological weapon: Medical and public health management." *JAMA* 281:2127 (1999).

7. C.W. Dixon. "Smallpox in Tripolitania, 1946: An epidemiological and clinical study of 500 cases, including trials of penicillin treatment." *J. Hyg.* 46:351–377 (1948).

8. C.W. Dixon. *Smallpox* (London: J & A Churchill Ltd., 1962), 1460.

9. A. Herrlich et al. "Experimental studies on transformation of the variola virus into the vaccinia virus." *Arch. Gesamte. Virusforschvag* 12:579–599 (1963).

10. U.S. Bureau of the Census. *Resident Population of the United States: Estimates, by Age and Sex* (Washington, DC: U.S. Bureau of the Census, 2002).

11. Centers for Disease Control and Prevention. *Protecting Americans: Smallpox Vaccination Program (CDC).* 13 December 2002. Available at: http://www.bt.cdc.gov/agent/smallpox/vaccination/vaccination-program-statement.asp. Accessed 11 February 2004.

12. S. Frey et al. "Clinical responses to undiluted and diluted smallpox vaccine" *N. Engl. J. Med.* 346:1265–74 (2002).

13. F. Fenner et al. *Smallpox and Its Eradication* (Geneva: World Health Organization, 1988). Available online at http://www.who.int/emc/diseases/smallpox/Smallpoxeradication.html.

14. A.W. Downie et al. "Virus and virus antigen in the blood of smallpox patients: Their significances in early diagnosis and prognosis." *Lancet* 2:164–166 (1953).

15. A.W. Downie and K. McCarthy. "The antibody response in man following infection with viruses of the pox group, III: Antibody response in smallpox." J. Hyg. 56:479–487 (1958).

16. E. Hammarlund et al. "Duration of antiviral immunity after smallpox vaccination." *Nat. Med.* 9:1131 (2003).

17. M.R. Albert. "Smallpox manifestations and survival during the Boston epidemic of 1901 to 1903." *Ann. Intern. Med.* 137:993 (2002).

18. T.M. Mack. "Smallpox in Europe, 1950–1971." *J. Infect. Dis.* 125:161–169 (1972).

19. S.M. Hsieh et al. "Age distribution for T-cell reactivity to vaccinia in a healthy population." *Clin. Infect. Dis.* 38:86–9 (2004).

20. A.R. Kemper, M.M. Davis and G.L. Freed. "Expected adverse events in a mass smallpox vaccination campaign." *Effective Clin. Pract.*, March–April, 2000. Available at http://www.acponline.org/journals/acp/marapr02/kemper.htm. Accessed 4/1/04.

21. Centers for Disease Control and Prevention. Draft recommendations for use of smallpox vaccine in a pre-event smallpox vaccination program: supplemental recommendations of the Advisory Committee on Immunization Practices (ACIP) and the Healthcare Infection Control Practices Advisory Committee (HICPAC). Available at: http://www.bt.cdc.gov/agent/smallpox/vaccination/acip-guidelines.asp.

22. J. Cherry et al. "Clinical and serologic study of four smallpox vaccines comparing variations of dose and route of administration: Primary percutaneous vaccination." *J. Infect. Dis.* 135:145–54 (1977).

23. S. Frey et al. "Clinical responses to undiluted and diluted smallpox vaccine." *N. Engl. J. Med.* 346:1265–74 (2002).

24. Centers for Disease Control and Prevention. "Update: Adverse events following smallpox vaccination: United States." *MMWR* 53:106 (2004).

25. J.M. Lane et al. "Complications of smallpox vaccination, 1968: National surveillance in the United States." *N. Eng. J. Med.* 281:1201–1208 (1969).

26. J.M. Lane et al. "Complications of smallpox vaccination, 1968: Results of ten statewide surveys." *J. Infect. Dis.* 122:303–309 (1970).

27. C.H. Kempe. "Studies on smallpox and complications of smallpox vaccination." *Pediatrics* 26:176–189 (1960).

28. J.W. Grabenstein W. Winkenwerder. "U.S. military smallpox vaccination program experience." *JAMA* 289:3278 (2003).

29. R.A. Good R.L. Varco. "A clinical and experimental study of agammaglobulinemia." *Lancet* 75:245–51 (1955).

29a. A.L. Naleway et al. "Eczematous skin disease and recall of past diagnoses: implications for smallpox vaccination." *Ann. Intern. Med.* 139;1 (2003).

30. J. Breman D. Henderson. "Diagnosis and management of smallpox." *N. Engl. J. Med.* 346:1300–8 (2002).

31. J.G. Bartlett et al. "Smallpox vaccination in 2003: Key information for clinicians." *Clin. Infect. Dis.* 36:883–902 (2003).

32. E. Freed, R. Duma and M. Escobar. "Vaccinia necrosum and its relationship to impaired immunologic responsiveness." *Am. J. Med.* 54:411–20 (1972).

33. V. Fulginiti et al. "Progressive vaccinia in immunologically deficient individuals." *Birth Defects Orig. Artic. Ser.* 4:129–45 (1968).

34. R. Redfield et al. "Disseminated vaccinia in a military recruit with human immunodeficiency virus (HIV) disease." *N. Engl. J. Med.* 316:673–6 (1987).

35. J. Lane et al. "Deaths attributable to smallpox vaccination, 1959 to 1966, and 1968." *JAMA* 212:441–4 (1970).

36. J. Neff et al. "Contact vaccinia-transmission of vaccinia from smallpox vaccination." *JAMA* 288;1901–5 (2002).

37. Centers for Disease Control and Prevention. "Secondary and tertiary transfer of vaccinia virus among U.S. military personnel: United States and worldwide, 2002–2004." *MMWR* 53:103 (2004).

38. J.S. Halsell et al. "Myopericarditis following smallpox vaccination among vaccinia-naïve U.S. military personnel." *JAMA* 289:3283 (2003).

39. J.G. Murphy, et al. "Eosinophilic-lymphocytic myocarditis after smallpox vaccination." *Lancet* 362:1378 (2003).

40. Centers for Disease Control and Prevention. "Cardiac deaths after a smallpox vaccination campaign-New York City, 1947." *MMWR* 52:933 (2003).

41. N.M. Ferguson et al. "Planning for smallpox outbreaks." *Nature* 425: 681–685 (2003).

Appendix B. The Treatment of Smallpox

There is no specific treatment for smallpox. Antiviral agents that have in vitro activity include cidofovir and ribavirin.[1–4] With the mouse model of orthopoxvirus infection cidofovir demonstrates benefit, but only if it is delivered prior to viral challenge. With regard to ribavirin, there is one case report of treatment of progressive vaccinia with this agent; but it is not possible to judge efficacy because it was a single case and because thepatient also received VIG.[5] Thus, the practical reality is that treatment is supportive with IV fluids and nutrition. Skin lesions do not usually contain bacteria and a secondary bacterial infection is unusual. In terms of the healthcare worker to provide this care, preference should be given to someone who is recently vaccination, but an alternative strategy is to vaccinate the potential care provider who can then begin work with direct contact almost immediately. The highest priority should be given to healthcare workers who have been previously vaccinated and have arm scars to indicate a take.

References (Treatment)

1. R.O. Baker, M. Bray, and J.W. Huggans. "Potential antiviral therapeautics for smallpox, monkeypox and other or orthopoxviruses." *Antiviral Res.* 57:13–23 (2003).

2. D.F. Smee, M. Bray and J.W. Huggans. "Antiviral activity and mode of action studies of ribavirin and mycophendit acid against orthopox viruses in vitro." *Antivir. Chem. Chemother.* 12:327–35 (2001).

3. D.F. Smee, K.W. Bailey and R.W. Sidwell. "Comparative effects of cidoforir and cyclic HPMPC on lethal cowpox and vaccinea virus respiratory infections in mice." *Chemotherapy* 49:126–31 (2003).

4. A.M. Kesson et al. "Progressive vaccinia treated rivavirin and vaccina immunoglobulum." *Clin. Infect. Dis.* 25:911–14 (1997).

Chapter 4

Smallpox: Recognition, Prevention of Spread, and Treatment

Raymond M. Fish, Ph.D., M.D., FACEP

Synopsis

The author would like to thank Neal R. Abarbanell, M.D. for his review of this paper and his helpful suggestions.

Part of this chapter was a revised version of "Special Presentation: Smallpox," by Raymond M. Fish, published in *Practical Reviews in Emergency Medicine* 27:9 (2003). The author would like to thank Oakstone Publishing, a division of Haights Cross Communications, for permission to republish this material.

The smallpox (variola) virus has killed more people than any other pathogen in the history of man. Routine vaccination has not been performed for many years, and persons previously vaccinated are susceptible to infection. Variola viral stocks have been kept in one laboratory at the CDC in Atlanta, and in one laboratory in the former Soviet Union. There are anecdotal reports that the former Soviet Union had produced larger quantities of smallpox virus and engineered biological weapons that involved smallpox, plague, anthrax, tularemia, and brucellosis. In Iraq during the Gulf War in 1991, stocks of camel pox virus were discovered. (Kawalek and Rudikoff 2002; Henderson 1999a).

There was widespread acceptance of the 1972 Bioweapons Convention Treaty. This treaty called for all countries to destroy their stocks of bioweapons and to cease research on offensive weapons. Nevertheless, it is believed that the virus is maintained in laboratories in Russia and possibly other countries as well (Kawalek and Rudikoff 2002; Henderson 1999a).

The last case of naturally acquired smallpox occurred in Somalia in 1977, and the World Health Organization declared the global eradication of smallpox in 1980 (PBS 2004; WHO 1999). Even though smallpox was eradicated in the late 1970s, concern exists regarding the possible use of smallpox virus as an agent for bioterrorism (Henderson 1999b; Mack 2003; Constantin 2003; Suarez et al. 2002; Drazen 2002). If smallpox is spread as an act of terrorism, public health officials and physicians may be asked to deal effectively with smallpox, despite the fact that most have never seen a patient with the condition.

There are two morphologically indistinguishable forms of smallpox virus: variola major, the classical form of the disease with a mortality of 10–30 percent (3 percent in vaccinated populations), and variola minor, with a mortality rate of about 1 percent. Variola minor is a mild form of smallpox caused by a less virulent strain of the virus.

Most survivors of smallpox will have disfiguring scars, with blindness occurring in up to 10 percent of survivors.

4.1 Smallpox Transmission

It is thought that smallpox could be deliberately introduced into susceptible civilian populations through aerosols, infected volunteer carriers, and by fomites (inanimate objects that can transfer pathogens). Infected carriers in the most infectious stage of smallpox would be ill, making deliberate person-to-person transmission a suicide mission. Although monkeys have been infected with smallpox, there are no known natural animal or insect vectors or reservoirs for smallpox (Kawalek and Rudikoff 2002; Henderson 1999a).

A. Aerosols versus larger droplets

Smallpox is spread from one person to another by small aerosolized particles and also by larger droplets. The aerosols and larger droplets are both able to contaminate the mucosal membranes of other persons. Only the aerosols remain in the air for hours and travel relatively long distances without assistance from ventilation systems.

It is thought by some authors that person-to-person transmission of smallpox is usually not by tiny aerosols, but rather by larger saliva droplets that do not remain suspended in the air for long time periods as aerosols do. Relatively large airborne droplets are thought to be infective for only a matter of minutes (Mack 2003).

Others do believe that coughing and sneezing are often a significant factor, and the associated infective "droplet nuclei" can be transported by air currents away from the immediate vicinity of the smallpox patient (Fenner et al.1988, 189).

B. Fomites

Direct contact with skin lesions and fomites can lead to transmission of smallpox. Fomites can spread infection if they are not properly disposed of. Fomites include blankets and clothing.

C. Factors affecting transmission

There are several factors that tend to limit transmission. These factors will make efforts to contain the secondary spread of smallpox more successful. Most virus shedding and transmission occur during the first week of marked rash and rapidly evolving symptoms. At this time, the physical appearance of an unvaccinated person with smallpox is quite alarming, and symptoms are usually severe enough that the person will stay in bed. Most transmissions have been at the bedside, and to family members. None of the 945 cases in a study of a smallpox outbreak were contracted on an airplane, train, or bus. There has been spread in hospitals, possibly due to infected linens and spread through ventilation system from one room to others. There is a one to three week interval between exposure and infectiousness, allowing time for contacts to be identified, isolated, and given immunization (Mack 2003).

Table 4.1
Factors Affecting the Secondary Spread of Smallpox

1. Person-to-person viral transmission may more commonly result from large saliva droplets rather than from tiny aerosolized droplets
   a. Transmission distance of larger droplets is limited
   b. Transmission distance can be increased by ventilation systems
2. Most virus shedding and transmission occur during the first week when the infected person should be identifiable and immobile because:
   a. The rash is quite noticeable
   b. The symptoms are debilitating, leading to bed rest and medical consultation
3. A 1-to-3 week interval from exposure to infectiousness allows contacts to be identified and treated
4. Fomites can transmit the infection, but this should be preventable

4.2 Clinical Presentation and Diagnosis

A. Types of smallpox

There are four clinical types of smallpox: ordinary, modified (due to previous vaccination), flat-type, and hemorrhagic. Persons who have been vaccinated many years earlier may develop the modified form of smallpox, which is milder than the ordinary form. The modified form will evolve more rapidly and have a limited skin eruption. The flat and hemorrhagic forms of smallpox both have high fatality rates. Flat-type smallpox is characterized by severe toxemia and the delayed appearance and slow

Table 4.2
Types of Smallpox

1. Ordinary, with three subtypes:
   a. Confluent. The face and forearms have a confluent rash, meaning that lesions meet or run together
   b. Semiconfluent. The rash is confluent on the face, but discrete elsewhere
   c. Discrete. There are areas of normal skin between pustules on the face and elsewhere
2. Modified
   a. Modification is due to previous vaccination or maternal antibodies in infants
   b. The course of the disease is milder than the ordinary case of smallpox
   c. There is usually no fever when the generalized skin rash develops
   d. The course evolves more rapidly and has a limited skin eruption
3. Flat-type, or malignant smallpox
   a. High mortality rate
   b. More common in children
   c. Severe toxemia
   d. Delayed appearance and slow development of soft, flat skin legions
   e. "Velvety" to the touch
   f. Sections of the skin may slough off
4. Hemorrhagic
   a. High mortality rate with early death
   b. Occurs in less than 3% of patients
   c. Severe toxemia
   d. Hemorrhage may occur in the ocular conjunctiva, gums, nose, gastrointestinal tract, lungs, urinary tract, and vagina
   e. Thrombocytopenia (low platelets) and sometimes other coagulation abnormalities occur

development of soft, flat skin lesions. Hemorrhagic smallpox occurs in less than 3 percent of patients and is characterized by severe toxemia, conjunctival, mucosal, and gastrointestinal hemorrhage, and early death (Kawalek and Rudikoff 2002; Fenner 1988).

B. Clinical course of smallpox (Rao 1972)

The clinical course of smallpox varies greatly from one patient to another and also from one clinical type to another. Perhaps the best description of individual patients and of the clinical types of smallpox was given by Rao (1972). This section summarizes some of his observations.

1. Ordinary smallpox

There are usually two to three days of pre-eruptive fever with varying severity of constitutional symptoms. Symptoms become less severe with onset of the focal rash. In some cases, lesions first appear on the mucous membranes of the tongue and palate. This rash consists of tiny red spots, coming a few hours to a day before the appearance of the skin rash. The rash usually comes on day 3 or 4. The rash most often appears at first on the face and takes the form of fleabite-like macules (flat lesions). Lesions of smallpox are more deeply embedded in the skin than those of varicella (chickenpox). Loss of fluid results in a dimpling at the apex of the lesion, an appearance referred to as umbilication.

Following the appearance of the facial rash, lesions appear on the proximal extremities, trunk, and lastly on the distal extremities. This rapid progression is completed within twenty-four hours, and most patients will not notice the order of lesion development. By day six the small macules become papular (raised) and vesicular (sack-like). These break down and discharge large amounts of virus, as does the patient's saliva.

In ordinary smallpox, fever usually drops on day 4 or 5 when the rash appears and rises on day 7 or 8. The fever remains high during the vesicular and pustular stages, after which scabs form over the lesions. Viral and bacterial respiratory problems are more common in the unvaccinated and develop around day 8. In fatal cases, death usually occurs between the twelfth and eighteenth day of fever. In survivors, scabs separate between days 25 to 30. Scabs on palms and soles often have to be separated with a needle.

Table 4.3
Stages of the Ordinary Type of Smallpox

1. Incubation phase
   a. Usually 10 to 14 days (rarely as short as 7 or as long as 19 days)
   b. The patient is asymptomatic and rarely infectious
2. The pre-eruptive (prodromal) phase of 2 to 3 days may include
   a. Pharyngitis, bronchitis
   b. Sudden fever of 101–105 degrees, chills
   c. Prostration
   d. Headache
   e. Backache
   f. Delirium and/or seizures
   g. Abdominal pain, nausea, diarrhea and/or vomiting
3. Infectious eruptive phase
   a. Enanthem (an eruption on palatal and pharyngeal mucous membranes) precedes skin rash by a day
   b. Highly infectious period is from day 1 of the rash, lasting 7 to 10 days.
   c. Infectious state ends when all the scabs have been shed, usually 3 to 4 weeks after onset of rash

Kawalek and Rudikoff 2002; Suarez and Hankins 2002; Fenner et al. 1988

2. Modified variety of smallpox

The modified type of smallpox is not fatal and usually occurs in persons who have been vaccinated. In the modified variety, pre-eruptive symptoms last two to three days with high fever and mild constitutional symptoms. Rash is uncommon. The skin rash may not appear at all, but if it does, macules rapidly become papular and then vesicular, and scab by day 10 or before, without having a pustular stage. The distribution of lesions may not follow the classical pattern. The lesions are more superficial than normal and may be pleomorphic (having different forms). The lesions do not umbilicate, and form superficial scabs that usually separate before day 14. Scars tend to be superficial and may not be permanent.

3. Flat type

In the flat variety, lesions flatten out and remain more or less flush with the skin rather than forming vesicles. Constitutional symptoms are fairly severe and continue after appearance of skin rash. An enanthem (eruption) on the tongue and palate may be confluent. A severe rash may also develop on the rectal mucosa and elsewhere. Most lesions will have hemorrhages into their bases, with a dark black or purple center with surrounding erythema. The lesions have little fluids and do not have umbilication. The rash may not follow the usual centrifugal (face first) pattern. The course is toxic and febrile, with viral pneumonitis and possibly pneumonia developing on day 7 or 8. Previous vaccination makes survival more likely. In fatal cases, usually involving unvaccinated persons, there is development of an acute dilation of the stomach and an ashen grey color of skin lesions one or two days before death. Death usually occurs between days 8 and 12.

4. Hemorrhagic smallpox

There are two varieties of hemorrhagic smallpox. In the early form, hemorrhage into skin and/or mucous membranes appears before the skin rash. In the late form, hemorrhage occurs after the onset of skin rash. Both forms of hemorrhagic smallpox are usually fatal.

Hemorrhagic smallpox is more common in adults and women, especially in pregnancy. Even apparently successful vaccination does not seem to offer as much protection against hemorrhagic smallpox as it does with other types of smallpox. In one study of the contacts of 385 cases, not one case of hemorrhagic smallpox occurred. These observations have suggested that a different or a more virulent variola virus strain may be involved in hemorrhagic smallpox.

In hemorrhagic smallpox, the pre-eruptive stage is usually prolonged to four or five days, and the symptoms are more severe. Skin rash may be preceded by hemorrhages into the skin or mucous membranes. In some cases focal skin lesions may never develop. Bleeding may occur in the ocular conjunctiva, gums, nose, gastrointestinal tract, lungs, urinary tract, and vagina. Bleeding is associated with thrombocytopenia (a low platelet count) and sometimes other coagulation abnormalities.

C. Differential diagnosis

1. Chickenpox

The most characteristic finding of smallpox is its rash. Lesions are generally in the same stage of development with smallpox. In contrast, with chickenpox, lesions in various stages of development can be seen at

Table 4.4
Comparison of Chickenpox and Smallpox

Feature	Chickenpox	Smallpox
Prodromal phase symptoms	Minimal symptoms	Sudden high fever, severe aching, prostration
Prodromal phase duration	0–2 days	2–4 days
Development of rash: synchrony	Lesions in various stages of development	Lesions are generally in the same stage of development
Time from onset of rash until peak of eruption	3–5 days	7–10 days
Initial skin lesions	Primarily central	Centrifugal (face and forearms)
Lesions on palms and soles	Almost never	There may be
Density of rash on trunk as compared to elsewhere	The rash in chickenpox is more dense over the trunk (the reverse of smallpox)	Less dense on the trunk than elsewhere
Serologic findings	Increased antibody to varicella virus	Increased antibody to variola virus
Antigen or nucleic acid detection	Varicella-zoster virus	Variola virus

Kawalek and Rudikoff 2002; Henderson 1999a; Suarez and Hankins DV 2002; Breman and Henderson 2002

the same time. Thus, in chickenpox, scabs, vesicles, and pustules may be seen simultaneously on adjacent areas of skin. The smallpox rash starts on the face and forearms and then spreads to other areas. The rash starts as pink macules and develops over several days into papules, vesicles, pustules, and then crusts. Pustules (also referred to as pocks) are round, firm, umbilicated, and deeply embedded in the dermis. Lesions may occur on the palms and soles. Crusts begin to form around the eighth or ninth day of the rash. The scabs eventually separate, leaving depigmented, pitted scarring (Kawalek and Rudikoff 2002; Suarez and Hankins 2002).

The most characteristic features in smallpox that help distinguish it from other diseases are the greater number of lesions on the face and distal extremities, and the appearance of lesions in the same stage of development in different body areas.

2. Other diseases

Several conditions that may be confused with smallpox should be mentioned (Kawalek and Rudikoff 2002):

- Severe varicella (chickenpox), especially in immunocompromised patients
- Disseminated herpes simplex infection
- Extensive, secondarily infected molluscum contagiosum lesions in an HIV patient with fever from another cause.
- The hemorrhagic form of smallpox can be similar in appearance to:
    - meningococcemia
    - Stevens Johnson syndrome
    - leukemia

4.3 Smallpox in Pregnancy

Vaccination in pregnancy is discussed in the section on vaccination below.

The pregnant patient with smallpox tends to have a high rate of premature termination of pregnancy and a high fetal and maternal death rate. Pregnant women tend to develop the often-lethal hemorrhagic type of smallpox. In one study, vaccinated pregnant women who developed smallpox had a 27 percent fatality rate, and unvaccinated women had a 61-percent fatality rate. Thus, vaccination was not nearly as effective in pregnant women as in other persons. Of women who developed smallpox in the first twenty-five weeks of gestation, 72 percent had fetal loss. Women who developed smallpox after twenty-five weeks of gestation, 48.6 percent had fetal loss (Rao 1972).

4.4 Treatment of Smallpox (Breman and Henderson 2002)

A. Notification

When the diagnosis of smallpox is likely, the physician should notify hospital infection control personnel, state and local health departments, and the CDC (Centers for Disease Control and Prevention at http://www.bt.cdc.gov/).

B. Immunization

Smallpox patients should be vaccinated, especially if the illness is in an early stage.

C. Isolation

Strict respiratory and contact isolation is important.

Multiple patients should ideally be kept in an isolation hospital or other facility.

If possible, a person with smallpox should be managed in a negative-pressure room.

Visitors should be healthy, vaccinated, and aware of isolation procedures. Pregnant women should not visit smallpox patients. The reason for this is that pregnant women, regardless of vaccination status, tend to get severe and frequently fatal types of smallpox (Rao 1972, 120).

In Germany, seventeen people on three floors of a hospital contracted smallpox from one patient; this was thought to be due to the patient's cough, low humidity levels, and hospital air currents (Henderson 1999b).

Isolation of contacts. Patient contacts (including medical personnel) that occurred up to seventeen days before the onset of symptoms should remain in isolation until the diagnosis of smallpox is confirmed or disproved. If the diagnosis of smallpox is confirmed, vaccination and quarantine for seventeen days are required (Suarez and Hankins 2002, 89).

D. Supportive care

Hydration and nutrition are important because fluids and protein are lost by febrile persons with weeping lesions.

E. Secondary infection of lesions

Secondary infection of smallpox lesions can be treated with penicillinase-resistant antibiotics.

F. Eye involvement

Daily eye rinsing is required in severe cases. Although not proven effective for smallpox, corneal lesions may be benefited by topical idoxuridine (Dendrid, Herplex, or Stoxil).

4.5 Treatment of Cowpox, Vaccinia, and Monkeypox

A. Possible effectiveness of Cidofovir

Animal studies have suggested that cidofovir and its cyclic analogues may be beneficial for cowpox, vaccinia, and monkeypox if given at the time of exposure or immediately afterward (Breman and Henderson 2002).

B. The CDC recommends smallpox vaccination for monkeypox

In June 2003, the Centers for Disease Control and Prevention (CDC) issued interim guidance advising that "persons investigating monkeypox outbreaks and involved in caring for infected individuals or animals should receive a smallpox vaccination to protect against the possibility of contracting monkeypox. CDC is also recommending that persons who have had close or intimate contact with individuals or animals confirmed to have monkeypox should also be vaccinated. They can be vaccinated up to fourteen days post-exposure. Since the smallpox vaccine is not an approved vaccine for monkeypox, the smallpox vaccine for this CDC recommended use is being distributed under FDA special procedures to allow such emergency use in association with individual patient informed consent and approval by an institutional review board (ethics committee). CDC is not recommending smallpox vaccination for veterinarians, veterinary staff or animal control officers who have not been exposed. However, the public health agency does encourage such personnel to use standard infection control measures to prevent contact or airborne transmission of the virus if they are involved in investigation or treatment of ill animals." (CDC 2003a)

4.6 Vaccination

As of January 2004, there is enough smallpox vaccine for every man, woman, and child in the United States (Ridge 2004).

A. Vaccine efficacy in various settings

The smallpox vaccine contains a live-virus preparation of the infectious vaccinia virus. The vaccine itself is not perfect. Successful vaccination two to three years preceding exposure reduces the attack rate to under 10 percent and the mortality to under 1 percent. If given in the first four days following exposure, the attack rate can be as high as 50 percent, with the severity of the disease being decreased. The efficacy of diluted vaccine is being studied (Kawalek and Rudikoff 2002).

Smallpox infection provides the patient with lifelong immunity, but the same cannot be said for vaccines. With Jenner's original vaccine in the nineteenth century, death rates were lower if revaccination was performed every ten years. Persons living in endemic areas who had been vaccinated over twenty years earlier were found to have a protection rate of 80 percent. However this protection is thought to be due to the combined effect of vaccination and later subclinical smallpox infections that prolonged the period of immunity. A study of the 1902 smallpox outbreak in England suggested that 93 percent of people aged fifty or greater who had been vaccinated once years earlier avoided severe disease and death (Kawalek and Rudikoff 2002).

B. Vaccine administration procedure and local response

Smallpox vaccine is usually given in the deltoid area intracutaneously with a bifurcated needle that has been dipped into the vaccine solution. The vaccine droplet remains between the prongs and is introduced into the dermis by puncture or scratch. Five to fifteen superficial punctures are done to cause penetration of the vaccine. A successful primary smallpox vaccination, or a "take," produces a Jennerian vesicle. Three to four days after being vaccinated, there is itching and redness at the site. A papule surrounded by a red halo forms at two to five days and develops into a vesicle that becomes umbilicated. By the tenth day the vesicle should be pustular and maximum in size. The papule dries and becomes crusted by the third week. The scab will fall off, leaving a scar. If this series of events does not occur, the person should be revaccinated. Persons who have been previously vaccinated who develop erythema and edema have had an equivocal reaction and should be revaccinated (Kawalek and Rudikoff 2002).

C. Viral shedding from the vaccination site

Viral shedding from the vaccination site is maximum from four to fourteen days, but the vaccinia virus can be recovered from the skin until the scab separates from the skin. Spread of the vaccinia virus to other body sites is referred to as autoinoculation. The virus can also be spread to other persons. Some of these other persons may have contraindications to receiving the vaccinia virus and may have adverse reactions.

D. Ring vaccination

Because of the risk involved with giving the vaccine, universal immunization is not a generally agreed-upon solution to the threat of smallpox that terrorism has raised. One immunization strategy that may limit the spread of smallpox is ring vaccination. Ring vaccination includes isolation of confirmed and suspected smallpox cases with tracing, vaccination, and close surveillance of contacts to these cases as well as vaccination of the household contacts of the contacts.

E. People likely to benefit from immunization because they are at high risk of developing smallpox

The following are considered high risk groups and should be prioritized for vaccination in a smallpox outbreak (CDC 2001):

1. Face-to-face close contacts (< 6.5 feet or two meters), and household contacts to smallpox patients after the onset of the smallpox patient's fever.
2. People exposed to the initial release of the virus
3. Household members of smallpox patient contacts who do not have contraindications to vaccination
4. People involved in the direct medical care, public health evaluation, or transportation of confirmed or suspected smallpox patients
5. Laboratory personnel
6. Others who have a high likelihood of exposure to infectious materials (e.g., personnel responsible for hospital waste disposal and disinfection)
7. Personnel involved in contact tracing and vaccination, or quarantine/isolation or enforcement, or law-enforcement interviews of suspected smallpox patients
8. People permitted to enter any facilities designated for the evaluation, treatment, or isolation of confirmed or suspected smallpox patients
9. Those present in a facility or conveyance with a smallpox case if fine-particle aerosol transmission was likely during the time the case was present (e.g. hemorrhagic smallpox case and/or case with active coughing)

F. People are at higher than usual risk for developing post-vaccination complications

Before 1972, smallpox vaccination was recommended for all children in the United States at the age of one year. Most states required vaccination before the child could enter school.

In addition to children under the age of one year, others who have a greater than usual risk of complications include persons who have any of the following conditions (CDC 2001; Henderson 1999b):

- eczema (or a history of eczema)
- other forms of chronic dermatitis
- pregnancy
- hereditary immune deficiency disorders
- altered immune states, including
  - HIV, AIDS
  - leukemia
  - lymphoma
  - current use of alkylating agents, antimetabolites, radiation, or large doses of corticosteroids, including many patients with transplants

Those with the above conditions who have been in close contact with a smallpox patient or who have significant risk for occupational reasons, may be given vaccinia immune globulin (VIG) at the time of vaccination in a dose of 0.3 mL/kg body weight. VIG does not reduce vaccine efficacy. If VIG is not available, vaccination may still be indicated, as there is more chance of morbidity and mortality from smallpox than there is from vaccination (Henderson 1999b).

G. Smallpox vaccination complications (CDC 2004; Henderson 1999b; *MMWR* 2001)

1 Postvaccinial encephalitis

Postvaccinial encephalitis ooccurs in one of 300,000 persons receiving their primary (first) smallpox vaccination. A quarter of these cases are fatal, and some survivors will have permanent neurological sequelae such as paralysis or other CNS problems. Postvaccinial encephalitis presents eight to fifteen days after vaccination. Encephalitic symptoms may include fever, headache, vomiting, drowsiness, spastic paralysis, meningitic signs, coma, and seizures. CSF usually has a pleocytosis. Treatment is supportive. VIG is not effective for postvaccinial encephalitis (Henderson 1999b).

2. Progressive vaccinia

Progressive vaccinia has also been called vaccinia gangrenosa and vaccinia necrosum. Progressive vaccinia is frequently fatal in persons with immune deficiency disorders. With progressive vaccinia, vaccinial lesions fail to heal and progress to involve adjacent skin with necrosis of tissue. The condition can spread to bones and viscera. Vaccinia immune globulin and ribavirin have been used experimentally to treat progressive vaccinia (Henderson 1999b).

3. Eczema vaccinatum

Eczema vaccinatum occurs in persons who currently or in the past have had eczema or other chronic or exfoliative skin conditions, such as atopic dermatitis. Vaccinial lesions may extend to cover all areas covered (or previously covered) by the chronic or previous skin condition. Eczema vaccinatum is usually mild and self-limited, but can be severe and even fatal. VIG is therapeutic and is indicated in severe cases. Severe cases of eczema vaccinatum have been observed in contacts of those who have been vaccinated (*MMWR* 2001, 8; (Henderson 1999b).

4. Generalized vaccinia

Generalized vaccinia occurs with blood-borne dissemination of the vaccinia virus. Lesions appear six to nine days after vaccination. VIG is the treatment for patients who are ill or have serious underlying disease (*MMWR* 2001, 8; Henderson 1999b).

5. Inadvertent inoculation

Inadvertent inoculation of self and others occurs when there is transmission to other persons or to other sites on the person who has been vaccinated, which is termed autoinoculation.

Frequent hand washing and proper care of the vaccination site can reduce spread of the virus from the vaccination site. In general, the vaccination site can be left uncovered or can be loosely covered with a porous bandage such as gauze until the scab has separated. An occlusive bandage may lead to maceration of the site. Bandages should be changed every day or two to prevent maceration due to fluid buildup. Bandages should be placed in sealed plastic bags before disposal. Decontamination of clothes is with hot water laundering using bleach. The vaccination site should be kept dry, although bathing can continue. No salves or ointments should be used.

Tertiary contact vaccinia occurred in one recent case after a man received primary smallpox vaccination. Despite observing precautions to avoid household spread, his wife, who was breastfeeding, developed vesicles on both areolas. Twenty-five days after the father was vaccinated, the infant developed a papule on her upper lip. Culture and polymerase chain reaction confirmed contact vaccinia in both the mother and child. The authors of this case report suggest that vaccine recipients should not sleep in the same bed as a breastfeeding mother, the breastfeeding mother should wash her hands before breastfeeding, and that breastfeeding be temporarily stopped if skin lesions do develop (Garde et al. 2004).

6. Autoinoculation sites

Autoinoculation can occur when a person touches the vaccination site and then touches another side on his (or her) body or face. Spread of the vaccinia virus has led to lesions on the face, eyelids, mouth, nose, rectum, and genitalia. Most lesions heal without treatment, but VIG may be needed in cases of periocular implantation. However, if vaccinial keratits is present, VIG is contraindicated because it might increase corneal scarring. For possible ocular involvement, look for cornea opacities and then examine the cornea with fluorescein staining. If any lesions are seen, consult an ophthalmologist. A rather large flow chart is available on the Internet describing the treatment of vaccinia and smallpox eye lesions (CDC 2003b).

7. Cellulitis at the inoculation site

Cellulitis at the inoculation site was seen in 10.2 percent of people receiving vaccine in one study, a rate about three times as high as the usually noted 3.9 percent in the clinic involved. This increased incidence may have been due to using a scratch method of inoculation (which was part of an investigational-new-drug protocol), and to the use of occlusive dressings (Sauri 2002).

8. Other cutaneous reactions

Other cutaneous reactions have resulted from smallpox vaccination. These have included erythema multiforme, and a variety of urticarial, maculopapular, and blotchy erythematous eruptions. These generally clear without therapy. In general, one should avoid steroids in such cases.

9. Fever

Approximately 70 percent of children have a temperature over 100° F at four to fourteen days after primary vaccination. Fifteen to 20 percent of children will have a temperature of 102° or more. Incidence of fever is less common in adults and after revaccination in children.

H. Vaccination in pregnancy

Pregnant women should be counseled to avoid direct exposure to any individual who has been recently vaccinated because of the possibility of secondary transmission of vaccinia virus.

Smallpox vaccine is not recommended for pregnant women for routine or non-emergency indications. Smallpox vaccine is contraindicated for women who are breastfeeding and for women who might become pregnant within three months of vaccination. Because the smallpox vaccine is a live attenuated vaccine, it is contraindicated three months prior to conception. However, if vaccination is inadvertently performed in early pregnancy, termination is not indicated.

Concerning smallpox exposure in pregnancy, the CDC says, "If there is a smallpox outbreak, recommendations on who should get vaccinated will change. Anyone who is exposed to smallpox should get vaccinated, because they will be at greater risk from the disease than they are from the vaccine. Public health authorities will recommend who should be vaccinated at that time and what measures people can take to protect themselves from smallpox." (CDC 2004).

4.7 Vaccinia Immune Globulin (VIG)

A. Uses: Prophylaxis and treatment of vaccination complications

As mentioned in the sections of this chapter discussing various complications of vaccination, VIG is sometimes administered with smallpox vaccination to reduce the risk of developing certain complications. VIG is also given to treat certain types of complications that do occur. The efficacy and recommendations for administration of VIG are discussed in the section below on smallpox vaccination complications.

B. Dosages (check CDC website for latest recommendation)

1. Prophylactic

This might be given, for example, to a person with eczema who has had contact with a smallpox patient. Treatment involves giving VIG simultaneously with vaccination. The VIG dose is 0.3 mL/kg body weight. This will not reduce vaccine efficacy. If VIG is not available, the vaccine may still be given if smallpox infection is likely.

2. Treatment of vaccination complications

This involves repeated doses of VIG. VIG is useful in treating patients with progressive vaccinia, eczema vaccinatum, severe generalized vaccinia, and periocular infections that are secondary to inadvertent inoculation. For these persons, VIG is given in a dose of 0.6 mL/kg body weight in divided doses over a 24–36 hour period. This is done because the volume is so great: 42 mL for a 70-kg person! If there is no improvement in two or three days, VIG may be repeated. VIG is scarce, available in the United States only from the CDC (Henderson 1999b).

According to the MMWR June 22, 2001, there are no contraindications to smallpox vaccination during a smallpox emergency when a person has had exposure to the smallpox virus. However, if there is no emergency situation and there has been no smallpox exposure, persons described above as being more likely to have complications should not receive smallpox vaccine.

Unless there is an emergency situation with actual smallpox exposure, the vaccine is also not recommended for persons who live in a household with persons with the above-mentioned skin conditions, immunosuppression, or pregnancy.

Live viral vaccines in general are contraindicated during pregnancy, so vaccinia vaccine should not be given to pregnant women for nonemergency indications. Vaccinia vaccine has not caused congenital malformations, but has resulted in fetal death and death soon after birth in a number of cases.

4.8 Conclusions

The management of smallpox is complex. If smallpox infection is introduced into modern society, new information will develop because of the large numbers of people with transplants, cancer therapy, HIV, and other conditions. Therefore, treating physicians should consult up-to-date resources on the Internet when clinical cases are encountered. Internet access should be available in emergency departments and other medical practice settings.

If you vaccinate persons, be aware that household and other contacts with contraindications to exposure to the vaccinia virus must be taken into account. These contacts would include persons who are pregnant, immunosuppressed, under one year of age, and members of the other groups discussed above.

References

Breman and Henderson. "Current concepts: Diagnosis and management of smallpox." *NEJM* 346(17):1300–1308 (2002)

Centers for Disease Control (CDC). *Interim Smallpox Response Plan and Guidelines*, Draft 2.0, 11/21/01. Previously (11/21/01) online via http://www.cdc.gov/nip/smallpox/. (2001).

———. *CDC Recommends Smallpox Vaccination to Protect Persons Exposed to Monkeypox*. Press release, June 11, 2003. http://www.cdc.gov/od/oc/media/pressrel/r030611.htm on 1/21/2004. (2003a).

———. *Clinical Evaluation Tool for Smallpox Vaccine Adverse Reactions Ophthalmologic Reactions/Inadvertent Innoculation in a Vaccinee (or in a Close Contact).* www.bt.cdc.gov/agent/smallpox/vaccination/clineval (03-12-2003 version). (2003b).

———. *Smallpox Fact Sheet: Smallpox Vaccination Information for Women Who Are Pregnant or Breastfeeding*. January 16, 2004 http://www.bt.cdc.gov/agent/smallpox/vaccination/preg-factsheet.asp. (2004).

Constantin, C.M. et al. "Smallpox a disease of the past? Consideration for midwives." *Journal of Midwifery & Women's Health* 48(4):258–267 (2003).

Drazen, J. "Smallpox and bioterrorism." *NEJM* 346(17):1262–1263 (2002).

Fenner, F. et al. *Smallpox and Its Eradication* (Geneva: World Health Organization, 1988). Book available for viewing at http://www.who.int/emc/diseases/smallpox/Smallpoxeradication.html.

Garde, V., D. Harper and M.P. Fairchok. "Tertiary contact vaccinia in a breast-feeding infant." *JAMA* 291:725–727 (2004).

Henderson, D.A. "Smallpox: Clinical and epidemiologic features." *Emerging Infectious Diseases* 5(4):537–539 (1999a).

Henderson, D.A. et al. "Smallpox as a biological weapon: Consensus statement." *JAMA* 281(22):2127–2137 (1999b).

Mack, T. "A different view of smallpox and vaccination." *NEJM* 348(5):460–3 (2003).

Kawalek and Rudikoff, found in *Clinics in Dermatology,* vol. 20, pages 376–387, 2002.

MMWR (CDC *Morbidity and Mortality Weekly Report*). Vaccinia (Smallpox) Vaccine. Recommendations of the Advisory Committee on Immunization Practices (ACIP), 2001. Vol. 50 / No. RR-10 June 22, 2001

PBS. World Health Organization declares smallpox eradicated 1980. 1/18/2004 http://www.pbs.org/wgbh/aso/databank/entries/dm79sp.html .

Ridge, Tom. Remarks by Secretary Tom Ridge at the Caucus for Producers, Writers and Directors, Thursday Jan. 15, 2004 U.S. Department of Homeland Security Website, January 16, 2004. http://www.dhs.gov/dhspublic/display?content=2908

Rao, A.R. *Smallpox* (Bombay: Kothari Book Depot, 1972).

Sauri, M.A. "Responses to smallpox vaccine." *NEJM* 347(9):689–690 (2002).

Suarez, V.R. and G.D. Hankins. "Smallpox and pregnancy: From eradicated disease to bioterrorist threat." *Obstet. Gynecol.* 100(1):87–93 (2002).

World Health Organization. Smallpox eradication: Destruction of variola virus stocks. Report by the Secretariat. 15 April 1999. Available January 18, 2004 at www.who.int/gb/EB_WHA/PDF/WHA52/ew5.pdf

Chapter 5

Terrorist Bombings: Injury Mechanisms and Characteristics

Raymond M. Fish, Ph.D., M.D., FACEP

Synopsis

5.1 Multiple Mechanisms of Injury in Terrorist Bombings

The variety of injury mechanisms associated with blast injuries are listed in Table 5.1. Terrorist bombings are designed to inflict as much injury and suffering as possible through a variety of mechanisms. A relatively close-range exposure to a bomb that contains nails or other objects can produce a combination of penetrating wounds, blast injury, blunt trauma, and severe burns.

The author would like to thank Neal R. Abarbanell, M.D., for his review of this chapter and his helpful suggestions.

Some of the material in this chapter is derived from the chapter "Characteristics and Mechanisms of Blast Injury" in the book *Medical and Bioengineering Aspects of Electrical Injuries* (2003), by R.M. Fish and L.A. Geddes. The author thanks Lawyers & Judges Publishing for permission to reprint this material. Figures 5.1 and 5.2 are reprinted from Steele 2002, with permission of Worldnetdaily.com (http://www.worldnetdaily.com/).

Table 5.1
Classification of Blast Injury Mechanisms

Type of Blast Injury	Characteristics
Primary	The blast wave travels through air or water to impact the body. Internal injury may occur with no visible external signs.
Secondary	The blast wave propels objects or fragments that impact the body to cause injury.
Tertiary	The blast wave displaces the body. Injury occurs when the body impacts other objects.
Other	1. Exposures: inhalation, eye, and dermal exposure to: a. toxic chemicals b. dust (both radioactive and nonradioactive) 2. Thermal burns from the explosion itself and from blast-ignited fires 3. Mechanical trauma, as from collapse of structures
Injury mechanisms that may be exacerbated by terrorist bombing methods	1. **Severe burns** due to • Close proximity of suicide bombers to victims • Confinement in a closed space such as a building or vehicle 2. Injury from materials near, or mixed with, the explosive: • **Penetrating injury** involving up to several hundred metallic objects in one victim • **Chemical warfare** agents such as cyanide and warfarin • **Biological warfare** resulting from a suicide bomber infected with hepatitis or AIDS • **Radiological warfare** resulting from "dirty bombs" containing radioactive material

Elsayed 1997; Stapczynski 1982; Phillips 1986; Mayorga 1997.

A. Penetrating injury

X-rays taken from victims of suicide bombings have revealed pieces of metallic fragments embedded in, bones, muscles, the brain, and body organs. Bombs are sometimes packed with spikes, nails, screws, nuts, bullets, and ball bearings. One goal of terrorists is to do as much damage as possible and destroy functional life where they fail to actually kill. Their result is that often those who live and their relatives may suffer more than those who die. Treating victims of terror for mental and physical health problems has presented a whole new set of medical challenges. Some patients have had up to 300 individual metallic fragments, measuring from millimeters to centimeters, imbedded literally from head to toe. Injuries have included punctured colon, pneumothorax, and lacerations of the liver, kidney, and brain. Victims have suffered amputated limbs, fractures, lacerations, paralysis, deafness and blindness. Sometimes the fragments will cause more damage if they are taken out, so removal is not always indicated (Steele 2002).

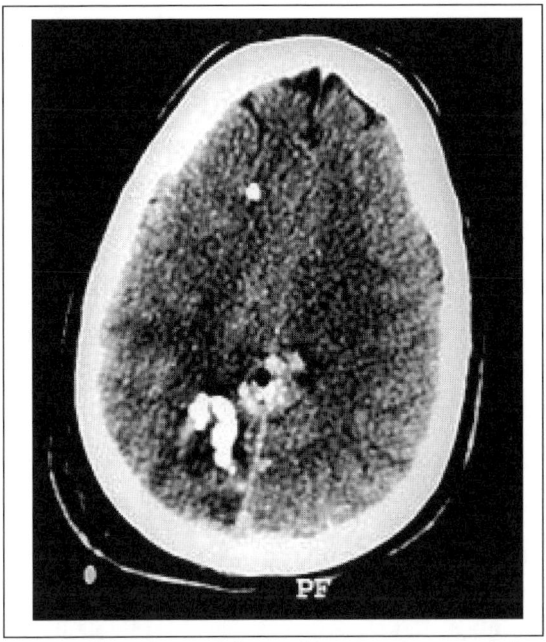

Figure 5.1 *CT scan of head. Metal, bone, blood and air are within normal brain tissue. Reprinted from Steele, 2000, with permission of worldnetdaily.com.*

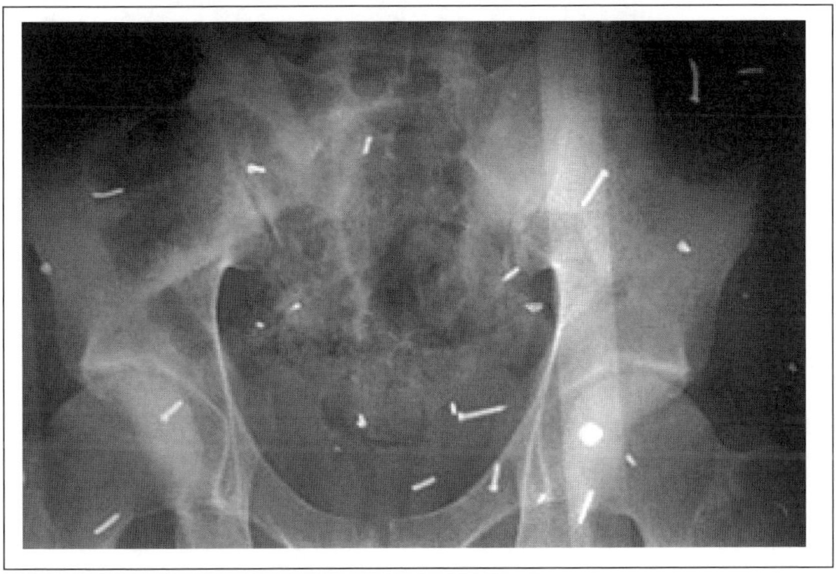

Figure 5.2 *Front view of a pelvis imbedded with nails and metal fragments. Reprinted from Steele, 2000, with permission of worldnetdaily.com.*

B. Chemical warfare

Chemical warfare has entered the picture with reports of cyanide being added to materials mixed with the explosives carried by suicide bombers. Attempts have been made to have cyanide gas released when a bomb is detonated (Findlay 2002).

Although it is sometimes thought that the heat of a blast will inactivate chemicals, a rat poison-anticoagulant has reportedly resulted in bleeding problems in terrorist bombing victims. Pesticides have also been used in terrorist bombings. So far, nails in bombs have caused more injuries than chemicals. The use of chemicals by terrorists is a harbinger of things to come, and there are chemicals that will be more effective if used (Chang 2003).

C. Biological warfare

Bone fragments from suicide bombers have been known to penetrate bombing victims, and it is feared that the fragments may transmit infection. Suicide bombers have been found to be infected with hepatitis B (Chang 2003). Routine immunization of suicide bombing victims for hepatitis B has been recommended by some (Siegel-Itzkovich 2001). At least one suicide bomber has had AIDS (Stein and Hirshberg 2003, 390).

D. Dirty bombs

"Dirty bombs" containing radioactive material are also a threat. Depending on the amount, type, and dispersion of the radioactive material, the psychological effects of a dirty bomb may be more significant than the physical effects. The last section of Table 5.1 summarizes the injury mechanisms sometimes exacerbated by terrorist bombing methods.

5.2 The Nature of Blast Waves

Explosions lead to what is referred to as a blast wave. An explosion heats and accelerates air molecules. The resultant steep rise in the atmospheric pressure at the site of the explosion is propagated in all directions. The rise in pressure over the normal ambient atmospheric pressure is referred to as overpressure.

Overpresssure is formed by compression of air in front of the blast wave. Blast wave overpressure has also been called high-energy impulse noise. Such blast wave overpressure is a sharp, rapid rise in ambient atmospheric pressure that follows detonation of munitions, firing of some weapons, explosions, and electrical arcs. Exposure to air blast can cause fatal injury with no apparent external signs of injury. Classifications of injury mechanisms that follow blasts are listed in Table 5.1.

Figure 5.3 shows an idealized waveform resulting from air blast, often referred to as a Friedlander waveform. This has a rapid rise to a peak value, followed by an exponential decay that may go below ambient pressure before returning to the steady state ambient pressure. Both the positive (overpressure) and negative (underpressure) portions of pressure variations can contribute to injury. The peak value of underpressure cannot exceed one atmosphere of pressure, while overpressure is often many times this amount (Zhang et al. 1996). The duration of the overpressure (duration of the pressure rise above steady state ambient pressure) can be extremely short, but can be very destructive. Overpressure times are usually measured in milliseconds or microseconds (Elsayed 1997). If a blast occurs within an enclosure, such as a building, the pressure-time graph appears somewhat different than the idealized Friedlander waveform be-

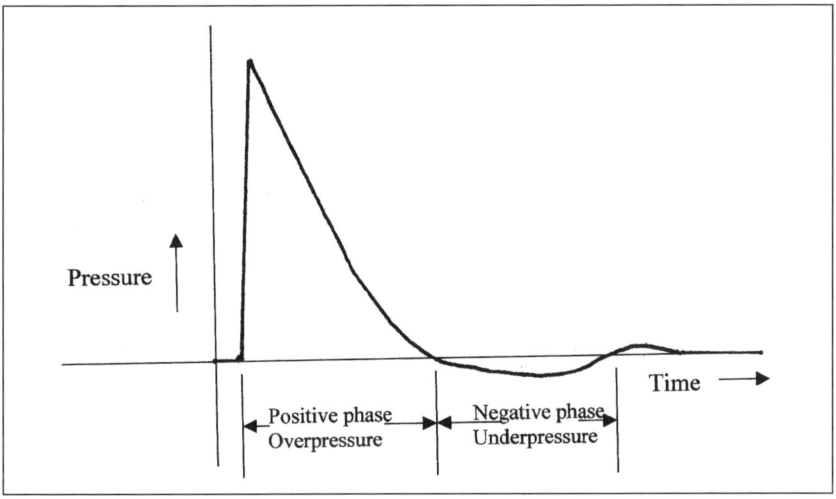

Figure 5.3 *An idealized drawing of the changes in air pressure that result from an explosion, often referred to as a Friedlander waveform. Reprinted with permission from the chapter "Characteristics and Mechanisms of Blast Injury" in the book Medical and Bioengineering Aspects of Electrical Injuries, by R.M. Fish and L.A. Geddes, Lawyers & Judges Publishing, 2003.*

cause of wave reflections off of surfaces within the enclosure (Mayorga 1997). For complex waveforms, the impulse (integral of pressure over time) is of importance, in addition to the maximum peak overpressure value. Other factors determining the effect of the blast include duration of overpressure, distance from the pressure source, and body orientation toward the blast (Elsayed 1997).

5.3 Factors Affecting Severity of Blast Injury

The velocity of the shock wave and duration of the positive pressure component are determined by the energy of the explosive force, the surrounding medium (air or water), and the distance from the explosion (Stapczynski 1982; Kryter 1965; Sudderth 1974).

A. Blast exposure in water

In water, pressure waves lose energy less quickly with distance. The lethal radius around an explosion in water is about three times what it would be in air (Phillips 1986). Explosive forces transmitted to patients in water sometimes result in transient lower extremity weakness. Such weakness may last seconds to minutes.

If a blast results in tears of lung tissue, hemoptysis (coughing of up blood) and air emboli sometimes result. Leakage of air from the alveoli into the blood and systemic circulation can lead to ischemic tissue injury in the body and brain. Head and body orientation toward the blast will also have a significant influence on blast effects (Elsayed 1997).

B. Nearby structures and enclosed spaces

Blast pressure is significantly affected by nearby structures. A shock wave reflected from a vertical surface, such as the wall of a building, can double peak pressure (Corey 1946, 626). Multiple reflections of a shock wave off of walls, people, pillars, and doors can create complex blast waveforms (Cooper 1983, 955; Treadwell, 1989). Therefore blast injury effects are increased in enclosed spaces, such as buildings and vehicles.

C. Spalling

Gas-containing organs, especially the ear, gastrointestinal tract, and respiratory system are most often injured with blast exposure. When a blast shock wave travels from one medium to another that has less density (e.g.

tissue to air), local physical tensions are created in the first medium. This would occur when the blast shock wave moves from tissue fluid to air in the lung alveoli. This production of local tissue tension is called spalling, and it produces microscopic and macroscopic tears of the tissue at the interface (Stein and Hirshberg 1999, 1540).

5.4 Specific Blast Injuries

A. Ear injury

Tympanic membrane rupture can result in pain, conductive hearing loss, hemorrhage, and dizziness. Inner ear injury can result in tinnitus and hearing loss of up to 100 db. An ear facing a blast may receive overpressures several times that which would result from a face-on blast. Therefore similar explosions can result in injuries of very different severities, depending on the orientation of the ear canal to the incident wave (Garth 1995, 364). The human eardrum may rupture at pressures as low as 14 kiloPascals (kPa), which is 2 psi. At 345 kPa (50 psi), about 50% of eardrums will be ruptured (Richmond et al. 1989). Chandler and Edmond (1997) report that tympanic membrane rupture will occur in 50 percent of

Table 5.2
Blast Injury to Various Organs

Organ	Nature of Possible Blast Injuries
Airway	The upper respiratory tract can have petechiae, ecchymosis, edema, and bleeding. Airway obstruction is uncommon.
Brain Direct injury	Concussion syndrome, cognitive difficulties, cerebral contusion, subdural hematoma, epidural hematoma, cerebral hemorrhage, and brain edema.
Brain Indirect injury	Cerebral infarction (stroke) from air emboli. This can be from multiple small emboli or a few large ones. Secondary brain injury, especially that due to hypoxia and hypotension following physical trauma
Ear	Tympanic membrane rupture, serous otitis, fractures of ossicles, displacement of stapes, inner ear injury, persistent pain, tinnitus, dizziness.
Eye	Conjunctival hemorrhage (most common) Air emboli Orbital bone fractures with high energy overpressures.
Heart	Coronary artery emboli leading to infarction or sudden death Dysrhythmias. Myocardial tears
Lung	Toxic effects from inhalation of combustion gases Pulmonary contusion and edema Tears of the lung tissue producing: a. Hemoptysis b. Hemorrhage, which is usually lethal if it involves over 61% of lung parenchyma. c. Air emboli (leakage of air from the alveoli into the blood and systemic circulation)
Skin	Thermal injury from radiation, hot gases, or fires

Elsayed 1997; Mayorga 1997; Murthy 1979; Phillips 1986; Phillips and Zajtchuk 1989; Stapczynski 1982.

adults at noise levels over 185 dB peak. These pressures are roughly a billion times the auditory threshold. One pound per square inch approximately equals 7 kPa (Phillips, 1986).

B. Gastrointestinal injury

Spalling also occurs in the walls of other hollow organs, such as the bowel. In the alimentary tract, one sometimes finds hemorrhages beneath the visceral peritoneum that can extend into the mesentery. This occurs mainly in the cecum and colon. Bowel perforations sometimes occur. Such perforations can develop up to forty-eight hours after the blast (Stein and Hirshberg 1999, 1542).

C. Blast lung injury

Spalling leads to hemorrhage and edema in the lung. The largest morbidity and mortality from blast injury itself results from lung damage, as judged from military experience and terror attacks on civilians. Microscopically in the lung there are alveolar microhemorrhages with perivascular and peribronchial distributions, tears of alveolar walls, and the development of blood-filled emphysematous spaces. Alveolar pulmonary-venous fistulae may develop and lead to systemic air embolism. Rib fractures and significant chest wall injury are uncommon in the absence of secondary or tertiary explosion effects. An overpressure of about 40 PSI is required to cause primary lung blast injury. Unless protective measures are taken, over 50 percent of victims with pulmonary injury from overpressures of 80 PSI, and all exposed to 200 PSI overpressures, will die (Stein and Hirshberg 1999, 1542).

D. Air emboli

Lung injury can introduce air into the circulatory system. Air emboli in the arterial circulation are responsible for most of the early mortality from primary blast injury (Phillips 1986, 1447).

Air emboli are thought to originate in the lungs when there are tissue disruptions between the alveoli (small airway spaces) and the intralobular venules (small veins). A connection between these structures is referred to as alveolar rupture, or alveolar-pulmonary fistula (Phillips 1986). Alveolar rupture allows air to leak into the blood and be carried to tissues in the body and brain. Air embolism may involve one or more large emboli, or many small emboli. The emboli may travel to the brain and create strokes, such as cerebral and other infarctions (Mayorga 1997). In some cases, showers of air emboli synchronous with respiration may be detected by Doppler flow monitoring of the carotid arteries that supply blood to the brain (Phillips 1986, 1449–1450). Air emboli are well known to give permanent strokes (cerebrovascular accidents) in divers (Greer 1992).

References

Chandler, D.W. and C.V. Edmond. "Effects of blast overpressure on the ear: Case reports." *J. Am. Acad. Audiol.* 8(2):81–8 (1997).

Chang, A. "Bombs and bioterror." ABCNEWS.com. August 6, 2003. http://abcnews.go.com/sections/world/DailyNews/poisonbomb020806.html

Cooper, G.J., R.H. Chait and J.T. Zajtchuk. "Casualties from terrorist bombings." *J. Trauma* 3:955–67 (1983).

Corey, E.L. "Medical aspects of blast." *U.S. Naval Medical Bulletin* 46(5):623–53 (1946).

Elsayed, N.M. "Toxicology of blast overpressure." *Toxicology* 121:1–15 (1997).

Findlay, G. "Attack and retaliation." ABCNEWS.com. June 5, 2002. http://abcnews.go.com/sections/world/DailyNews/mideast020605.html

Garth, R.J.N. "Blast injury of the ear: An overview and guide to management." *Injury* 26(6):363–6 (1995).

Greer, H.D. and E.W. Massey. "Neurologic injury from undersea diving." *Neurol. Clin.* 10:1031–45 (1992).

Kryter, K. and G.R. Garinther. "Auditory effects of acoustic impulses from firearms." *Acta Otolaryngol.* Suppl;211:1–22 (1965).

Mayorga, M.A. "The pathology of primary blast overpressure injury." *Toxicology* 121:17–28 (1997).

Murthy, J.M., J.S. Chopra and D.R. Gulati. "Subdural hematoma in an adult following a blast injury: Case report." *J. Neurosurg.* 50:260–1 (1979).

Phillips, Y.Y. "Primary blast injury." *Ann. Emerg. Med.* 15:1446–50 (1986).

Phillips, Y.Y. and J.T. Zajtchuk "Blast injuries of the ear in military operations." *Ann. Otol. Rhinol. Laryngol.* Suppl. 140:3–4 (1989).

Richmond, D.R. et al. "Physical correlates of eardrum rupture." *Ann. Otol. Rhinol. Laryngol.* Suppl. 140:35–41 (1989).

Siegel-Itzkovich, J. "Israeli minister orders hepatitis B vaccine for survivors of suicide bomb attacks." *B.M.J.*, August 25, 2001, page 417

Stein, M. and A. Hirshberg. "Medical consequences of terrorism: The conventional weapon threat." *Surg. Clin. North Am.* 79(6):1537–52 (1999).

Stapczynski, J.S. "Blast injuries." *Ann. Emerg. Med.* 11:687–94 (1982).

Steele, Mandi. "Survivors face agony in suicide attacks. Anti-personnel bombs wreak havoc on human bodies." WorldNetDaily May 30, 2002. http://www.worldnetdaily.com/news/article.asp?ARTICLE_ID=27778.

Stein, M. and A. Hirshberg. "Limited mass casualties due to conventional weapons." In *Terror and Medicine*, J. Shemer and Y. Shoenfeld, eds. (Miami: Pabst Science Publishers, 2003), 378–393. (http://www.pabst-science-publishers.us/medicine/m_books/3899670183.htm).

Sudderth, M.E. "Tympanoplasty in blast-induced perforation." *Arch. Otolaryngol.* 99:157–9 (1974).

Treadwell, I. "Effects of blasts on the human body." *Nursing RSA* 4:32–6 (1989).

Zhang, J.K. et al. "Studies on lung injuries caused by blast underpressure." *J. Trauma* 40(3):S77–S80 (1996).

Chapter 6

Terrorist Bombings: Injury Diagnosis and Treatment

Raymond M. Fish, Ph.D., M.D., FACEP

Synopsis

The author would like to thank Neal R. Abarbanell, M.D. for his review of this paper and his helpful suggestions.Figure 6.1 is reprinted from Steele 2002, with permission of Worldnetdaily.com (http:// www. worldnetdaily.com/).

6.1 The Accident Scene

A. Phases of care-giving at a mass casualty bombing scene

Certain patterns of rescuer behavior and medical care-giving tend to occur at the scene of terrorist bombings. These phases are described in Table 6.1 (derived from the text of Stein and Hirshberg 2003).

B. Aspects of bombing scene and ambulance treatment

(This section is adapted from the text of Stein and Hirshberg 2003.)

1. "Stay-and-Play" versus "Load-and-Go"

Scoop and run, with little treatment at the accident scene is appropriate and life-saving for many patients. Hypovolemic shock (significant blood loss) benefits most from rapid transport to the hospital where surgery can stop the bleeding. Therefore, delaying transport to the hospital to start IVs is generally not helpful, especially if the transport time is short. Intravenous lines can be started en route to the hospital. However, if transport is delayed to start IVs, valuable time is lost.

2. Amputation of body parts

In most cases, patients with amputated body parts from blast injury will not survive. Persons with traumatic amputation from a blast who are not moving or breathing overtly, have no palpable pulse, and have dilated pupils should be considered to be dead.

3. CPR

Respiratory assistance is an effective intervention, as discussed below. However, in the pulseless patient, CPR (respiratory support plus chest compressions) in the field has not been successful following blast injury, and it delays treatment of others who might benefit from EMS (emergency medical system) intervention.

4. Effective treatments at the accident scene

Airway control. The treatment that has probably saved the most lives is airway control with cervical spine immobilization. The unconscious patient may have an inadequate airway or inadequate ventilation. Oxygenation can be improved with oxygen given by mask and a

Table 6.1
Phases of Events at the Scene of Terrorist Bombings

Phase and Its Duration	Characteristics and Events
First phase: the chaotic phase. Lasts 15–25 minutes.	Ambulatory victims will evacuate to the nearest hospital, sometimes by means of civilian transportation. The first phase ends with the arrival of an EMS officer who can act as leader.
Second phase: the reorganization phase. Lasts 15 minutes to one hour.	The second phase starts when the EMS officer assumes control at the scene. Medical decision making and care will influence survival and morbidity. The first medical goal at the scene is to identify patients with an immediate life-threat. All EMS personnel should assist in this task. The EMS officer must halt the random evacuation that may occur, and provide for the more urgent casualties to be transported to the hospital first. This is often a difficult task.
Third phase: the site-clearing phase. Lasts up to three hours from the time of the initial explosion.	The surrounding area is searched for victims who were missed during the initial two phases. Victims may be trapped in vehicles or buildings, hidden under debris or located some distance from most of the other victims.
The fourth phase: the late phase. Occurs between the clearing of the site of live victims, until one or two days after the event.	Victim classification is expanded in this phase. Persons with apparently minor injuries may recognize them only after going home. Examples are abrasions, tinnitus, and emotional distress.
DURING ALL PHASES: Work with the bomb squad.	A second bomb may explode. This is most common in the first two phases at the scene of a terrorist bombing, usually coming 10 to 30 minutes after the first detonation. EMS personnel should work closely with police bomb squad personnel.

EMS = Emergency Medical System

Derived from the text of Stein and A. Hirshberg 2003.

rebreathing reservoir along with nasal or oral airways as needed. Positive pressure ventilation may be necessary and is often life-saving. However, ventilation should be done with the least possible pressure, as patients with blast lung injury tend to develop pneumothoraces and air emboli. If a tension pneumothorax is suspected, some form of chest drainage (needle decompression or chest tube) is needed prior to arrival to the hospital, whether or not positive pressure ventilation has been used.

Hemorrhage control in the field is limited to external bleeding, mainly from extremities. Tourniquet application is indicated only if direct pressure fails to control bleeding. IV fluid administration should not delay transport to definitive surgery.

Skeletal fracture alignment is important in field management. With an overwhelming number of patients, there may not be enough backboards and splints. Prior to hospital arrival, limb-to-limb splinting and the use of tape to secure the patient to a stretcher will often be adequate.

6.2 Initial Emergency Department and Hospital Treatment Priorities

In contrast to the usual battlefield situation, patients will often not have the best baseline physical condition and may include very young children, older adults, and pregnant women. Severe internal injury may exist with little in the way of external findings.

Treatment ABCs. A patient with a history of blast injury exposure should be managed with attention to the ABCs of ATLS (the Advanced Trauma Life Support program of the American College of Surgeons). Blunt trauma may result from persons being physically thrown, falling or having objects or parts of a building impact them. Penetrating injury and burns are also common. Positive pressure ventilation should be provided with the minimum necessary pressure (Guy et al. 1998; Mayorga 1997; Phillips 1986; Stapczynski 1982).

A. Airway

Airway hemorrhage and edema may occur, though this usually does not cause airway compromise. Signs of airway obstruction should be sought. Intubation is indicated for respiratory insufficiency.

B. Breathing

1. Respiratory distress

Respiratory distress should be treated with supplemental oxygen.

2. Positive pressure ventilation: Use only if necessary

Positive airway pressure may enlarge a small pneumothorax and facilitate air embolism. Therefore, modalities such as positive end expiratory pressure (PEEP) should be administered only if necessary. General anesthesia sometimes results in sudden death during the first forty-eight hours after blast injury of the lung, possibly because of air emboli. If possible, surgery should be delayed or done with another method of anesthesia (Phillips 1986).

When ventilation is necessary, techniques such as limited peak inspiratory pressure and permissive hypercapnia may be helpful (Stein and Hirshberg 1999).

3. Apnea

A brief or prolonged period of apnea may follow blast injury. Positive pressure ventilation will be necessary in such cases (as with Ambu bag or mouth-to-mouth), but the smallest effective airway pressures should be used.

4. Signs of respiratory injury

Early morbidity and mortality are often correlated with pulmonary injury. Signs and symptoms include chest tightness, chest pain, tachypnea (rapid breathing), use of accessory muscles of respiration, hemoptysis (coughing up blood), and respiratory insufficiency related to pulmonary hemorrhage, edema, or mechanical lung disruption including pneumothorax. Air emboli can present as brain or cardiac dysfunction. Supplemental oxygen (with nasal prongs or mask) is useful because of the possibility of worsening of pulmonary function over time, sometimes with development of the adult respiratory distress syndrome (ARDS).

Pneumothorax may present as a unilateral hyperresonance to chest-wall percussion and decreased breath sounds. With increased pressure in the pneumothorax (tension pneumothorax), a shift of the trachea and mediastinum to the side opposite the pneumothorax, severe shortness of breath, and eventually hypotension may occur. The trachea, palpated at the base of the neck anteriorly in the suprasternal notch, may be found to be deviated (pushed by the increased pressure) away from the side of the tension pneumothorax.

Leakage of air into various tissues is sometimes evidenced by subcutaneous emphysema (air under the skin causing in some cases visible swelling or a crunchy feeling of the tissues), or by a precordial systolic crunch (sounds synchronous with the heart beat due to air in the mediastinum or pericardium).

Even a tiny pneumothorax should be treated with a chest tube or equivalent device in patients who may need to receive positive pressure ventilation. This is because positive-pressure ventilation may force air into the pneumothorax, making it larger and possibly creating a tension pneumothorax (Stein and Hirshberg 1999).

5. Pulmonary radiographic findings

Chest radiographs may indicate pulmonary and cardiac injury and dysfunction. Hemorrhage and edema may produce infiltrates that are linear, patchy, or diffuse. These may be seen immediately following the explosion. Worsening afterward may be due to development of infection or ARDS (adult respiratory distress syndrome). Pulmonary consolidation may be indicative of pulmonary contusion (bruise of the lung) or of a hemothorax (blood between the chest wall and the lung).

A butterfly pattern may appear on plain chest x-ray films because pulmonary infiltrates and contusions sometimes develop initially around the pulmonary hila, with the periphery of the lungs being relatively spared. This can produce a dark halo around the lungs on radiographs. With worsening of the patient, complete whitening of the lung fields may occur, simulating the appearance of late-stage ARDS.

6. Radiographic findings of pneumoperitoneum

Positive pressure ventilation, especially if high pressures are used, can force air to leak through the fascial layers of the mediastinum into the abdomen, resulting in a pneumoperitoneum. Pneumoperitoneum is generally harmless, unless the pressure increases enough to displace the diaphragm, in which case the pneumoperitoneum may need to be drained of air.

The real danger when one sees an apparent pneumoperitoneum is to assume that it is due to air dissection from the mediastinum and miss the fact that there has been a hollow viscus perforation in the abdomen (such as a bowel perforation). A bowel or other perforation requires prompt sur-

Table 6.2
Air under the Diaphragm: Pneumoperitoneum

Source of Air in the Peritoneum	Treatment
Air leak associated with high pressure ventilation.	If the pressure increases enough to displace the diaphragm, the pneumoperitoneum may need to be drained of air
Bowel or other abdominal hollow viscus perforation (may occur up to 48 hours post-blast).	Prompt surgical intervention to prevent death from peritonitis and other complications

gery to prevent death from peritonitis and other complications (Stein and Hirshberg, 1999).

7. Severe blast lung injury and its treatment

Blast lung injury is a leading cause of death in terrorist bombings. Severe blast lung injury and its treatment is reviewed by Pizov et al. (1999). In his study, fifteen patients with primary blast lung injury from explosions on two civilian buses were reviewed, as summarized below. His study gives perspective, as well as specific information, on the treatment of this condition that few civilian physicians have managed.

Primary blast lung injury means that the lung injury was due to the blast wave traveling to, and impacting, the body. This is in contrast to secondary injury, in which objects are propelled, and the objects impact the body. Tertiary injury occurs when the blast wave displaces the body, which in turn impacts an object. In primary blast lung injury, pressure differentials disrupt the alveolar walls and damage the alveolar-capillary interface. This results in large emphysematous blood-filled spaces. Lining cells of air passages, the airway epithelium may be injured or stripped away. These lesions allow air to enter into the pleura (the lining around the lung) and into the mediastinum (the space between the lungs, containing the heart and large blood vessels). Physical signs associated with blast lung injury include hemoptysis (coughing up of blood) and barotrauma to the ears (damaged or ruptured eardrums).

An explosion in a bus, restaurant, or other enclosed area produces more injury than would occur with the same bomb in an open area. There are several reasons for the increased injury severity. First, the bomb is relatively close to the victims. Second, in an enclosed space blast waves are reflected off the walls of the bus or room, and then to the victims, rather than traveling off into the distance. Reflected blast waves increase the number and strength of blast forces that strike each bus passenger. Lastly, many persons are unable to escape from the burning vehicle or building, and thus receive burns that are often lethal.

Of the fifteen patients in the Pizov study, ten were extremely hypoxic on admission, with the arterial partial pressure of oxygen (pO_2) being under 65 mmHg with oxygen supplementation. Although older articles have suggested that blast lung injury can develop after 24–48 hours, there were no such cases seen in this study. Lung findings occurring days later may be due to infection or ARDS (adult respiratory distress syndrome). In this study, patients who had blast lung injury presented with the blast lung injury being apparent on presentation to the ED.

Initial treatment for hypoxia was mechanical ventilation and drainage of pneumothoraces (air surrounding the lung with partial or total collapse of the lung). Following this initial treatment, only four patients remained severely hypoxic. Initial chest x-rays showed bilateral lung opacities of various sizes in twelve patients (80 percent), bilateral pneumothoraces in seven patients (47 percent), and a unilateral pneumothorax in two patients. There was evidence of significant bronchopleural fistulae (connection and air leak between the larger airways the pleural space surrounding the lungs) in five patients (33 percent). Ten of the patients (67 percent) had hemoptysis (coughing up blood). All of the patients had eardrum perforation. Nine patients (60 percent) had burns. Four patients had splenic tears. Two patients had vascular lesions, four had bone fractures, and two had head injuries. One patient developed a fatal hemispheric stroke on the second day after the explosion.

All but one patient was intubated, with intubations being done at the scene of the explosions or in the admitting area of the Trauma Unit. Indications for intubation were unconsciousness, respiratory failure, or the need for emergency surgery. Arterial blood gases were repeated at least every six hours. Chest x-rays were taken on arrival, with more taken later. All patients were admitted to the ICU and monitored with invasive blood pressure measurements and CVP (central venous catheter) and/or pulmonary artery catheter. Volume resuscitation (intravenous fluid) was given.

To assist breathing with the least possible airway pressures, ventilators were set to use pressure-controlled, inverse-ratio ventilation with an inspiratory/expiratory ratio of 2:1, and to lower the PEEP (positive end-expiratory pressure) as much as possible. One patient received independent lung ventilation because of a large unilateral broncho-pleural fistula. Ventilation with volume-controlled or pressure support ventilation was used for patients with less severe lung injury.

Five patients developed ARDS, and no patient with mild blast lung injury developed any form of lasting lung injury. All three patients with severe blast lung injury who survived the first twenty-four hours did develop ARDS, as did 33 percent of the patients with moderate blast lung injury. Prolonged mechanical ventilation and ICU care were required for patients with respiratory failure. Respiratory management included positive pressure ventilation for fourteen of the patients. Overall, eleven of the fifteen patients survived.

C. Circulation

1. Tourniquets to control bleeding are not usually needed

At the accident scene, hemorrhage control is usually possible only if it is confined to external bleeding, as from the extremities. A tourniquet proximal to the bleeding site should be applied only if direct pressure on the bleeding site fails to control the bleeding adequately.

2. Intravenous fluids: "Load and Go" beats "Stay and Play"

Delays in transport will be fatal to some patients who are bleeding. The amount of intravenous fluids that can be given during transport is usually not enough to make a difference in the patient who is bleeding severely. If bleeding is not a severe problem, IV fluids are not needed. Therefore, transport to surgery should not be delayed by starting intravenous lines. If lines are started during transport without delaying the transport, that is fine.

3. Bradycardia

Blast overpressure has been associated with asystole, tachycardia, and ventricular fibrillation. Protracted bradycardia sometimes occurs in humans after blast injury. In experimental animals, bradycardia has been found to occur almost instantaneously and varies from a slight slowing to a reduction of more than 50 percent (Guy et al. 1998).

4. Myocardial lacerations

High levels of blast overpressure can cause myocardial lacerations. Myocardial ischemia and infarction can be the result of air or fibrinous emboli and are thought to be a major cause of death. Hypotension may be due to blood loss, dysrhythmias, myocardial ischemia from air emboli, or acute cor pulmonale (dilation and failure of the right side of the heart).

D. Disability: Neurological

A concussion syndrome may be secondary to mechanical head trauma or (possibly unrecognized) air emboli. The concussion syndrome may be suggested by minor mental status changes. Focal neurological findings may be due to systemic air emboli, although air emboli can also lead to generalized evidence of cerebral dysfunction, such as an altered affect, confusion, or disorientation (Phillips 1986, 1449). Therefore patients with focal or generalized neurological abnormalities should be worked up for mechanical head trauma as well as for air emboli.

Hyperbaric oxygen therapy is a specific treatment for air embolism. Hyperbaric therapy is sometimes useful many hours after onset of neurological and other problems due to air emboli.

Computed tomography (CT) has detected air embolism in some cases in the early course of cerebral air embolism. However, early CT findings do not correlate with clinical presentation, EEG, or histological manifestations of cerebral air embolism (Annane et al. 1995). CT findings will change over time. Infarcts due to the air emboli may become visible on CT several days later (Hirabuki al. 1988).

6.3 Specific Injuries

The most important specific injury, blast lung injury, is described in Section 6.2

A. Fractures and dislocations

In the field, as well as in early emergency department care, alignment of fractures is important (Stein and Hirshberg 1999). Reduction of joint dislocations as soon as possible is often helpful in providing immediate pain reduction, as well as in reducing vascular compromise, skin breakdown, and other complications.

B. Open wounds

In the field, covering of open wounds with sterile dressings, or even with makeshift cloth, is desirable (Stein and Hirshberg, 1999).

C. Abdominal injury

Hollow viscous abdominal organs are injured more frequently than solid abdominal organs. Blast injury can result in edema, hemorrhage, perforation, and laceration. The signs and symptoms associated with such lesions will vary considerably depending on the location of the lesions and the presence of other injuries. Reported signs and symptoms have included abdominal pain and tenderness, nausea, vomiting, an urge to defecate, and rectal bleeding. Contused bowel may necrose and perforate several days after injury, leading to significant morbidity and mortality (Stein and Hirshberg 1999).

D. Air emboli

Arterial gas embolism involves extravasation of air into the arterial system and may cause stroke-like brain injury. Definitive treatment includes administration of oxygen and recompression in a chamber. Permanent neurologic injury may result (Greer and Massey 1992). Hyperbaric therapy is effective to some extent in treating cerebral air emboli, even up to eleven hours after the acute event (Stapczynski 1982). However, earlier treatment, especially within six hours is more effective (Blanc et al. 2002). Mannitol may be used as an adjunctive treatment for air embolism, but should not delay or replace recompression.

Air emboli can sometimes be visualized in the retinal vessels or on computerized axial tomography studies of the brain (Hirabuki et al. 1988; Hwang et al. 1983). A patchy blanching of the tongue is also suggestive of arterial air emboli. Myocardial ischemia and dysrhythmias are often associated with coronary artery emboli. Arterial emboli to other vascular beds may give a clinical picture similar to that seen in the embolic aspects of decompression illness. Showers of air emboli synchronous with respiration may be detected by Doppler flow monitoring of the carotid arteries (Phillips 1986, 1449–1450). Definitive treatment for air emboli is hyperbaric oxygen. If hyperbaric therapy is not available, positioning the patient supine with the left side down and the body inclined so the head is lower than the feet has been recommended. This position theoretically causes venous air to accumulate at the right atrium where a central venous catheter can be used to remove it. The efficacy of this procedure has not been clearly demonstrated, and the harm done by air emboli is often so rapid that it is too late to do anything by the time the problem has shown itself. Hyperbaric therapy is sometimes useful many hours after onset of neurological and other problems due to air emboli.

E. The ear

Blast injury to the ear is sometimes associated with immediate pain and impairment of function, although in some cases patients have been noted to be unaware of the injury (Richmond et al. 1989, 37). A tympanic membrane ruptured by a pressure wave and unaccompanied by deeper injury will have incapacitating pain or balance disturbance in less than 5 percent of cases. Most will heal without intervention unless infection occurs. Between 10–20 percent will require surgical closure, and a small percentage of patients will develop chronic problems from infection or cholesteatoma (a growth in the middle ear containing cells and cholesterol). (Phillips and Zajtchuk 1989).

Blast injury can cause hearing deficits that are conductive, sensorineural, or mixed. Conductive loss from blast injury can involve tympanic membrane rupture, ossicular damage, and serous otitis (Kerr and Byrne 1975). Sensorineural hearing losses from inner ear damage may range from temporary threshold shifts, likely due to transient disruption of cochlear function, to a more permanent loss from labyrinthine fistulas, basilar membrane ruptures, or other injuries. Sensorineural hearing loss frequently is reported after blast injury and is often accompanied by tinnitus. Sensorineural hearing loss is more prevalent in the high frequencies and may also affect speech frequencies. Temporary threshold shift is thought to be due to a reversible biochemical cochlear dysfunction. Causes of sensorineural hearing loss that is likely to be permanent include perilymphatic fistula, loss of hair cell integrity, and rupture of labyrinthine membranes (Casler et al. 1989). There is little evidence to support treating sensorineural hearing loss with steroids, vasodilators, or vitamins, but such treatment is not generally harmful (Garth 1995).

Posterior-superior tympanic membrane perforations are associated with retraction pockets and cholesteatoma formation. Perforations larger than 30 percent of the total tympanic membrane surface have a low rate (0 percent to 22 percent) of spontaneous healing. Healing occurs at the rate of about 10 percent per month. Some studies have shown that spontaneous healing is unlikely to occur if there has been no healing in ten to fifteen days, though some suggest waiting six months for spontaneous healing to occur (Casler et al. 1989).

Acutely, if eardrum rupture is thought to have occurred, gentle clearing of debris from the external ear canal can be done using suction under a microscope, and no irrigation should be attempted (Stein and Hirshberg 1999; Phillips 1986). A tympanic membrane rupture is an indication that some damage may have occurred in the cochlea. There may be loss of hearing that lasts minutes to hours, or is permanent. It is thought that noise avoidance and use of hearing protection can be helpful (Phillips and Zajtchuk 1989).

F. Penetrating injury and retained foreign bodies

With suicide bombings, even more than with other types of bombings, a variety of foreign bodies are thrown with great force, often penetrating nearby victims. These penetrating objects include nails, screws, and other objects deliberately packed around the bomb.

A patient may have a foreign body located anywhere in the head or body. Initial presentations may be subtle because entrance wounds can be difficult to see and the patient may initially be asymptomatic, or focused on more painful injuries. Nails have been found in the brains of initially alert patients, and cardiac penetration has occurred with no early hemodynamic compromise. Penetrating injury tends to produce permanent deficits when it involves the eyes, brain, or spinal cord. There is no consensus on the need for whole-body (and head) x-ray to search for unsuspected foreign bodies. As suggested by Figure 6.1, multiple injuries to the bowel and other organs may occur.

Bone fragments of suicide bombers with viral contamination have penetrated victims' bodies. Testing of bone fragments from one victim detected hepatitis B, leading to immunizations being routinely given to many bombing victims. Therefore, routine hepatitis B immunization has been given to bombing victims prophylactically, though there is no established consensus concerning the need for this. At least one suicide bomber

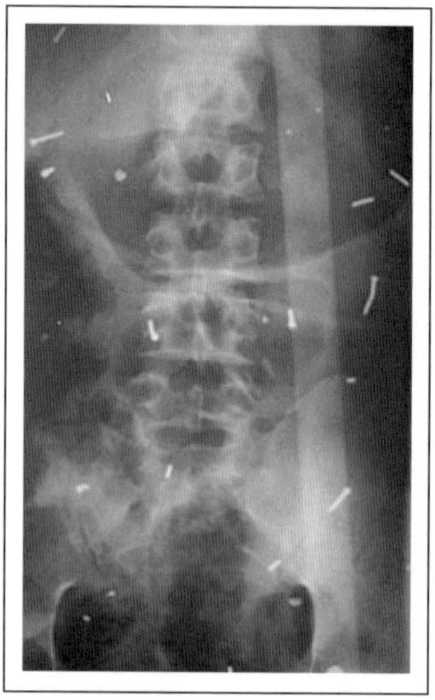

Figure 6.1 *Front view of an abdomen imbedded with nails and metal fragments. Injury of the spinal cord, intra-abdominal organs, and vascular structures would be expected. Reprinted from Steele 2000, with permission of worldnetdaily.com.*

has had AIDS (Stein and Hirshberg 2003, 390), though hepatitis B is more commonly found in the bombers.

Two injuries frequently missed in patients are tympanic membrane injury from the blast force, and penetrating eye injuries from flying debris.

References

American College of Surgeons. *Advanced Trauma Life Support for Doctors* (Chicago: American College of Surgeons, 1997).

Annane, D. et al. "Kinetics of elimination and acute consequences of cerebral air embolism." *J. Neuroimag.* 5:183–9 (1995).

Blanc, P., A. Boussuges and K. Henriette. "Iatrogenic cerebral air embolism: Importance of an early hyperbaric oxygenation." *Intensive Care Med.* 28:559–563 (2002).

Casler, J.D., R.H. Chait and J.T. Zajtchuk. "Treatment of blast injury to the ear." *Ann. Otol. Rhinol. Laryngol.* 98:13–16 (1989).

Garth, R.J.N. "Blast injury of the ear: An overview and guide to management." *Injury* 26(6):363–6 (1995).

Greer, H.D. and E.W. Massey. "Neurologic injury from undersea diving." *Neurol. Clin.* 0:1031–45 (1992).

Guy, R.J. et al. "Physiologic responses to primary blast." *J. Trauma* 45:983–7 (1998).

Hirabuki, N. et al. "Changes of cerebral air embolism shown by computed tomography." *Br. J. Radiol.* 61:252–5 (1988).

Hwang, T.L. et al. *Ann. Neurol.* 13:214–5 (1983).

Kerr, A.G. and J.E. Byrne. "Concussive effects of bomb blast on the ear." *J. Laryngol. Otol.* 89:131–43 (1975).

Mayorga, M.A. The pathology of primary blast overpressure injury. *Toxicology* 121:17–28 (1997).

Phillips, Y.Y. "Primary blast injury." *Ann. Emerg. Med.* 15:1446–50 (1986).

Phillips, Y.Y. and J.T. Zajtchuk. "Blast injuries of the ear in military operations." *Ann. Otol. Rhinol. Laryngol.* Suppl. 140:3–4 (1989).

Pizov, R. et al. "Blast lung injury from an explosion on a civilian bus." *Chest* 115:165–172 (1999).

Richmond, D.R. et al. "Physical correlates of eardrum rupture." *Ann. Oto. Rhinol. Laryngol.* 98:3–41 (1989).

Stapczynski, J.S. "Blast injuries." *Ann. Emerg. Med.* 11:687–94 (1982).

Steele, Mandi. "Survivors face agony in suicide attacks: Anti-personnel bombs wreak havoc on human bodies." May 30, 2002. As found at: http://www.worldnetdaily.com/news/article.asp?ARTICLE_ID=27778

Stein, M. and A. Hirshberg. "Medical consequences of terrorism: The conventional weapon threat." *Surgical Clinics of North America* 79(6):1737–52 (1999).

Stein, M. and A. Hirshberg. "Limited mass casualties due to conventional weapons." In *Terror and Medicine*, J. Shemer and Y. Shoenfeld, eds. (Miami: Pabst Science Publishers, 2003), 378–393. (http://www.pabst-science-publishers.us/medicine/m_books/3899670183.htm).

Chapter 7

Chemical Warfare and Terrorism Agents

Fredric Rieders, Ph.D., and Michael Rieders, Ph.D.

Synopsis

7.1 Introduction

The main purpose of this chapter is to make the topic of chemical warfare and terrorism agents accessible and understandable to the nonscientist. The term "chemical agents" or the abbreviation "CA" may also be used. The content of this chapter is aimed first at laymen as a technical introduction to this worrisome field. It will also be thought provoking and instructive to first responders, including medical, fire, rescue and law enforcement personnel, as well as to investigators, lawyers, adjudicators and administrators having to deal with the era of a growing panoply of ruthless, nihilistic terrorism.

Most chemical agents are simple substances that, even in relatively small amounts, are poisonous (i.e., toxic) to people. They may also be poison to other animals and to plants. Chemical agents are not infectious like viruses and bacteria. The ingredients that are needed to make chemical agents are often both inexpensive and readily available. These weapons have been called the "poor man's atomic bomb" because of their relatively low cost and their ability to inflict pain, suffering and death on large numbers of people.

Synthetic or man-made chemical agents, as well as natural poisons, can be dispersed in the form of a gas, liquid or solid, depending on the chemical nature of the agent and the way it is made into a weapon. The International Chemical Weapons Convention is an agreement among nations prohibiting toxic chemical use in warfare, containing a definition of toxic chemical agents used as weapons. The definition is very broad and includes any chemical that may cause the loss of ability to perform normal functions, or produce permanent injury to, or death of people and animals. Currently, a limited group of viruses (such as smallpox) and bacteria (such as anthrax) are considered biological warfare agents. Unfortunately, genetic engineering and a more sophisticated understanding of the science of disease may one day create new, even more lethal infectious biological agents, expanding the armament of infectious weapons. Unlike the short list of infectious biological agents, there is an ever-expanding list of chemical agents usable as terror and mass murder weapons. New, highly toxic, chemical substances are being synthesized by the thousands and tested as pharmaceutical drugs to fight cancer and other diseases, or to be used as pesticides.[1] The same approach to finding potential cures for deadly disease can be used as the basis for making and testing new toxic chemical agents. Even common household cleaning products can be fashioned into poisoning agents. Presently, there are over 21 million chemical substances registered in the U.S. Whether or not a substance is a chemical agent depends on its intended use and ability to produce harm.

The tables at the end of the chapter provide selected facts about chemical agents. Table 7.1 is a list of precursors which are chemical ingredients that are used to make CA. They can thus be footprints of contact with, possession or use of CA. A caveat is added by showing what non-nefarious origins and uses for the agents exist—in medicine, manufacturing and commerce. Table 7.2 is a summary of various industrial chemicals which can or already have been air dispersed with fatal results.

7.2 Historical Use of Chemical Agents

Knowledge of the use of chemical agents to cause individual and mass homicide is not a modern concept. Chemical poisoning as a means of murder has its roots in ancient human civilizations. The Sumerians, Egyptians, Hebrews, Asians, Indians, Greeks and Romans had written about deadly toxic substances, which could be used to sicken and kill their enemies. In Italy in the Middle Ages the science and art of poisoning was taught in schools in Venice and Rome. A secret armament of poison weapons was created in sixteenth century Venice by a group called the Council of Ten who commissioned professional poison murders for a fee. One famous family of poisoners known as the Borgia clan, terrified their fellow citizens with sophisticated and extensive use of poisons. People knew that dining with the Borgias could be their last meal.[2] Perhaps the Borgia family could be considered the first chemical terrorist group.

Fast forward to the twentieth century and World War I when poison gas was used by Germany in 1915 to kill hundreds of French troops and injure thousands more. Tons of chlorine gases were discharged into the wind, which then blew into the unprepared and unsuspecting troops who were battling the German Army near Ypres, Belgium. This attack using chemical weapons shattered the long-respected mutual understanding that poisonous chemicals were not to be used in warfare between so-called civilized armies. Once the unwritten rule was broken, the chemical weapons arms race escalated with both sides developing and using artillery shells and mortars filled with caustic and deadly poison liquids and gases. Tens of thousands of soldiers were severely injured and incapacitated by chemical agents but a relatively small percent of the casualties were killed by the immediate effects of the poison gas attacks.

Even after the horror of chemical warfare use in World War I, chemical weapons were unleashed on civilian and military targets in the decades that followed.[3] They were used to kill soldiers and noncombatants between 1918 and 1920 in Russia's bloody civil war. Chemical arms were first used in Iraq in the 1920s by the British Army and, over eighty years later, the British Army feared that Iraq would use them against their soldiers during Operation Iraqi Freedom. Chemical weapons were also used in 1935–36 when Italy invaded Ethiopia and by the Japanese during the period 1937–1942 against the Chinese forces. In many of these battles, the use of chemical weapons was one-sided with the opposing forces unprepared and unable to counterattack with the same type of weapon. Shifting winds and accidents while transporting, loading and handling toxic chemicals also produced injurious and fatal exposure to soldiers who were fielding them.

Although chemical weapons used in previous wars were stockpiled by the opposing armies and were available for use in World War II, only Japan used them in combat with China. Because of the fear of retaliation, major chemical warfare attacks were not launched between the Allied and Axis powers. German military scientists secretly continued to develop chemical warfare agents, although the military never used them. At the end of World War II, it was revealed that the Germans had developed extremely lethal nerve gas, that could swiftly paralyze its victims leaving them to suffocate and die.

When the United States and the Soviet Union emerged as superpowers after World War II, their military scientists engaged in extensive research and production of nerve gases along with more sophisticated delivery mechanisms. In 1952, British scientists developed a new nerve agent which became a major contribution to the chemical arms race. During the Cold War, large supplies of varying nerve gases were produced and stockpiled by the superpowers, but they remained unused following the collapse of the Soviet Union. One of the major challenges today is how to safely destroy the thousands of tons of ultra-deadly chemical agents produced during the Cold War.

Egypt used chemical weapons in the 1963–1967 Yemen civil war. Iraq launched chemical attacks in 1980–1988 during its war with Iran, and in 1988 it used chemical weapons against its own Kurdish people in order to suppress a rebellion. In June of 1994 and again March of 1995, nerve gas was used in terrorist attacks in Japan by a cult group called Aum Shinrikyo. The attacks, which stunned the people and government of Japan, killed fewer than twenty people but sickened thousands.

The terrorist use of chemical weapons against civilian targets is an event that has brought about extensive worldwide preparations and has incited a great deal of fear among all nations that this pattern will be repeated.

7.3 Recognition of Chemical Agent (CA) Effects

Chemical agents may have an immediate or delayed effect on people who are exposed to them, depending on the specific chemical agent used and the amount that gets into the individual. Terrorist attacks using chemical weapons are generally expected to have a rapid, overt effect with casualties at the scene.[4] Experience with chemical attacks such as the nerve gas release in a Tokyo, Japan subway, has borne out the expectation that chemical agent attacks produce an immediate impact. Biological attacks using infectious agents have a different time and spread profile because exposed victims may be unaware that they are infected, due to the long incubation period between exposure and illness.

The larger the amount of CA that gets into a victim, the faster the onset of poisoning symptoms and the more likely that the exposure will be lethal. Chemical agents typically have immediate harmful effects within minutes of exposure so victims know that they have been impacted by a toxic substance which causes them to seek medical help right away.

Another type of CA is the stealth CA that does not have an immediately obvious effect. Once it gets inside the body, stealth CA must be changed into toxic form to be harmful. This change may take hours or even days before the victims show symptoms of poisoning. Since they do not show overt harmful effects at the time of exposure, victims of stealth CA will leave the location where they were exposed without knowing that they have been poisoned. The pattern of stealth CA victims becoming sickened may be more similar to mass food poisoning or biological agent attack, because there is an incubation period before the onset of symptoms of poisoning.

7.4 Smell as a Warning of Chemical Agent Exposure

A person's sense of smell, coupled with knowledge of what the smell could be, can alert him to avoid an imminent danger of chemical exposure. Many chemical agents have a distinct odor while others have a faint smell or are odorless. Substances that are mixed with a chemical agent to make it more toxic may produce a strong odor that masks the agent or creates a mixed odor. Certain animals, dogs for example, have an exquisite sense of smell far superior to that of humans. The ability to perceive certain odors such as cyanide gas, varies from person to person, based on genetically inherited traits. A person with active allergies or a cold will have a diminished or absent ability to smell unless the odor is very strong.

Usually, when odor is perceived from smoke in the house, rotten food in the refrigerator or from a gas leak, it triggers the use of the sense of smell for finding the source of the odor. In the case of a chemical agent odor, deliberate opposite action is required: one must rapidly move upwind and away from the odor.

If the odor is perceived indoors, one needs to determine whether it is coming from inside or outside of the room or building. If the source appears to be in the building, one should head outdoors along a path away from the source. If trapped in a room by a source in an exit, sealing the door should be attempted, preferably with plastic sheeting and adhesive tape. In this situation air vents should also be sealed. These steps provide only temporary protection and need to be followed shortly by ventilation or neutralization of the chemical agents.

Generally, if the chemical agent has been deployed outdoors, one needs to seek shelter by going indoors and turning off all fans and ventilators, which pull air in from the outside. All outside doors and windows need to be closed. To stop air infiltration from the outdoor source, remaining openings should be sealed with duct tape and plastic sheeting; if this material is not at hand wet toweling can be stuffed into openings. After these measures one needs to move away from windows and doors to a more "inner location" such as a closet or an inner room.[5] These are basic actions to minimize exposure while the chemical agents dissipate or until rescue arrives. However, depending on the nature of the chemical agent (e.g., if it appears to be flammable or explosive), it may still be best to try and leave the building.

Not all, but many chemical agents have characteristic odors with odor thresholds low enough to serve as a timely warning.[6] For example, hydrocyanic acid (hydrogen cyanide, "cyanide gas," HCN) has an odor described as "bitter almond" (also as "lye or soup like"), with the ability to detect its smell an inherited trait.[7] HCN has an odor "threshold" range of 1 to 10 mg HCN/m^3 air while its immediately dangerous to life and health concentration (IDLH) is reported as approximately 55 mg HCN/m^3 air.

Thus, detection of HCN release by odor is a reasonably feasible early enough warning for escape or other defensive measures.

Phosgene has an IDLH OF 8 mg/m^3 air, while its odor threshold (as "newly mowed" or "musty" hay) is 2 mg/m^3. Between the 2 and 8 mg/m^3 the odor of phosgene becomes "choking." Thus, it has also a possibly manageable margin for defensive action.

The nerve agents sarin, soman, tabun and VX have been described as clear, colorless and odorless in the pure state, but also as having fruity odors. Overall, their odor thresholds appear too high for adequate warning, relative to their estimated IDLHs.

For chlorine (Cl_2), the first chemical warfare agent used in WWII, the IDLH is approximately 30 mg Cl_2/m^3 air, while the odor threshold for different individuals is reported as 1 to 15 mg/m^3. This is probably too close for adequate warning especially since 10 mg/m^3 are already dangerously irritating.

7.5 General Classifications

Chemical agents are classified according to where they produce their toxic effects on the body, such as nerve agents, or by their intended use, such as riot control agents. Some chemical agents burn or damage any surface on the body they come in contact with. Others must be absorbed into the body to do harm. A few must first be absorbed and then changed by body chemistry to become toxic. Antidotes are available to treat victims for exposure to some chemical agents; others have no antidote and no effective way to reverse their harmful effects. Many victims of chemical agent poisoning have survived with minimal or no long-term health problems. Other survivors have suffered chronic, debilitating illness and premature death.

7.6 Chemical Agents by Category

(According to CDC Emergency Preparedness & Response, December, 2003.)

biotoxins. abrin, ricin, and strychnine

blister agents/vesicants

mustards. distilled mustard (HD), mustard gas (H) (sulfur mustard), mustard/lewisite (HL) mustard/T, nitrogen mustards (HN-1, HN-2, HN-3) sesqui mustard (half mustard), and sulfur mustard (H) (mustard gas)

lewisite/chloroarsine agents. lewisite (L, L-1, L-2, L-3), mustard/lewisite (HL)

phosgene oxime (CX)

blood agents.

arsine (SA)

cyanide. cyanogen chloride (CK), hydrogen cyanide (AC), cyanide salts, potassium cyanide (KCN), sodium cyanide (NaCN)

caustics (acids). hydrofluoric acid and hydrogen fluoride

choking/lung/pulmonary agents. ammonia (NH_3), chlorine (CL), and hydrogen chloride (HCl), phosphine (PH_3), and phosphorus elemental, white or yellow (P_4)

phosgene. diphosgene (DP), phosgene (CG),

incapacitating agents. BZ, fentanyls and other opioids

long-acting anticoagulants. super warfarin

metals. arsenic, mercury, and thallium

nerve agents.

G agents. sarin (GB), soman (GD), and tabun (GA)

V agents. VX

organic solvents. benzene

riot control agents/tear gas. bromobenzylcyanide (CA), chloroacetophenone (CN), chlorobenzylidene malonitrile (CS), chloropicrin (PS), and dibenzoxazepine (CR)

toxic alcohols. ethylene glycol

vomiting agents. adamsite

7.7 Personal Protection and Law Enforcement Agents

Chemical agents that are used for nonlethal purposes, such as riot control or in law enforcement, are still considered chemical weapons. These agents include capsaicin (pepper spray) and Mace®, which is a trade name for the chemical 1-chloroacetaphenone. Their painful effects are temporary and mostly wear off within an hour. In some people the effects may persist for two hours, depending on dose and individual sensitivity. Within seconds after exposure, there is severe irritation of the nose, eyes, mouth, lungs and skin. The chemical's effects are tears streaming down the cheeks, mucus flowing from the nose, saliva drooling from the mouth, the skin turning red with a burning sensation; lung irritation causing coughing, shortness of breath and chest tightness.[8]

7.8 Repellant Agents

Repellant agents are nonlethal weapons that spread a stench so foul and repulsive that people become sick, dizzy and nauseous, and are forced to flee the area.

There are many animals and plants that produce strong aromas for defense, to warn others to stay away. The skunk, with its potent and pungent scent and spray, is a widely recognized example of the success of this weapon in a natural setting. Repellant agents, which are also called malodorants, have many uses including riot control, property protection and perimeter marking. They create panic and mass hysteria in order to force a facility evacuation or to move people forcibly from one location to another. So called stink bombs, which are available commercially, may also be used in pranks or practical jokes and could have unintended consequences, such as causing a stampede resulting in injury or death. Under such circumstances, the perpetrator of the prank could face serious consequences, including prosecution as a terrorist.

7.9 Tranquilizing Agents

This type of chemical agent targets the brain producing sedation, sleepiness and unconsciousness. These types of chemical agents are intended to immobilize people to prevent them from taking some action. A type of tranquilizing agent, a knock out gas, was used by Russian Internal Security Police in an attempt to rescue hostages from terrorists who had taken over the Moscow Opera House. Although the effects of certain knockout gases can be reversed with drugs (these agents are not intended to be lethal), many hostages died from acute poisoning from the gas. These nonlethal agents can be just as deadly as poison gas agents when used in real antiterrorist hostage-release situations in which the dosage can't be accurately controlled. This was the case in the Moscow Opera hostage rescue attempt.

Tranquilizing agents can be potent narcotics, sedatives or anesthetic gases. If they can be readily absorbed through the skin, they can be used as a liquid spray. Ideally these agents would be odorless, colorless gases which act quickly and safely to sedate and render their targets immobile or unconscious, but allow for quick reversal of effects and full recovery with minimal risk of injury or death. They would be ideal for hostage rescue or for live capture of groups of terrorists or soldiers if they can be made reliable and safe in actual use.

Tranquilizing agents could also be used to calm and relax people in a tense standoff situation without rendering them unconscious. In some cases the calming effect of the agent may be simply a matter of delivering a low dose to the intended targets.

7.10 Nerve Agents[8]

These types of chemical agents attack the functions of the nerves and the brain. They interfere with normal nerve function by blocking the action of an enzyme, preventing it from making an essential chemical change. Nerve agents such as sarin or VX don't actually destroy the nervous system. They cause the nerves to keep transmitting a signal, which produces overactivity in the muscles, glands and organs. Because there is too much stimulation by the nerves, the body's muscles and glands malfunction, with twitching muscles and secretions flowing from the eyes, nose and mouth. Some prescription drugs and insecticides produce the same kind of nerve poisoning when a person is exposed to a high dose. However, chemical nerve agents are much more potent than most (but not all) pesticides, causing toxic effects at very small doses. Most nerve agent poisonings can be treated with effective antidotes, which help to restore normal nervous system function. Antidote treatment must be started quickly or the victim may die, since this type of poison rapidly causes the victim to stop breathing.

A. Sarin[10,11]

Sarin is a liquid poison that evaporates slowly, like water, at room temperature. The onset and initial effects of sarin nerve agent depends on whether it comes in contact with a person as a liquid on skin or is inhaled as a vapor. Even a tiny droplet on skin may produce sweating and muscle fasciculation or twitching where the droplet lands. The nerve agent is easily absorbed through intact skin and will then circulate through the body to produce systemic effects. Later on, nausea, vomiting and diarrhea may start. These systemic effects may begin quickly or may take up to about eighteen hours from very low-level exposure. A large drop on skin can cause unconsciousness, convulsions, muscle paralysis and inability to breath within thirty minutes of exposure. Sarin kills by disrupting normal nervous system function causing muscle paralysis and suffocation.

Toxic effects of nerve agent when it is in the vapor form can begin within seconds to a minute. The chemical vapor typically impacts the unprotected face of the victim, and the eyes, nose, mouth and lung mucus membrane surfaces are first to react. If the vapor concentration is low, the victim may display signs of pinpoint pupils, bloodshot eyes and vomiting, and describe symptoms such as eye pain, reduced and blurred vision and nausea. Due to increased secretions from the effects of poison vapor, they may have a runny nose, tearing eyes and saliva production with drooling. Victims may be coughing and have difficulty breathing, with shortness of breath and chest tightness. If victims are exposed to a high concentration of vapor, consciousness may be lost in seconds, followed by convulsions, flaccid paralysis, cessation of breathing and cardiac arrest. Some or all of the signs described in low concentration exposure may also be present.

B. VX

VX was developed as a chemical warfare nerve poisoning agent by British scientists in 1952. VX is similar to sarin and tabun, but it is many times more potent. In the human body, VX attaches to an enzyme in nerve tissue and prevents the enzyme from breaking down a nerve transmitter called acetylcholine. This allows the acetylcholine chemical transmitter to build up and cause muscles to twitch and glands to over secrete fluids like mucus and saliva. It is a skin penetrating poison that is persistent on surfaces and does not evaporate to form a gas as readily as the other two nerve agents. VX quickly absorbs through the skin of the uncovered head and neck areas, which are especially vulnerable and sensitive.

The chemical nature of this nerve agent allows it to remain as a liquid coating that is resistant to evaporation from surfaces. It is one of the most persistent chemical weapon agents capable of remaining active as a liquid poison for longer than twenty-four hours, depending on ambient temperature and wind speed. The higher the temperature and wind speed, the faster it evaporates. The type of surface on which it is in contact also affects the evaporation rate. Evaporation from a porous surface such as a rug, will be slower than on a glossy surface like linoleum. Because of its ability to remain on surfaces, VX can be applied to exposed surfaces in advance of expected mass human contact, where it may lie in wait for many hours for its victims.

In the early 1970s research was conducted on human subjects to study the effectiveness of antidotes to VX and to better understand the harmful effects. A fraction of a milligram of VX was administered to human volunteers in an oral ingestion experiment. The subjects experienced diarrhea and a brief passing feeling of nausea 3-4 hours after ingestion. A much smaller dose injected into the veins of volunteers caused them to be light-headed and dizzy within an hour, and some became nauseous and vomited. After three hours blood pressure and heart rate were increased. A red blood cell enzyme called cholinesterase was reduced in all of the subjects. Measurement of this cholinesterase enzyme activity is a very important and sensitive indicator of poisoning with nerve agents such as VX. Antidotes are used to reactivate the cholinesterase enzyme to allow it to perform its normal function. Although somewhat dangerous to the research subjects, these studies provided important medical treatment information that could save lives in a terrorist attack.

7.11 Blood Agents

Blood agents get their name from the effect they have on the color of blood in the blood vessels. Poisoning produces a change in the normal color of the skin because the blood is not able to carry out its function of delivering oxygen to the body's tissues and cells. Normally, veins carry blood back to the heart and lungs after it has already delivered oxygen to the body tissues. Blood agents prevent the transfer of oxygen to the tissues, causing the cells to die. Blood agents actually poison the body's cells by stopping their ability to use oxygen. The oxygen stays in the blood, producing a red color in veins, which normally have a blue color.

The toxic substance in blood agents is cyanaide.[12,13] When breathed as a gas or taken by mouth as a solid or liquid, it poisons the body by preventing the transfer of oxygen from blood to tissues. It causes the body's cells to suffocate because they can't use oxygen. There is normally a small amount of cyanide in the body from eating certain foods. Cigarette smoking increases the cyanide load in the body. Breathing in or eating a little cyanide may have no effect at all, unlike with nerve agents where even a tiny drop can have a toxic effect. Exposure to a small amount may cause a person to feel dizzy, weak and nauseous. If removed from exposure, the person will gradually feel better. When a person takes in a large amount of cyanide, severe toxic effects begin in seconds. They may suddenly become unconscious, begin convulsing, stop breathing and die. Cyanide gets its reputation as a deadly poison because it can so swiftly cause death. There are treatments and antidotes for cyanide poisoning if the victim survives long enough to come under medical care. Exposure to small amounts of cyanide over a period of time can also produce mild symptoms followed by permanent brain damage and muscle paralysis.

Cyanide gas does have a warning odor that smells like bitter almonds, but only about half of the population has the genetically inherited ability to smell it. Cyanide gas can be smelled at levels in air that are below those that will cause rapid death. Cyanide gas is lighter than air so it will quickly dissipate outdoors. It is a more effective poison in a confined space such as in a subway car or aircraft cabin.

7.12 Vesicants

Blister agents, which are also called vesicants, produce visible damage to the skin and mucus membranes (lining of mouth, nose and eyes), which looks like sunburn and blisters. These agents also damage the lungs and tissues inside the body that are responsible for making blood. The harmful effects begin on contact, but the appearance of pain and damage from exposure may take many hours. Certain blister agents damage DNA, which may have long-term health effects including cancer and birth defects. In general, depending on the extent of exposure and the swiftness and quality of medical treatment, these agents produce more pain, misery and physical damage than death.

Sulfur mustard,[14] also called mustard gas, gets its name from the mustard or garlic-like odor it produces. The toxic effects of exposure to this chemical agent are delayed for hours to days depending on the amount and route of exposure. When sulfur mustard is in the form of a gas or fog, it causes irritation and burning on the skin, eyes and mucus membranes lining the mouth, nose and lungs. Victims may be sneezing and coughing. Once the poison is absorbed into the body it attacks the nervous system, heart and digestive system. Victims often have teardrops streaming from their eyes, overproduced saliva in their mouths, they feel sick, they may vomit and have no appetite. They have trouble breathing and appear to be very excited with chest pain from heart muscle damage and coughing. Loss of sense of smell and taste followed by hoarseness or inability to speak and trouble swallowing can develop hours and then days after exposure. Not only does this chemical agent kill many cells by poisoning enzymes and disrupting normal function, it produces breaks in DNA. Long term damage to DNA potentially increasing the risk of cancer and genetic damage to offspring may result from the toxic effects of mustard gas at the cellular level.

While there are supportive treatments and methods for removing sulfur mustard from the surface of the skin, there is no antidote. Sulfur mustard is persistent and stays active on surfaces for long periods of time so re-exposure from contaminated clothes, food or environmental surfaces is a continuing concern.

7.13 Toxins

Some plants and animals produce poisons that can be separated from them and used as chemical agents. These types of poisons are called toxins because they come from a living biological source. They include substances such as ricin, which is found in castor beans and tetrodotoxin, which is produced by puffer fish. Toxins harm or kill living organisms not by infecting their cells and reproducing, but by penetrating cells and poisoning their enzymes, membranes or biochemical processes thereby causing cell dysfunction leading to illness and even death.

A. Ricin[15,16]

The common, ornamental castor bean plant, *Ricinus comunis*, contains the poison ricin, which is among the most toxic plant-derived substances readily available. Castor bean plants are grown all over the world as ornamental plants as well as commercially in large quantities to produce oil. The processing of castor beans to make castor oil leaves a waste mash, which contains the poisonous ricin. It is from this waste bean mash that ricin can be extracted, concentrated and used as a chemical agent. It can also be extracted from raw, unprocessed beans. Ricin is not readily broken down by extreme heat or cold conditions, therefore it is very stable. Because it is a biologically derived poison from plant material, it is classified as a toxin. Ricin is not digested and destroyed by stomach acids and enzymes after being taken by mouth. Some of it is absorbed into the body intact, where it exerts its toxic effects.

If you took a typical packet of sugar substitute, which weighs about a gram, and divided the contents up into ten equal parts, less than one of those little white piles of powder, if it were ricin, would be fatal to most adults after oral ingestion. This is equivalent to ingesting eight castor beans. Under some circumstances, even a single bean can be fatal.

Manifestations of ingested ricin poisoning start as gastroenteritis (a digestive disorder) that may be mild or severe, and lead to death from fluid loss and shock. Onset of mild poisoning symptoms, which may be delayed after ingestion for 1–4 hours or more, can include nausea and vomiting along with diarrhea and cramping pain. Poisoning victims may report symptoms similar to influenza such as weakness, fever and muscle and joint pain. These milder poisoning signs and symptoms can progress over 4–36 hours and become severe, with continuous vomiting and massive, even bloody diarrhea. The extensive fluid loss can cause dehydration and shock. Kidney and liver failure can occur as consequences of severe poisoning.

Exposure to this toxin can occur by ingesting or inhaling it, or by injection through the skin. Ricin is not an infectious agent, so it is not spread by person-to-person contact. Inhaling or injecting ricin into the body are the most severely toxic routes of exposure and are more likely to be lethal. Intentional terrorist contamination of food, drink and water supply is the simplest and most likely means of mass poisoning by the oral ingestion route.

Ricin was threatened to be used as a terrorist poison to target water supplies as recently as October, 2003.[17] A note with demands, along with a container with ricin were found in an envelope at a mail processing center in Greenville, South Carolina. After comprehensive medical and environmental surveillance, no ricin-related illness or exposure was identified. The source of the toxin has not yet been identified and eliminated. Ricin continues to be a significant threat to public health as a potential poisoning agent in the hands of terrorists.

B. Abrin[18,19]

Abrin is a poisonous protein that is found in an ornamental bean commonly called the Jequirity bean. This toxic protein can pass through the wall of the intestine intact and enter the blood and the circulatory system. Most proteins are broken down before they get through the digestive system into the body, but not abrin. Another poisonous bean, the castor bean contains the toxin called ricin. It causes poisoning in a similar manner as abrin. There is currently no effective antidote for this type of poison, and there is no way to enhance its elimination from the body once it is absorbed. An antitoxin called Jequiritol serum is no longer commercially available to use against abrin poisoning.

The plant that produces the bright red bean which has a black dot on one end, is called by the scientific name *Abrus precatorius*. The bright coloring and attractiveness of the Jequirity bean have resulted in children being poisoned after chewing and swallowing them. Even a single bean can be toxic. The plant grows in tropical regions and is used as an ornamental ground cover in such areas as southern Florida and the Keys. Although the most common bean is scarlet red with a jet black area covering one end of it, there are also white beans with the black "eye" on one end and black beans with a white eye. The seeds are periodically used in bead necklaces and jewelry, which may become attractive to and ingested by children.

Because of the natural abundance and availability of the Jequirity bean and the relative ease of extracting and concentrating abrin from it, it poses a terrorist threat as a biologically derived toxin. The toxin can be used as a mass poisoning agent by spreading it on food or in beverages where it would be ingested, or by spraying it in the air over a crowd or in a ventilation system where it would be inhaled into the lungs. Abrin is not an infectious agent and is not spread by person-to-person contact, unless a person is physically contaminated with the poisonous material and it is transferred and ingested or inhaled by another person.

Abrin poisoning causes severe stomach and intestinal pain and inflammation called gastroenteritis. Victims of poisoning develop vomiting, cramps and diarrhea, which may have blood in it. These effects are seen typically within a few hours after consumption, but may take two days and may continue for over a week to ten days. Bloody tears or bleeding from the retina of the eyes is a characteristic sign of poisoning. Death from abrin ingestion has been reported after 3–4 days of constant gastroenteritis, heavy loss of fluids and symptoms of shock, which include tiredness and confusion, cold, sweaty, pale blue skin, rapid breathing and sudden drops in blood pressure.

7.14 Cell Poisons

The cell is the most basic building block of living creatures. Cells contain biochemical and structural "machinery" that allow them to function, repair themselves and reproduce. Cell poisoning agents disrupt some part of the biological machinery causing the cell to malfunction or die. When enough cells are damaged or killed, the whole organism can no longer function and it may die.

A. Fluoroacetate[20,21]

Fluroacetate is a potent poison that has the appearance of crystalline or fine white powder which may resemble baking soda or sugar substitute. It is odorless and tasteless, and it easily dissolves in water. A dose the size of a baby aspirin pill can kill a 150-pound person, but as little as 1 milligram, an amount the size of a head of a pin, can cause significant toxic symptoms.

Fluoroacetate poisoning can occur by oral ingestion of contaminated food or drink, absorption through wounded skin and by inhaling airborne powder. Symptoms and signs of poisoning are not immediate because this agent must first be made toxic by the body's metabolism and energy production system.

Fluoroacetate is changed by a "lethal" synthesis into a new molecule called fluorocitrate that stops an enzyme from working. This poisoned enzyme, called aconitase, blocks the primary energy source used to maintain body function; it also causes stomach and intestinal problems, such as nausea, vomiting and diarrhea. Toxic effects on the brain include agitation, confusion, and seizures progressing to coma, inability to breathe and heart rhythm abnormalities. The delay between initial absorption and the appearance and feeling of poisoning can be thirty minutes to several hours. Death from heart failure or inability to breath has occurred as long as five days after swallowing a large dose.

Fluoroacetate poisoning may be mistakenly attributed to a stomach or intestinal disease, effects of a virus or a heart attack. Even after surviving the initial poisoning, victims may suffer kidney shutdown. There is no effective antidote to fluoroacetate poisoning.

Licensed pest control professionals have access to fluoroacetate, as well as people involved in the manufacturing and distribution of the poison. It is not as tightly controlled as are narcotic drugs, and diversion for terrorist use is a concern. Since it is used in industrial and outdoor settings to control rodents, insects and even predators like coyotes, it may be a target for theft from the bait site.

7.15 Learning from the Past: Future Chemical Agent Terrorism

The United States homeland has not been hit by a successful major chemical agent attack like the one that was perpetrated on the Japanese involving sarin nerve agent release in the Tokyo subway system at rush hour. In the 1993 bombing of the World Trade Center, suspicion was raised that a simultaneous attack with a cyanide chemical agent was attempted but did not succeed[22,23] because the bomb blast did not produce a cyanide gas cloud. This story emerged from statements made by the trial judge during sentencing of the terrorist bombers. In 1995, one hundred thirty grams of ricin, a deadly toxin, was seized from a suspect who then committed suicide while incarcerated.[24] The intended use of the ricin is unknown, but that quantity of ricin could kill thousands if it was dispensed as an inhalable aerosol or secreted into food or drink.

Terrorists have demonstrated their ability to creatively weaponize civilian transport systems—such as a jet aircraft filled with fuel, flown by trained suicidal murderers on a mission of mass destruction. The same mindset could be expected to attempt to unleash chemical agents on a civilian population by weaponizing chemical facilities and detonating them. On December 3, 1984 in Bhopal, India, a populous shanty town in the shadow of a giant chemical production plant suffered the deadly and debilitating effects of a massive chemical release. Thirty tons of toxic methylisocyanate vapor erupted from the plant killing and injuring countless thousands. Within hours, chemical exposure was fatal to around 3,000 and an estimated 200,000 suffered chemical burns, some with permanent disability. This chemical disaster, which was determined to be an accident, produced a toxic shroud of mucus membrane corroding chemical fog that turns to acid when it comes in contact with the sensitive tissues of the eyes, nose, mouth, throat and lungs. Those who survived this chemical cloud of death and tissue damage suffered vision loss from ulcerated eyes, chronic lung dysfunction and permanent trouble with breathing. Some had respiratory tissue that was so stiff and fibrotic, that over time their heart enlarged, in an effort to pump blood through their lungs. Many victims died much younger than would be expected if they had not been exposed to the chemical agent. There was also an increase in unborn infant deaths and many more babies of exposed mothers died at birth or shortly afterward than would be normally expected.[25]

This was all a result of a chemical plant accident. One can imagine what chemical catastrophe could be created by a well-planned and executed terrorist attack using a weaponized chemical facility. Based on past tactics, it could be expected that the attack would consist of simultaneous, multiple facility detonations. Terrorist tactics have exploited the power of orchestrating multiple surprise events to produce a tidal wave[26] of terror, doubt and uncertainty of what will happen next. The multiple civilian passenger jet weapon attacks on America on September 11, 2001 and the near simultaneous bombings in Madrid, Spain are examples of a planned series or bunch of closely timed events that took governments and their citizens by surprise and produced a magnified result strategically designed to influence, change or create a future event.

Table 7.1
Precursors of CWAs and Alternate Uses

Precursor (CAS Number) CAS-RN	Chemical Warfare Agents	Alternate Uses Commercial, Industrial, Domestic
ammonium bifluoride 1341-49-7	sarin (GB), soman (GD), cyclohexyl sarin, GF	manufacturing of magnesium alloy, glass; sterilizing food and beer equipment
arsenic trichloride 7784-34-1	arsine, lewisite, adomsite (DM)	manufacturing of pharmaceutic arsenicals and insecticides
benzilic acid 76-93-7	BZ	
2-chloroethanol 107-07-3	sulfur mustard (HD), sesqui mustard, nitrogen mustard (HN-1)	sprouting dormant potatoes; manufacturing of ethylene oxide, ethylene glycol, insecticides
3-hydroxy -1-methylpiperidine 3554-74-3	Psychoactives (e.g., BZ)	
3-quinuclidinol 1619-34-7	BZ	hypotensive
diethyl ethylphosphonte	ethyl sarin (GE)	
diethyl methylphosphonite 15715-41-0	VX	
diethyl N,N-dimethyl phosphoromidate 2404-03-7	tabun (GA)	
diethylaminoethanol 100-37-8	VG, VM	manufacturing of pharmaceuticals, crop protection agents, paper, leather and plastics
diethylphosphite 762-59-2	sarin (GB), VG, soman (GD), GF	
diesopropylamine 108-18-9	VX	manufacturing of catalysts, medication, pesticides
dimethyl ethylphorphonate 6163-75-3	ethyl sarin (GE)	
(DMPP) dimethyl methylphosphonate 756-79-6	sarin (GB), soman (GD), GF	flame retardant, gasoline additive, antifoam, plasticizer, textile conditioner
diethylamine 124-40-3	tabun (GA)	manufacturing of rubber, detergents, soaps, DMF, DMA; antioxidant; gasoline additive; pesticides; missile fuels; rubber vulcanizing; HCl
dimethylphophite 868-85-9	sarin (GB), soman (GD), GF	lubricant additive, fire proofing
ethylphosphonous dichloride 1498-40-4	VE, VS, ethyl sarin (GE)	
ethylphosphonous difluoride 430-78-4	VE, ethyl sarin (GE)	
ethylphosphonyl dichloride 1066-50-8	ethyl sarin (GE)	
ethylphosphonyl difluoride 753-98-0	ethyl sarin (GE)	
hydrogen fluoride 7664-39-3	sarin (GB), soman (GD), ethyl sarin (GE), GF	fluorination, liquid rocket fuel additive, uranium refining, metal cleaner, glass etching
methyl benzilate 76-89-1	BZ	tranquilizers

continued on next page

methylphosphonous dichloride 678-83-5	VX	
methylphosphonous difluoride 676-97-1	VX, VM, sarin (GB), soman (GD), GF	
methylphosphonyl diflouride 676-99-3	sarin (GB), soman (GD), GF	
N,N-diisopropyl-2-aminoethylchloride•HCl	VX	
N,N-diisopropyl-aminoethanethiol 5842-07-9	VX, VS	
N,N-diisopropyl-(_)-aminoethanol 96-80-0	VX	
N,N-diisopropyl-(_)-aminoethylchloride 96-79-7	VX, VS	
O-ethyl, 2-diisopropyl aminoethyl methylphosphonate (QL) 57856-11-8	VX	
phosphorus oxychloride 10025-87-3	tabun (GA)	plasticizers, gasoline additives, hydroulic fluids, insecticides, flame retardants
phosphorus pentachloride 10026-13-8	tabun (GA)	pesticides, plastics
phosphorus pentasulfide 1314-80-3	VG, VX	insecticide, mitocide, lubricant oil additive, pyrotechnics
phosphorus trichloride 7719-12-2	VG, tabun (GA), sarin (GB), soman (GD), GF, salt process, rearrangement process	insecticides, gasoline additive, plasticizer, dyestuffs
pinacolone 75-97-8	soman (GD)	
pinacolyl alcohol 464-07-3	soman (GD)	
potassium bifluoride 7789-29-9	soman (GD), sarin (GB), GF	fluorine production, alkylation catalyst, coal formation reduction, silver solder fluid
potassium cyanide 151-50-8	tabun (GA), hydrogen cyanide	pesticide, fumigant, electroplating
potassium fluoride 7789-23-3	sarin (GB), soman (GD), GF	fluorinating organics; cleaning and disinfecting food processing equipment, including brewery and dairy; glass and porcelain manufacturing
sodium bifluoride 1333-83-1	sarin (GB), soman (GD), GF	antiseptic, neutralizer in laundry, tin plate production
sodium cyanide 143-33-9	tabun (GA), HCN (AC), cyanogen chloride	gold and silver extraction from ores, fumigant, manufacturing of dyes and pigments, core hardening of metals, nylon production
sodium fluoride 7681-49-4	sarin (GB), soman (GD), GF	pesticide, disinfectant, dental prophylactic, glass and steel manufacturing
sodium sulfide 1313-82-2	sulfur mustard (HD)	paper manufacturing, rubber manufacturing, metal refining, dye manufacturing
sulfur dichloride 10545-99-0	sulfur mustard (HD)	rubber vulcanizing, insecticides, vulcanizing oils, chlorinating agent

continued on next page

sulfur (mono)chloride 10025-67-9	sulfur mustard (HD)	pharmaceuticals, sulfur dyes, insecticides, rubber vulcanizing, polymerization catalyst, hardening softwood, silver extraction from ores
thiodiglycol 111-48-8	sulfur mustard (HD), sesqui mustard (Q)	dycarrrier—textiles, lubricant additives, plastic manufacturing
thionyl chloride 7719-09-7	nitrogen mustard (HN-3)	chlorinating agent, catalyst, pesticides, engineering plastics
triethonolamine 102-71-6	nitrogen mustard (HN-3)	detergents, cosmetics, corrosion inhibitor, plasticizer, rubber accelerant
triethonolamine•HCl	nitrogen mustard (HN-3)	insecticides, surfactants, waxes, polishes, textile specialties, toiletries, lubricants, cement additive, petroleum demulsifier, synthetic resin
triethyl phosphite 122-52-1	VG	plasticizers, lubricant additives
trimethyl phosphite 121-45-9	DMMP molecular rearrangement	

Source: "Chemical Warfare Agents Precurser" CDC-NIOSH Hazardous Substances Database, Specialized Information Services.

Table 7.2
Industrial Chemicals That Can (Have Been) Air Dispersed with Fatal Results

IDLH = Immediately Dangerous to Life or Health; TWA = 8 Hour "Permissible Exposure"; ppm = parts agent/million parts per air					
IDLH				**TWA**	
ppm	**mg/m^3**	**Chemical Name**	**CAS No.**	**ppm**	**mg/m^3**
50	125	acetic acid	64-19-7	10	
2	5	acrolein	107-02-8	0.1	
300	210	NH_3	7664-01-07	50	35
3	10	arsine	7784-02-1	0.05	0.2
	4	beryllium	7440-41-7		0.5
3		bromine	7726-95-6	0.1	
	9	cadmium	7440-03-9		5
40,000		CO_2	124-38-9	5,000	
1,200		CO	630-08-0	35	40
10	30	chlorine gas n.b. also a CWA	7782-50-5	0.5	
5	15	chlorine dioxide	10049-04-4	0.1	0.3
	15	chloroacetophenone (Mace®)	532-27-4	0.05	0.3
	2	chlorobenzylidene-malononitrile	2698-41-1	0.05	0.4
	14	chloropicrin	76-06-02	0.1	0.7
2	15	decaborane	17702-41-9	0.3	0.05
	10	demeton (Systox®) (skin)	8065-48-3		0.1
2	4	diazomethane	334-88-3	0.2	0.4
15		diborane	19287-45-7	0.1	0.1
	5	dactin (DDH) (bleach)	118-52-5		0.2
7	35	dimethylsulfate	77-78-1	0.1	0.5
	5	dimnitro-o-cresol (DNOC) (skin)	534-52-1		0.2
	2	endrin (skin)	72-20-8		0.1
	5	EPN (skin)	2104-64-5		0.5
7		ethylene chlorohydrin (skin)	107-07-3	5	16
	0.2	Guthion® (solid)	86-50-0		10
50	55	hydrogen cyanide	74-90-8	10	11
25	30	hydrogen fluoride (HF)	7664-39-3	3	2.5
1	4	hydrogen selenide (H_2Se)	7783-07-5	0.05	0.2
100	150	hydrogen sulfide (H_2S)	7783-06-04	10	15
2	20	iodine	7553-56-2	0.1	1
5	9	ketene	463-51-4	0.5	0.9
	0.5	lithium hydride	7580-67-8	0	25
	2	methylmercury			0.1
3	7	methylisocyanate	624-83-9	0.02	0.05
2	14	nickelcarbonyl	13463-39-3	0.001	0.007
	5	nicotine (skin)	54-11-5	0.5	
25		nitric acid (HNO_3)	7697-37-2	2	5
20		nitropen dioxide	10102-44-0	1	2
0.1		osmium tetroxide		0.0002	0.002
0.5	5	oxygen difluoride	7783-41-7	0.05	0.1
5	10	ozone	10028-15-6	0.1	0.2

continued on next page

	1	paraquat (skin)	1910-42-5		0.5
	10	parathion (skin)	56-38-2		0.1
1	2	pentaborone	19624-22-7	0.005	0.01
	2.5	pentachlorophenol (skin)	87-86-5		0.5
15	60	phenylhydrazine	122-60-1	5	22
4		phosdrin (skin)	7786-34-7	0.1	
2	8	phosgene n.b. also a CWA	75-44-5	0.1	0.4
50	70	phosphine	7803-51-2	0.3	0.4
	5	phosphorus (white/yellow)	7723-14-0		0.1
	25	potassium cyanide	151-50-8	5	5
	1	selenium	7782-49-2		0.2
2	16	SeF_4	7783-79-1	0.05	0.4
	2.5	sodium fluoroacetate (skin)	62-74-8		0.05
	10	sodium hydroxide	1310-73-2		2
5	25	stibine (SbH_3)	7803-52-3	0.1	0.5
	3	strychnine	57-24-9		0.15
	15	sulfuric acid	7664-93-9		1
5	30	sulfur chloride	10025-67-9	1	6
1	10	sulfur pentafluoride (S_2F_{10})	5714-22-7	0.01	0.1
	10	TEDP (sulfotep) (skin)	3689-24-5		0.2
	25	sellurium	13494-80-9		0.1
1	10	sellurium hexafluoride	7783-80-4	0.02	0.2
	5	TEPP (Tetron®) (skin)	107-49-3		0.05
3	40	tetraethyl lead (TEL) (skin)	78-00-2		0.075
5	30	tetramethyl succinonitrile (skin)	3333-52-6	0.5	3
4	32	tetronitromethane	509-14-8	1	8
	15	thallium (soluble salts) (skin)			0.1
2.5	18	2,4TDI	584-84-9	0.02	0.14
30		tributyl phosphate	126-73-8	2.5	5
3	40	triorthocresyl phosphate (skin)	78-30-8	<0.01	0.1
	1,000	triphenyl phosphate	115-86-6		3
	10	uranium (metal)	74210-61-1		0.25
	50	zinc dichloride fume	7646-85-7		1

Source: NIOSH (CDC) *Pocket Guide to Chemical Hazards and DHHS* (NIOSH) Publications No. 94-116.

Endnotes

1. L.R. Ember. "Taking stock of clinical arms," *Chemical Engineering News*, pp. 23–24, September 10, 2001.

2. John Harns Trestrail, III. *Criminal Poisoning: Investigational Guide for Law Enforcement, Toxicologists, Forensic Scientists and Attorneys* (Totowa, NJ: Humana Press, 2000), p. 7.

3. www.nti.org/h_learnmore/cwtutorial/chapter02_02.html.

4. C. Kozlow and J. Sullivan. *Jane's Facility Security Handbook* (Alexandria, VA: Jane's Information Group, 2000), p. 281.

5. Matthew J. Ellenhorn. *Ellenhorn's Medical Toxicolgy: Diagnosis and Treatment of Human Poisoning*, 2nd ed. (Baltimore: Williams & Wilkins, 1997), p. 1285.

6. Ellenhorn, note 5, p. 1284.

7. As an undergraduate student taking analytical chemistry, one of the authors was able to smell HCN gas when it was accidentally produced during a chemistry laboratory titration experiment. The titration involved the use of an acid that was then discarded into a sink. Another student was repeating a previous experiment, using a potassium cyanide solution that was also being run off into the same sink. When the acid solution mixed with the potassium cyanide solution a small amount of HCN gas was liberated, just enough for the author to smell it and alert the instructor. The experiments were halted, exhaust hoods turned on, windows opened and the lab was evacuated. Fortunately no one was harmed. The HCN gas concentration was high enough to produce a warning odor to allow appropriate action before it reached a poisonous level.

8. F.R. Sidell, W.C. Patrick and T.R. Dashiell. *Jane's Chem-Bio Handbook* (Alexandria, VA: Jane's Information Group, 1998), p. 109.

9. Sidell, note 7, pp. 57, 68–70.

10. Ellenhorn, note 5, pp. 1281–1282.

11. Sidell, note 7, pp. 72–75.

12. R.C. Baselt. *Disposition of Toxic Drugs and Chemicals in Man*, 7th ed (Foster City, CA: Biomedical Publications, 2004), pp. 276–278.

13. Sidell, note 7, pp. 79, 84–88.

14. J.C. Dacre and M. Goldman. "Toxicology and pharmacology of the chemical warfare agent sulfur mustard," *Pharmacological Reviews* 48(2):289–326 (1996).

15. D. Frohne, and H.S. Pfander. *A Color Atlas of Poisonous Plants* (London: Wolf Publishing, Ltd., 1983), pp. 113–116.

16. Matthew J. Ellenhorn and Donald G. Barceloux. *Medical Toxicology: Diagnosis and Treatment of Human Poisoning*, 2nd ed. (NY: Elsevier, 1988), pp. 1847–1849

17. *Morbidity and Mortality Weekly Report*, 152(46):1129–1131 (2003).

18. Frohne, note 14, pp. 120, 126.

19. Ellenhorn, note 5, p. 1849.

20. Trestrail, note 2, pp. 113–114.

21. Baselt, note 11, pp. 470–471.

22. T. Post et al. "A cloud of terror—and suspicion," *Newsweek*, April 3, 1995.

23. B.E. Pate. *Reality Theory: A Means to Control the Public's Fear of Chemical Weapons Use,* Chemical Warfare Publication, Army War Course, 1997.

24. J.D. Robertus. "Identification and Structural Analysis of Ricin Inhibitors," December, 1996, p. 5. Available from the National Technical Information Service at http://www.ntis.gov/search/product.asp?ABBR=ADA322174.

25. Ellenhorn, note 5, p. 1237.

26. Alain Paul Martin. "Hitch-hiking on surprise events and tidal waves to create unique opportunities," in *Harnessing the Power of Intelligence, Counterintelligence and Surprise Events* (Ottawa: Executive.org, 2002).

Chapter 8

Chemical Warfare Agents: Analytical Methods

Ashraf Mozayani, Pharm.D., Ph.D., D-ABFT

Synopsis

8.1 Introduction

Defining the phrase "chemical warfare agents" (CWA) can be a somewhat daunting task. Humans evolved in an environment that is essentially composed of dilute mixtures of many chemicals in a few "solvents," primarily water and nitrogen. Virtually any of those dilute chemicals in its pure or concentrated form can be toxic if the intent is present and the chemical is properly deployed. It follows that any of those chemicals could be employed as a chemical warfare agent.

Similarly, many living organisms produce compounds intended to have an adverse effect on other organisms. Snakes produce venom, bacteria produce toxins, plants produce poisons and so forth.

8.2 Scope

This chapter is restricted to existing and proposed methods for the analysis of chemical warfare agents. Where possible, analytical methods for the parent substance in air or environmental matrices is included as well as the compound, its metabolites or other biological markers in human tissues and fluids.

The substances included in this chapter will be restricted to agents that have been used as chemical warfare agents in the past (e.g., chlorine, phosgene), substances that were (or are) produced specifically as chemical warfare agents (e.g., tabun, VX) and toxins produced by biological organisms that have been or may be used as chemical warfare agents (e.g., ricin, botulinum toxin). Specifically excluded are living organisms like smallpox and anthrax which more appropriately fall under the heading of biological warfare agents.

8.3 Specimen Handling

The analysis of human or environmental samples suspected of containing CWAs almost invariably fall under the heading of "forensic" samples, since the results of these analyses may reasonably be expected to appear as evidence in court, from civil actions to war crimes tribunals. As such, the samples must be collected, transported, handled and stored with an eye to good forensic practice. All contact with the specimen should be recorded.

As much detail as can be accurately obtained about the collection must be rigorously recorded, including such seemingly innocuous detail as weather conditions. Collected samples must be placed in appropriate containers and sealed in good forensic fashion. Refrigeration may be required and is rarely detrimental. A good rule of thumb is . . . when in doubt, refrigerate.

Transportation should also follow forensic standards and should be rapid and reliable. Insulated containers may be required to maintain storage temperatures.

After arrival at the laboratory, good laboratory practice should be followed. This includes documentation of all handling of the specimen, descriptions of the specimen and its condition, recording of all aliquots taken from the specimen and the conditions under which it is stored. Analytical procedures used on the specimen should be validated and appropriate blank, positive and negative controls should be run.

8.4 Classification of CWAs

Chemical warfare agents (CWAs) can be arranged in three broad categories based on their intended action on humans. Casualty agents are intended to kill or disable the target, while harassing agents are designed merely to temporarily disrupt the ability to function without totally incapacitating the individual. Toxins are biological products which have been adapted for chemical warfare purposes and may cause disability or death.

Casualty agents can be further classified based on the intended effect. Blood agents cause hemolysis or interfere with the oxygen transport process, while choking (or pulmonary) agents are primarily suffocating gases although significant tissue edema and other damage may also occur. Nerve agents interfere with nerve functioning, usually by irreversible binding to the enzyme acetylcholinesterase (AChE). Vesicants cause external tissue damage without inhalation. Incapacitating agents render the subject unable to function, either by causing unconsciousness, hallucinations, paranoia or other physical or psychological effects.

In any attempt to develop an analytical scheme for a series of chemical compounds, it is critical that the chemical structure be understood. Listed in the tables below are a number of the CWAs that are of concern in today's world, along with their chemical structures. This list is not meant to be comprehensive since, as stated above, virtually any chemical may be used as a CWA and new agents are not difficult to synthesize.

A. Casualty agents

1. Blood agents

Although cyanogen bromide and cyanogen chloride are included in lists of potential CWAs, practical considerations make their use unlikely. Both have relatively low toxicity and both are relatively unstable, making long-term storage difficult. Both compounds are irritants but the primary toxicity is due to the release of cyanide during hydrolysis. Cyanide stops

Table 8.1
Common Blood Agents

Blood Agent	Formula/Structure
cyanogen cyanide	Cl–C≡N
cyanogen bromide	Br–C≡N
hydrogen cyanide	H–C≡N
arsine	AsH_3

the normal utilization of oxygen by forming an inhibitory complex with cytochrome oxidase in cells. The median lethal concentration (LCt50) of cyanogen chloride is estimated to be 11 grams-min/m^3 (versus about 5 grams for hydrogen cyanide). The irritating effect of cyanogen chloride in humans has been measured at 0.0025 milligram per liter of air, primarily on the eyes causing severe pain and copious tearing.[1]

Hydrogen cyanide, although a liquid at room temperature, is difficult to use in a battlefield situation due to its high volatility which results in rapid dispersion and dilution. The median lethal concentration (LCt50) of hydrogen cyanide is estimated to be approximately 5 grams-min/m3.

a. Cyanogen chloride and cyanogen bromide. A number of techniques are applicable to the analysis of cyanogen halides in their bulk form, including gas chromatographic-mass spectrometric analysis (GC/MS).[2]

Cyanogen chloride and cyanogen bromide have been routinely detected in drinking water for many years. EPA method (EPA Method 551.1) uses a liquid/liquid microextraction and GC analysis for the detection of these compounds. A method using headspace solid-phase microextraction coupled with GC-electron capture detection has a sensitivity of about 1 μg/L.[3]

The analysis of cyanogen halides in biological specimens is focused primarily on the detection of the cyanide produced by hydrolysis of the compounds in aqueous media. The analysis of cyanide is discussed below.

b. Analysis of cyanides. Cyanide analysis is a routine procedure in most forensic toxicology labs and the literature on the analytical methodology is voluminous. One of the most common procedures utilizes the reaction between cyanide and barbituric acid in the presence of pyridine.

The reduction of palladium chloride to metallic palladium is common, while many labs employ gas chromatographic methods.[4,5]

Cyanide-specific electrodes for most pH/conductivity meters are commercially available. The literature describes a colorimetric method based on the cyanide-Cl_2 reaction,[6] and an analysis using a quartz crystal microbalance.[7]

c. Arsine. Arsine is the most acutely toxic form of arsenic. While most of the other arsenic compounds employed as CWAs are classified as vesicants, this simplest hydride of arsenic (AsH_3) causes rapid and severe hemolysis upon exposure. The mechanism of action is not known but appears to be dependent on membrane disruption by a mechanism other than hemoglobin oxidation.[8]

Traditionally, the analysis of biological samples for arsine has relied on standard methods for the determination of arsenic. Primarily these methods involve atomic absorption spectrometry after ashing of the biological sample,[9] although results using inductively coupled plasma mass spectrometry have also been reported.[253]

A search of the literature revealed one mention of the detection of arsine in biological matrices.[10] Arsenic analysis will be discussed in more detail in the section on vesicants, specifically the Lewisites.

2. Choking (pulmonary) agents

Chlorine is included in this discussion because of its historical significance (i.e., it was the first lethal gas used in modern chemical warfare). Chlorine is considered to be obsolete as a CWA and in fact is not listed as a scheduled substance in the Chemical Weapons Convention.

a. Chloropicrin (PS, trichloronitromethane). Chloropicrin is widely used in agriculture as fumigant for soils and stored grains. As with most of the CWA in this category, chloropicrin inhalation induces severe pulmonary edema.

Chloropicrin has been determined in drinking water,[11–15] soil, grains and air by a number of techniques including direct air analysis, purge and trap gas chromatography, GC-MS and colorimetric methods.

A method has been developed for the detection of chloropicrin in stimulated deliberate exposure situations using thermal desorption GC/MS.[16] Chloropicrin was detected and quantitated by GC and GC/MS (1.6 ng/g of wet weight) in the lung tissue of a homicide victim.[17]

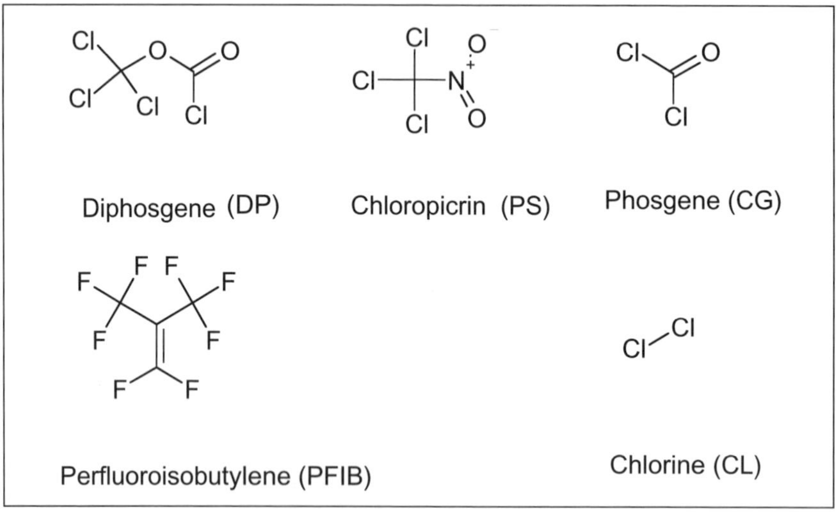

Figure 8.1 *Structures of choking agents*

b. Phosgene (CG, carbonyl chloride). Phosgene is widespread in the chemical industry and was responsible for an estimated 80 percent of the CWA deaths in World War I, although some of those deaths may have been due to diphosgene (q.v.). Phosgene is not considered to be a significant modern CW threat due to its gaseous nature, difficulty in handling and relatively low toxicity when compared to other agents. The median lethal concentration of phosgene in humans is about 3.2 grams-min/m^3, and the and the median incapacitating dose (ICt50) is estimated at about 1.6 grams-min/m^3.

Phosgene is slowly hydrolyzed by water to form hydrochloric and phosphoric acids, which are significant contributors to the delayed edema seen in individuals who have inhaled low concentrations of the gas. Unfortunately for the analyst, this hydrolysis leaves precious little unique residue on which to base an identification or quantitation.

Phosgene may be detected in air by the human nose (the gas has a smell reminiscent of freshly mown hay), although toxic amounts may be inhaled when the concentration in air is too low to be detected by the sense of smell. More precise analytical methods rely on GC and GC/MS procedures.[18–20]

Phosgene undergoes a reaction with a mixture of p-dimethylaminobenzaldehyde and diphenylamine to form a yellow to orange color in the presence of dangerous amounts of phosgene. These and similar reactions are the basis of the phosgene warning badges worn by workers in chemical industry who may be exposed to the gas.[21]

The detection of phosgene in biological fluids or tissues has not been reported.

c. Diphosgene (DP, trichloromethyl chloroformate). The toxic effects of diphosgene are almost identical to those of phosgene. DP was used in World War I primarily because its higher boiling point made it easier to handle, although rapid dispersion was still a problem. Diphosgene is not considered to be a significant threat in modern CW. The median lethal concentration of phosgene in humans is approximately 3.2 grams-min/m^3, and the median incapacitating dose (ICt50) is also the same as phosgene at 1.6 grams-min/m^3.

The analysis of diphosgene is identical to that of phosgene.

3. Nerve agents

All of the compounds used as nerve agents in modern CW are acetylcholinesterase (AChE) inhibitors. These agents act by bonding to AChE

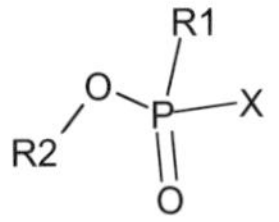

Nerve agent	Military Name	X	R_1	R_2
		"G" series		
Tabun	GA	-CN	$-N(CH_3)_2$	$-C_2H_5$
Sarin	GB	-F	$-CH_3$	$-CH(CH_3)_2$
Soman	GD	-F	$-CH_3$	$-CH(CH_3)C(CH_3)_3$
	GE	-F	$-CH_2\,CH_3$	$-CH(CH_3)_2$
Cyclosarin	GF	-F	$-CH_3$	-cyclohexyl
		"V" series		
	VE	$-S(CH_2)_2N(CH_2CH_3)_2$	$-CH_2\,CH_3$	$-CH_2\,CH_3$
	VG	$-S(CH_2)_2N(CH_2CH_3)_2$	$-O\,CH_2\,CH_3$	$-CH_2\,CH_3$
Amiton	VM	$-S(CH_2)_2N(CH_2CH_3)_2$	$-CH_3$	$-CH_2\,CH_3$
	VX	$-S(CH_2)_2N(CH[CH_3]_2)_2$	$-CH_3$	$-CH_2\,CH_3$
	V-gas	$-S(CH_2)_2N(CH_2CH_3)_2$	$-CH_2CH(CH_3)_2$	$-CH_2\,CH_3$

***Figure 8.2** Structures of organophosphorus nerve agents*

causing the enzyme to be inhibited. The exposed individual experiences a buildup of the neurotransmitter acetylcholine, resulting in increased levels of bodily secretions, muscle twitching and significant effects on the cardiovascular and central nervous systems.

All of the modern CW nerve agents are organophosphorus compounds and are chemically related to the common organophosphorus insecticides, although the toxicity of the CW agents is much greater. The NATO abbreviations of the "G" series are the order in which these agents were developed by Germany in the years before World War II.

Since the nerve agents are structurally similar, many of the analytical methods developed over the years have the ability to detect most of the common agents. The early methods depended on the inhibition of AChE.[22,23] More recently, methods using gas chromatography, mass spectrometry or both have been developed for the detection of nerve agents in soil,[24–31] concrete,[32] aqueous solutions,[33–38] brain[39] and blood and urine.[40–49]

Matrix-assisted laser desorption ionization mass spectrometry (MALDI-TOF/MS) has been used to detect the altered proteins that are produced as a result of the alkylating properties of many nerve agents.[50]

Badges based on fluorescence induction by living photosynthetic tissue have been developed for the detection of airborne nerve agents[51] and field test kits to detect exposure to nerve agents by measuring AChE activity have had some success.[52]

Enzyme methods and ELISA techniques using monoclonal antibodies have had success in detecting soman (GD) in human serum, animal serum, milk, and tap water in concentrations between 1.3×10^{-6} and $2.0 \times {}^{10\text{-}6}$ mol/L.[53–56]

A number of other devices have been developed to detect nerve agent breakdown products.[57–61]

The analysis of sarin is covered in a recent review article[62] which also includes a discussion of historical exposures to the agent, long-term physical effects of exposure and synergistic effects when sarin exposure is concomitant with certain other agents. The authors conclude that much work still needs to be done on the physiological actions and effects of this agent.

4. Vesicants

The primary effects of vesicants on exposed individuals occur initially on the skin, but not immediately. Symptoms may not appear for several hours and include pain and tissue damage, extreme irritation, formation of blisters, and slow-healing injuries. Permanent injury to the eyes is also possible and death from exposure is often a result of extreme irritation in the upper respiratory tract with the formation of pulmonary edema.

There are three fundamental groups of compounds which are used as vesicants in chemical warfare. The first is the original mustard gas (bis(2-chloroethyl)sulfide, or HD) and its analogs such as sesquimustard. The second group of vesicants are the nitrogen analogs of mustard gas, commonly referred to as the "nitrogen mustards." The third group of vesicants are the "arsenicals," three of which (the lewisites) can be thought of as arsenic analogs of mustard gas. Another compound which may cause blisters and is usually included in the vesicants category but which fails to fall

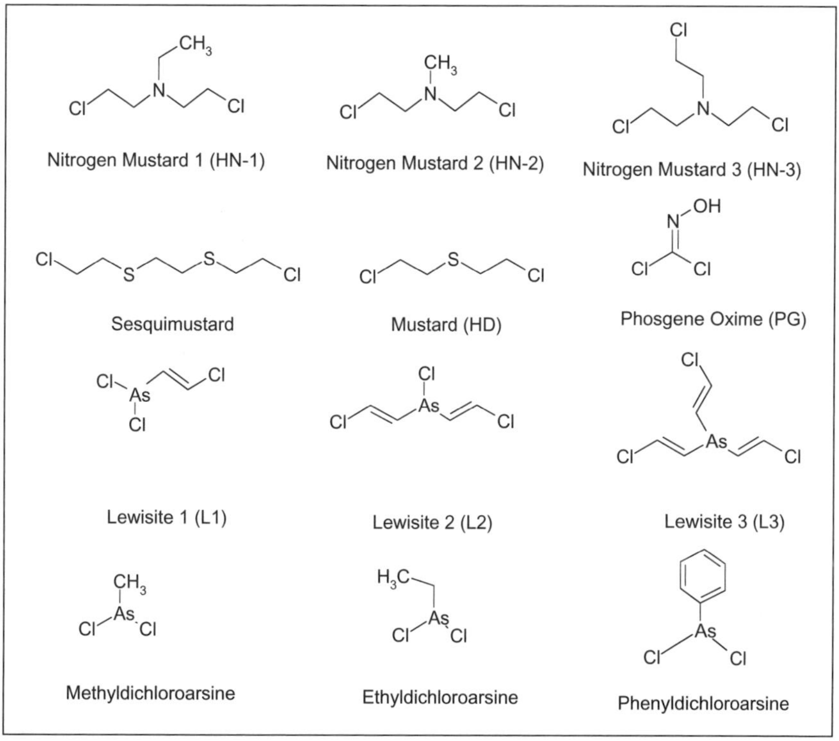

Figure 8.3 *Vessicants*

into the above three groups is phosgene oxime (CX). Phosgene oxime's effect on the skin is different from that of the mustards or arsenicals, producing immediate and extremely painful irritation to skin, eyes, and respiratory system. A rash covering the entire body may result from even limited contact with phosgene oxime and may develop into sores and necrotic lesions on the skin.

a. Sulfur mustards (HD). Sulfur mustard (HD) undergoes metabolic hydrolysis to form thiodiglycol sulfoxide and thiodiglycol as its primary metabolites. The usefulness of the sulfoxide as a marker for sulfur mustard exposure is limited due to the presence of low levels of the compound in normal human urine. Other metabolites detected in urine include 1,1'-sulphonylbis [2-S-(N-acetylcysteinyl)ethane]), (1,1-sulphonylbis[2-(methyl-sulphinyl)ethane] and 1-methylsulphinyl-2-[2-(methylthio)ethylsulphonyl]ethane],[63–65] N7-(2-hydroxyethylthioethyl)guanine[66] and N1-(2-hydroxyethylthioethyl)-4-methyl imidazole.[67]

Since thiodiglycol sulfoxide and thiodiglycol are the metabolites present in the greatest concentration, many of the methods developed to detect mustard exposure rely on the detection of these metabolites.[68–73] Methods have been developed to detect some of the other sulfur mustard metabolites in urine, however.[74–77]

The detection of sulfur mustard in blood and serum has also been accomplished.[78–80] Some of the more interesting work has been to identify the adducts formed between hemoglobin and sulfur mustard after exposure to the gas.[81–83]

Chromatographic and biological methods have been developed for the detection of sulfur mustards, their metabolites or their breakdown products in water, air, soil or other nonbiological matrices.[16,51,84–95] In addition to the hemoglobin adducts, identification has been made of adducts with valine, cysteine, keratin and DNA[96–101] and in tissues from exposure victims.[102]

Two older reviews of detection methods for sulfur mustard are somewhat outdated technologically but still contain some relevant information concerning the detection and identification of mustard gas in biological matrices.[103,104]

b. Nitrogen mustards (HN-1, HN-2, HN-3). The nitrogen mustards can be viewed as sulfur mustard in which the sulfur atom has been replaced by a nitrogen. The effects of the nitrogen mustards are almost identical to those of sulfur mustard. HN-2 is also known by the synonym mechlorethamine and is used clinically as treatment for several malignancies, including lymphoma. In addition to HN-2, several analogs that are not considered to be CWA have been synthesized and are in use as anticancer agents.

The nitrogen mustards are readily metabolized in the human body and the metabolites are relatively simple to detect. HN-1 produces N-ethyldiethanolamine, HN-2 produces N-methyldiethanolamine and HN-3 produces triethanolamine as their primary metabolites. Lemire et al. have developed a method for the quantitation of these metabolites.[105]

The method for the detection of anticancer nitrogen mustards in blood after derivatization may be applicable to other mustards as well.[106] As was the case with sulfur mustard, the nitrogen mustards form adducts with heme and other proteins. These adducts have been studied extensively and detection of these adducts may indicate exposure to chemical warfare agents. However, in these cases care must be taken to rule out the possibility of exposure to anticancer nitrogen mustards.[107–112]

Devices and methodologies have also been developed for the detection of nitrogen mustards in air and on contaminated environmental samples[113,114] and monitoring protocols have been developed to monitor worker exposure.[115,116]

c. Arsenicals. Unlike the nitrogen and sulfur mustards, lewisite was developed by America near the end of World War I. Also unlike the mustards, clinical symptoms begin almost immediately on exposure to lewisite. Even though the arsenicals can cause blindness, the rapid onset of symptoms tends to alert the victim to the presence of a CWA and allows time to take protective action before substantial injury occurs.

Analytically, the analysis of the arsenicals are complicated by the fact that in many weaponized forms, the agent is dissolved in a complex hydrocarbon mixture such as diesel oil. Chromatographically, this results in a forest of peaks which can be difficult to resolve. Muir et al. have developed a derivatization scheme which helps resolve this problem.[117] Ion mobility increment spectrometry has been reported as a practical method for the rapid detection of lewisite and other CWAs.[118]

The chromatographic detection and identification of lewisite or its degradation products in the environment has been reported.[119–121]

In vivo, the lewisites either hydrolyze to 2-chlorovinylarsonous acid which is excreted in the urine, or bind to proteins in the blood. A mass spectrometric method for the detection of the urinary metabolite has been reported[122,123] while a method for biomonitoring exposure to the compounds by detecting hemoglobin adducts is applicable to blood.[123]

Literature reports on the analysis of phenyldichloroarsine, ethyldichloroarsine and methyldichloroarsine are scarce. It would appear that the metabolism of these species would result in quite simple residues and the usefulness of identification of these compounds by the detection of metabolites would be difficult. It is quite possible that these arsenicals form adducts with hemoglobin and glutathione as do the lewisites and the identification of the adducts might provide a route to their detection. In fact, Dill et al. have looked at phenyldichloroarsine binding to glutathione[124] and to lipoic acid.[125]

Phosgene oxime is a rather obscure candidate for use in CW. Its chemical structure suggests that it would readily hydrolyze to phosgene in vivo and any analysis would likely be similar to the search for phosgene. Early literature reports suggest that the Bulgarians looked at the clinical aspects of this compound in the 1950s and a colorimetric method is mentioned by Malatesta et al.[126,127]

B. Harassing agents

The harassing agents can be used as CWAs but are encountered more frequently when used as riot control agents by civilian authorities. As the name implies, their function is not to disable an individual but to encourage him to leave the area. Many attempts have been made to make the standard "tear gases" more effective, but the more recent additions of CS and CR (see Figure 8.4) to the arsenal have provided increased effectiveness with reduced toxicity.

It should be mentioned that these compounds are all liquids or solids at room temperature and would be more accurately referred to as "finely dispersed aerosols" or an equivalent phrase, since they are not true gases.

The two basic types of harassing agents are the lachrymators (tear gases) and the sternutators (vomiting agents). The newest member of the lachrymator family is OC (oleoresin capsicum), commonly known as pepper spray.

1. Lachrymators

Several articles have been published outlining methods for the chromatographic identification of the earlier lachrymators, with the methods varying from thin layer to GC/MS.[128–135] Fung et al. have characterized the components of pepper spray and identified several different capsaicinoids.[136]

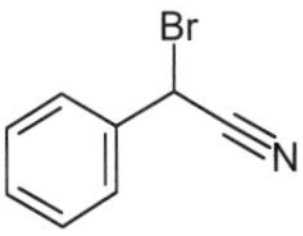

a-Bromobenzyl cyanide (CA)

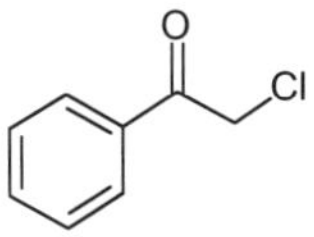

2-Chloroacetophenone (CN)

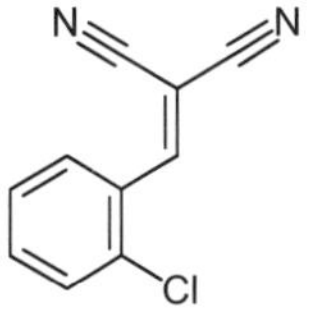

o-Chlorobenzylidenemalonitrile (CS)

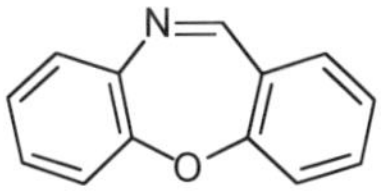

Dibenz-(b,f)-1,4-oxazepine (CR)

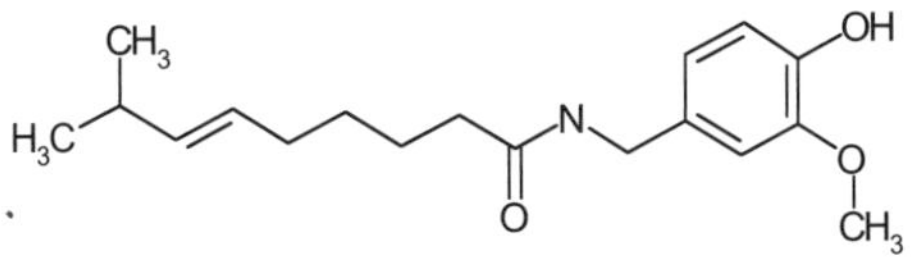

Capsaicin (Pepper Spray)

CNB is a mixture of CN, CCl_4 and benzene
CNC is a mixture of CN and $CHCl_3$
CNS is a mixture of CN, $CHCl_3$ and chloropicrin

Figure 8.4 *Harrassing agents*

The metabolism of lachrymators has been studied in humans and rats and should provide helpful information for those attempting to determine exposure from biological samples.[137–139] A series of articles outlining the investigation of the complex metabolism of CR has been published.[140–142]

Doring et al. have concluded that blood samples should be analyzed for CN as soon as possible after collection since CN reacts relatively quickly with blood. The chloro- and chlorofluorocarbon solvents could be detected in the blood of experimental animals for several weeks in stored blood and may provide a better marker for lachrymator exposure than the lachrymator itself,[143] although some researchers have reported the detection of the lachrymators themselves in tissue samples and on skin and clothing.[144,145]

2. Sternutators (vomiting agents)

The sternutators have been used as riot control agents, although such use is rare. When used as CWAs, the intended purpose is to induce nausea and vomiting, which encourages the affected individual to remove any protective clothing and renders him more susceptible to other agents. The symptoms have a slower onset than the lachrymators.

A method has been developed for the analysis of DM in soils[146] and in plants.[147] It may be possible to extend the experimental parameters in these two studies to other matrices.

C. Incapacitating agents

Incapacitating agents are generally common drugs which have been adapted for use as CW agents. Dispersal and delivery systems are designed to distribute the substances so that the largest number of individuals may be affected. A recent example of the use of an incapacitating agent

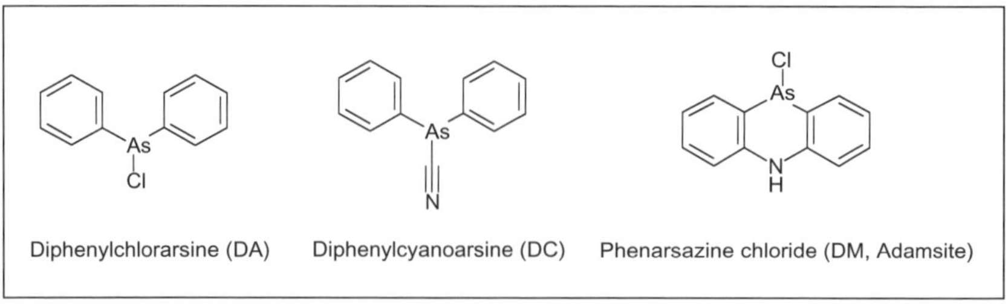

Figure 8.5 *Sternutators (vomiting agents)*

was the theater hostage situation in Moscow, where fentanyl (or an analog —the exact identity of the substance is still being debated) was dispersed into the theater through the air conditioning and heating ducts.[148]

Incapacitating agents may be divided into three broad categories: depressants, stimulants and psychoactive drugs. These drugs are routinely analyzed in modern toxicology labs and the methods for their analysis are well reviewed. No attempt will be made to undertake a complete review of this literature here. An excellent source for methods of analysis of these drugs is the book by Baselt.[149]

Examples of drugs that have been used or adapted as CW agents are listed in Table 8.2. This list is not conclusive and many analogs to these drugs have also been synthesized and may find a use as CWAs.

D. Toxins

Toxins are plentiful in the natural environment, existing in snakes, fish, scorpions, spiders, fungi, bacteria, insects and plants. The food processing industry has developed numerous products and methods to detect and quantitate these toxins in order to assure the quality of food products. As a result, relatively more methods are available and numerous commercial kits also exist.

Three of the most commonly cited toxins applicable for use as CWAs are aflatoxin, botulinum toxin and ricin. Aflatoxin is produced by a family of fungi (e.g., *Aspergillus flavus* and *Aspergillus parasiticus*) which are common inhabitants of soil throughout the world. Aflatoxins are routinely found on root crops like peanuts. Botulinum toxin is produced by the bacteria *Clostridium botulinum* while ricin is the toxic component of the fruit of the castor plant, *Ricinus communis* (the castor bean). Less well known are saxitoxin and trichothecene mycotoxin. Saxitoxin is the toxic prin-

Table 8.2
Drugs that Have Been Used or Adapted as CW Agents

Depressants	Psychoactive drugs	Stimulants
Morphine	LSD	Amphetamine
Fentanyl	Mescaline	Cocaine
	Phencyclidine	
	Psilocybin	

ciple produced by the algae (*Gonyaulax sp.*) responsible for "red tide." Trichothecene mycotoxin (T2), found in the CWA "yellow rain," is a toxin produced by the Fusarium species of fungi.

Laboratory synthesis is impractical for many of the toxins since they are complex proteins or complex molecules with multiple chiral centers which prohibit efficient, high-yield synthesis. The simplest, saxitoxin, with only four chiral centers and a molecular weight of only 299, has been referred to as "one of the most toxic non-protein substances known."[150]

The toxins selected for inclusion in this section are based somewhat on their notoriety. Certainly the list of toxins which are possible CWAs is much longer. Space and time limit the number of these substances which can be included here.

1. Ricin

The possibility of toxins such as ricin being dispersed in populated areas has triggered a search for sensors capable of rapidly detecting their presence. A number of different approaches have been reported in the literature and sensors have been developed for the simultaneous detection of multiple analytes.[151–161] The mass spectrometric characterization of ricin from different subspecies of Ricinus has been reported.[162]

The mass spectrometric identification of large proteinaceous molecules like ricin generally requires advanced instrumentation such as matrix assisted laser desorption ionization mass spectrometry (MALDI-TOF). For laboratories that don't have access to such instrumentation, a number of ELISA (enzyme-linked immunosorbant assay) and other immunoassay techniques may provide presumptive identification of ricin in biological samples.[163–166]

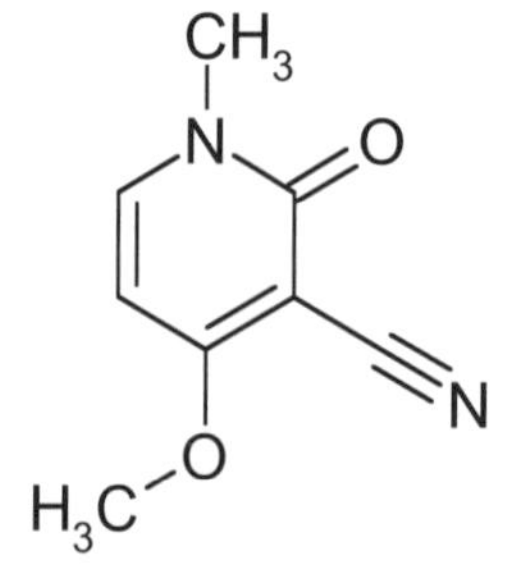

Figure 8.6 *Ricinine*

In addition to ricin, the castor plant contains a number of other toxic principles. One of these, ricinine (Figure 8.7) is a simple molecule which is amenable to GC/MS analysis[167] and has been used as a marker in samples suspected of containing ricin. The detection of ricinine by GC/MS is a much faster procedure than identifying ricin itself. The detection of ricinine or its metabolites in biological fluids might provide a means of detecting ricin exposure.

2. Aflatoxins

Rather than a single substance, the aflatoxins are actually a series of closely related compounds produced by some Aspergillus species of fungi. The specific aflatoxins are labeled with a designating letter, e.g., aflatoxin B1 and also include aflatoxins B2, B2a, G1, G2, G2a, M1, M2, and Q1. A great deal of literature exists on the detection of aflatoxins in foodstuffs and commercial ELISA kits are available.

Aflatoxins form adducts with amino acids, DNA, albumin and guanine. The detection of these adducts in urine,[168–174] blood[172,175–178] and tissue[179] has been used to assess aflatoxin exposure. Other methods for the detection of aflatoxin and its metabolites rely on instrumental chromatographic analysis preceded by an immunoaffinity chromatography purification step[180–184] immunoassay,[185,186] traditional chromatography [187–191] or mass spectrometry.[192]

Methods have also been developed for the detection of aflatoxins in air and on food.[193–195]

3. Botulinum toxin

Botulinum toxin is a paralytic poison that has found use in modern cosmetic procedures such as Botox. Several serotypes of the botulinum

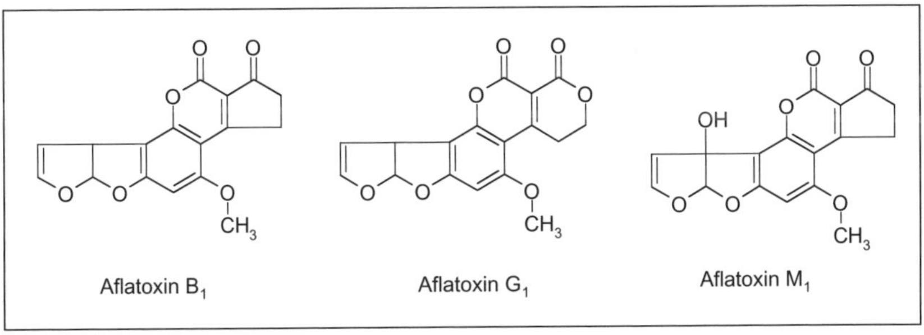

Figure 8.7 *Aflatoxins*

neurotoxin are known, including A, B, E and F. The toxin is also believed to have been mass produced and weaponized for use as a CWA. Methods have been developed to detect weaponized botulinum toxin in air.[196–198]

The detection of botulinum toxin in biological fluids has relied primarily on immunoassay techniques[199–205] although some work has been done on using polymerase chain reaction (PCR) to detect the toxin in food and soil.[206]

4. Saxitoxin

Saxitoxin is a toxin produced by certain algae and is responsible for the "red tide." Most traditional human exposure to saxitoxin is related to eating shellfish from contaminated water during times of algal blooms. Urinary metabolites of saxitoxin include neosaxitoxin and decarbamoyl-saxitoxin and the analysis of urine from a poisoning victim detected parent saxitoxin as well.[207] Saxitoxin has been detected in biological fluids by immunoassay,[208–211] receptor binding assay,[212] mass spectrometry,[213,214] and by high-pressure liquid chromiatography (HPLC).[215–218]

5. Trichothecene mycotoxin

Trichothecene mycotoxin (T2) from the Fusarium species of fungi is a complex molecule with a molecular weight of 466 and eight chiral centers. Fusarium fungi are commonly found on cereal grains in the Northern Hemisphere and may produce a number of trichothecene related toxins including nivalenol and deoxynivalenol. The detection of any of these three substance is indicative of exposure to the trichothecenes and methods have been developed to detect all of them. A recent study of retail infant cereals in Canada revealed the presence of deoxynivalenol in 63 per-

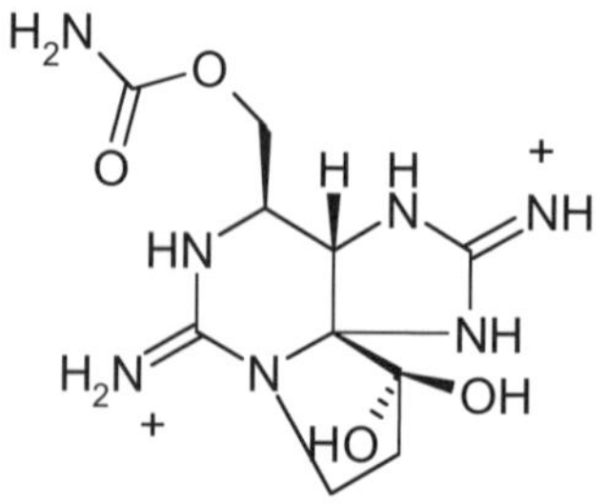

Figure 8.8 *Saxitoxin*

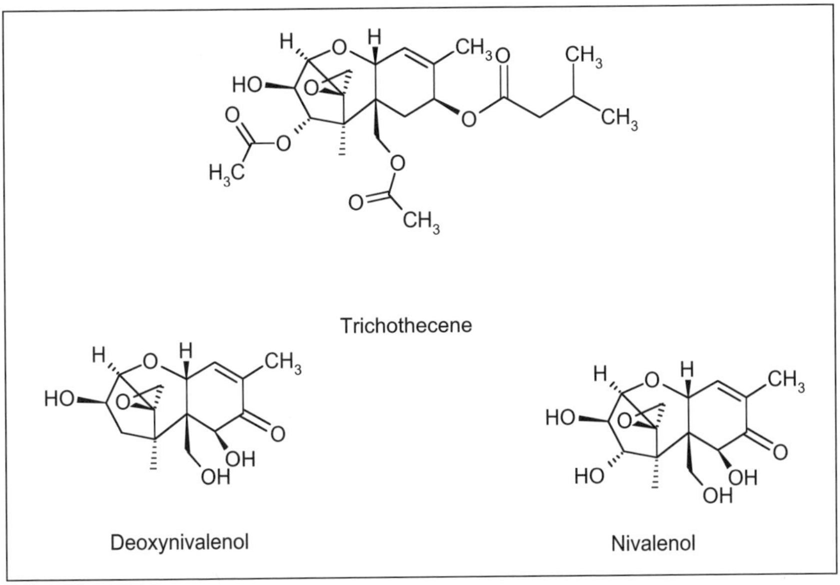

Figure 8.9 *Trichothecenes*

cent of the samples.[219] Deoxynivalenol is excreted to a large extent as a glucuronide in urine and pretreatment with a glucuronidase may increase the sensitivity of assays. Given the structural similarities among the several trichothecene mycotoxins, glucuronide formation may be the preferred metabolic pathway.[220]

Detection of trichothecene in biological matrices has been accomplished by HPLC,[221] gas chromatography,[222–228] mass spectrometry,[229–235] and immunoassays.[236–240]

A number of methods have been developed for the detection of the trichothecene mycotoxins in foods and environmental samples, including immunoassays,[230,241–245] HPLC,[246–248] and mass spectrometry.[249–252]

8.5 Conclusion

The number of substances which have been investigated for use as chemical warfare agents is quite large and ranges from the chemically simple (e.g., chlorine) to the extremely complex (e.g., botulinum toxin). Even more alarming is the number of potential chemical warfare agents that are available. The toxicologist must be imaginative, open-minded yet very cautious when attempting to detect CWA exposure. Care must be taken, especially with the naturally occurring toxins, that detection of the substance in biological fluids is due to CWA exposure and not to normal dietary, environmental or occupational exposure. A good quality assurance program as outlined by LeBeau[254] is an essential part of this determination.

Endnotes

1. http://www.nti.org/e_research/profiles/NK/Chemical/1090.html.

2. Eckenrode, B.A. *J. of the American Society for Mass Spectrometry*, 2001, 12:6:683–693.

3. Cancho, B., Ventura, F. and Galceran, M.T. *J. of Chromatography A* 2000, 897:1–2:307–315.

4. Odoul, M. et al. *J. Anal. Toxicol.* 1994 Jul–Aug;18(4):205–7.

5. Shiono, H. et al. *Am. J. Forensic Med. Pathol.* 1991 Mar;12(1):50–3.

6. Gülçin Gümü_, Birsen Demirata and Re_at TALANTA 2000, 53:2:305–315.

7. A. Mirmohseni and A. Alipour, Sensors and Actuators B: Chemical 2002, 84:23:245–251.

8. Winski, S.L. et al. *Fundam. Appl. Toxicol.* 1997 Aug;38(2):123–8.

9. Freeman, H., Uthe, J.F. and Flemming, B. *At. Abs. Newsl.* 15 (1976), 49–50.

10. Thomas, J. and Kristensen, L.V., *Ugeskr Laeger*. 1967 Apr 27;129(17):553–5.

11. Golfinopoulos, S.K., Nikolaou, A.D. and Lekkas, T.D. *Environ. Sci. Pollut. Res. Int.* 2003;10(6):368–72.

12. Kampioti, A.A. and Stephanou, E.G. *J. Chromatogr. A*. 1999 Oct 1;857 (1–2):217–29.

13. Guo, M. et al. *Environ. Sci. Technol.* 2003 May 1;37(9):1844–9.

14. Daft, J.L. *J. Assoc. Off. Anal. Chem.* 1983 Mar;66(2) 228–33.

15. Kallio H, Shibamoto T. *J Chromatogr.* 1988 Nov 11;454:392–7.

16. Carrick, W.A., Cooper, D.B. and Muir, B. *J. Chromatogr. A*. 2001 Aug 3;925

(1-2):241–9.

17. Gonmori, K. et al. *Am. J. Forensic Med. Pathol.* 1987 Jun;8(2):135–8.

18. Dangwal, S.K. *Ind. Health.* 1994;32(1):41–7.

19. Hendershott, J.P. *Am. Ind. Hyg. Assoc. J.* 1986 Dec;47(12):742–6.

20. Tuggle, R.M. et al. *Am. Ind. Hyg. Assoc. J.* 1979 May;40(5):387–94.

21. Cabot, C. et al. *J. Toxicol. Clin. Exp.* 1992 Oct–Nov;12(4-5):267–73.

22. Reiner, E. et al. *Arh. Hig. Rada. Toksikol.* 1993 Jun;44(2):159–62.

23. Hammond, P.S. and Forster, J.S. *Anal. Biochem.* 1989 Aug 1;180(2):380–3; Sipponen, K.B. *J. Chromatogr.* 1987 Feb 27;389(1):87–94.

24. Kataoka, M. et al. *Environ. Sci. Technol.* 2001 May 1;35(9):1823–9.

25. Hook, G.L et al. *J. Chromatogr. A.* 2003 Apr 11;992(1–2):1–9.

26. Groenewold, G.S. et al. *Anal. Chem.* 1999 Jul 1;71(13):2318–23.

27. Kataoka, M. et al. *J. Chromatogr. A.* 1998 Oct 23;824(2):211–21.

28. Rosso, T.E. and Bossle, P.C. *J. Chromatogr. A.* 1998 Oct 16;824(1):125–34.

29. Vermillion, W.D. and Crenshaw, M.D. *J. Chromatogr. A.* 1997 May 16; 770(1–2):253–60.

30. Black, R.M. et al. *J. Chromatogr. A.* 1994 Feb 25;662(2):301–21.

31. Borrett, V.T. et al. *J. Chromatogr. A.* 2003 Jun 27;1003(1–2):143–55.

32. Groenewold, G.S. et al. *Environ. Sci. Technol.* 2002 Nov 15;36(22):4790–4.

33. D'Agostino, P.A., Hancock, J.R. and Provost, L.R. *J. Chromatogr. A.* 1999 Apr 30;840(2):289–94.

34. Degenhardt-Langelaan, C.E. and Kientz, C.E. *J. Chromatogr. A.* 1996 Feb 2;723(1):210–4.

35. Schneider, J.F., Boparai, A.S. and Reed, L.L. *J. Chromatogr. Sci.* 2001 Oct;39(10):420–4.

36 Sega, G.A., Tomkins, B.A. and Griest, W.H. *J. Chromatogr. A*. 1997 Nov 28;790(1–2):143–52.

37 O'Neill, H.J. et al. *J. Chromatogr. A*. 2002 Jul 12;962(1-2):183–95.

38. D'Agostino, P.A., Chenier, C.L. and Hancock, J.R. *J. Chromatogr. A*. 2002 Mar 15;950(1–2):149–56.

39. Matsuda, Y. et al. *Toxicol. Appl. Pharmacol.* 1998 Jun;150(2):310–20.

40. Tsuchihashi, H. et al. *J. Anal. Toxicol.* 1998 Sep;22(5):383–8.

41. Bonierbale, E., Debordes, L. and Coppet, L. *J. Chromatogr. B. Biomed. Sci. Appl.* 1997 Jan 24;688(2):255–64.

42. van der Schans, M.J. et al. *Toxicol. Appl. Pharmacol.* 2003 Aug 15; 191(1):48–62.

43. Noort, D. et al. *Arch. Toxicol.* 1998 Oct;72(10):671–5.

44. Driskell, W.J. et al. *J. Anal. Toxicol.* 2002 Jan–Feb;26(1):6–10.

45. Miki, A. et al. *J. Anal. Toxicol.* 1999 Mar-Apr;23(2):86–93.

46. Nakajima, T. et al. *Arch. Toxicol.* 1998 Sep;72(9):601–3.

47. Shih, M.L. et al. *Biol. Mass. Spectrom.* 1991 Nov;20(11):717–23.

48. Goransson-Nyberg, A. et al. *Arch. Toxicol.* 1998 Jul–Aug;72(8):459–67.

49. Nagao, M. et al. *Toxicol. Appl. Pharmacol.* 1997 May;144(1):198–203.

50. Smith, J.R. et al. *J. Appl. Toxicol.* 2001 Dec;21 Suppl 1:S35–41.

51. Sanders, C.A., Rodriguez, M. Jr. and Greenbaum, E. *Biosens. Bioelectron.* 2001 Sep;16(7–8):439–46.

52. Taylor, P.W. et al. *Mil. Med.* 2003 Apr;168(4):314–9.

53. Erhard, M.H. et al. *Arch. Toxicol.* 1990;64(7):580–5.

54. Loke, W.K. et al. *Anal. Biochem.* 1998 Mar 1;257(1):12–9.

55. Zhou, Y.X. et al. *Arch. Toxicol.* 1995;69(9):644–8.

56. Miller, J.K. and Lenz, D.E. *J. Appl. Toxicol.* 2001 Dec;21 Suppl 1:S23–6.

57. Wang, J. et al. *Anal. Chem.* 2002 Dec 1;74(23):6121–5.

58. Steiner, W.E. et al. *Anal. Chem.* 2002 Sep 1;74(17):4343–52.

59. Wang, J. et al. *Anal. Chem.* 2002 Mar 1;74(5):1187–91.

60. Hopkins, A.R. and Lewis, N.S. *Anal. Chem.* 2001 Mar 1;73(5):884–92.

61. Nassar, A.E. et al. *Anal. Chem.* 1998 Mar 15;70(6):1085–91.

62. Abu-Qare, A.W. and Abou-Donia, M.B. *Food Chem. Toxicol.* 2002 Oct; 40(10):1327–33.

63. Black, R.M. and Read, R.W. *Xenobiotica.* 1995 Feb;25(2):167–73.

64. Black, R.M. et al. *Xenobiotica.* 1992 Apr;22(4):405–18.

65. Black, R.M. et al. *J. Anal. Toxicol.* 1992 Mar–Apr;16(2):79–84.

65. Fidder, A. et al. *Arch, Toxicol.* 1996;70(12):854–5.

67. Sandelowsky, I. et al. *Arch. Toxicol.* 1992;66(4):296–7.

68. Graham, J.S. et al. *J Appl Toxicol.* 2000 Dec;20 Suppl 1:S161–72.

69. Black, R.M. and Read, R.W. *J. Chromatogr. B. Biomed. Appl.* 1995 Mar 10;665(1):97–105.

70. Black, R.M. and Read, R.W. *J. Chromatogr.* 1991 Oct 11;558(2):393–404.

71. Wils, E.R. et al. *J. Anal. Toxicol.* 1985 Nov–Dec.

72. Jakubowski, E.M. et al. *J. Chromatogr.* 1990 Jun 8;528(1):184–90.

73. Wils, E.R., Hulst, A.G. and van Laar. J. *J. Anal. Toxicol.* 1988 Jan–Feb;12(1):15–9.

74. Black, R.M., Clarke, R.J. and Read, R.W. *J. Chromatogr.* 1991 Oct 11;558 (2):405–14.

75. Vycudilik, W. *Forensic Sci. Int.* 1987 Sep;35(1):67–71.

76. Vycudilik, W. *Forensic Sci. Int.* 1985 Jun–Jul;28(2):131–6.

77. Munavalli, S. and Pannella, M. *J. Chromatogr.* 1988 Mar 25;437(2):423–8.

78. Dangi, R.S. et al. *J. Chromatogr. B. Biomed. Appl.* 1994 Nov 18;661(2):341–5.

79. Hambrook, J.L., Howells, D.J. and Schock, C. *Xenobiotica.* 1993 May; 23(5):537–61.

80. Maisonneuve, A. et al. *J. Chromatogr.* 1992 Dec 2;583(2):155–65.

81. Noort, D. et al. *Arch. Toxicol.* 1997;71(3):171–8.

82. Fidder, A. et al. *Chem. Res. Toxicol.* 1996 Jun;9(4):788–92.

83. Noort, D. et al. *Chem. Res. Toxicol.* 1996 Jun;9(4):781–7.

84. Noort, D. et al. *J. Appl. Toxicol.* 2000 Dec;20 Suppl 1:S187–92.

85. Kimm, G.L., Hook, G.L. and Smith, P.A. *J. Chromatogr. A.* 2002 Sep 20;971(1–2):185–91.

86. Smith, J.R. and Shih, M.L. *J. Appl. Toxicol.* 2001 Dec;21 Suppl 1:S27–34.

87. Hooijschuur, E.W. Kientz, C.E. and Brinkman, U.A. *J. Chromatogr. A.* 2001 Sep 14;928(2):187–99.

88. Mazurek, M. et al. *J. Chromatogr. A.* 2001 Jun 1;919(1):133–45.

89. Beck, N.V. et al. *J. Chromatogr. A.* 2001 Jan 12;907(1–2):221–7.

90. Hooijschuur, E.W., Kientz, C.E. and Brinkman, U.A. *J. Chromatogr. A.* 1999 Jul 23;849(2):433–44.

91. Black, R.M. et al. *J. Chromatogr. A.* 1994 Feb 25;662(2):301–21.

92. Griest, W.H. et al. *J. Chromatogr.* 1992 May 29;600(2):273–7.

93. Fowler, W.K. and Smith, J.E. Jr. *J. Chromatogr. Sci.* 1990 Mar;28(3):118–22.

94. Heyndrickx, A., De Puydt, H. and Cordonnier, J. *Arch. Belg.* 1984; Suppl:61–8.

95. Albrio, P.W. and Fishbein, L. *J. Chromatogr.* 1970 Jan 21;46(2):202–3.

96. Smith, J.R. et al. *J. Appl. Toxicol.* 2001 Dec;21 Suppl 1:S35–41.

97. Noort, D. et al. *Chem. Res. Toxicol.* 1999 Aug;12(8):715–21.

98. Benschop, H.P. et al. *J. Anal. Toxicol.* 1997 Jul-Aug;21(4):249–51.

99. Ludlum, D.B. et al. *Chem. Biol. Interact.* 1994 Apr;91(1):39–49.

100. Fidder A. et al. *Chem. Res. Toxicol.* 1994 Mar–Apr;7(2):199–204.

101. Noort, D. et al. *J. Appl. Toxicol.* 2000 Dec;20 Suppl 1:S187–92.

102. Drasch, G. et al. *J. Forensic Sci.* 1987 Nov;32(6):1788–93.

103. Machata, G. and Vycudilik, W. *Arch. Belg.* 1984;Suppl:53–5.

104. Heyndrickx, A., Cordonnier, J. and De Bock A. *Arch. Belg.* 1984;Suppl: 102–9.

105. Lemire, S.W., Ashley, D.L. and Calafat, A.M. *J. Anal. Toxicol.* 2003 Jan–Feb;27(1):1–6.

106. Cummings, J. et al. *Anal. Chem.* 1991 Aug 1;63(15):1514–9.

107. Noort, D., Hulst, A.G. and Jansen, R. *Arch. Toxicol.* 2002 Mar;76(2):83–8.

108. Sperry, M.L., Skanchy, D. and Marino, M.T. *J. Chromatogr. B. Biomed. Sci. Appl.* 1998 Sep 25;716(1–2):187–93.

109. Thulin, H. et al. *Chem. Biol. Interact.* 1996 Jan 5;99(1-3):263–75.

110. Osborne, M.R., Wilman, D.E. and Lawley, P.D. *Chem. Res. Toxicol.* 1995 Mar;8(2):316–20.

111. Kohn, K.W., Hartley, J.A. and Mattes, W.B. *Nucleic Acids Res.* 1987 Dec 23;15(24):10531–49.

112. Albrecht, G. et al. *Naunyn Schmiedebergs Arch. Pharmacol.* 1976 Aug;2 94(2):179–85.

113. Stuff, J.R. et al. *J. Chromatogr. A.* 1999 Jul 23;849(2):529–40.

114. Gresham, G.L., Groenewold, G.S. and Olson, J.E. *J. Mass Spectrom.* 2000 Dec;35(12):1460–9.

115. Thulin, H. et al. *Toxicol. Ind. Health.* 1995 Jan–Feb;11(1):89–97.

116. D'Agostino, P.A. and Provost, L.R. *J. Chromatogr.* 1988 Feb 19;436(3): 399–411.

117. Muir, B. et al. *J. Chromatogr. A.* 2004 Mar 5;1028(2):313–20.

118. Buryakov, I.A. *J. Chromatogr. B. Analyt. Technol. Biomed. Life Sci.* 2004 Feb 5;800(1–2):75–82.

119. Tomkins, B.A., Sega, G.A. and Ho, C.H. *J. Chromatogr. A.* 2001 Feb 9;909(1):13–28.

120. Chaudot, X., Tambute, A. and Caude M. *J. Chromatogr A.* 2000 Aug 4;888(1–2):327–33.

121. Szostek, B. and Aldstadt, J.H. *J. Chromatogr A.* 1998 May 22;807(2):253–63.

122. Wooten, J.V., Ashley, D.L. and Calafat, A.M. *J. Chromatogr. B. Analyt. Technol. Biomed. Life Sci.* 2002 May 25;772(1):147–53.

123. Fidder, A. et al. *Arch. Toxicol.* 2000 Jul;74(4–5):207–14.

124. Dill, K. et al. *Arch. Biochem. Biophys.* 1987 Sep;257(2):293–301.

125. Dill, K. et al. *Chem. Res. Toxicol.* 1989 May–Jun;2(3):181–5.

126. Malatesta, P., Bianchi, B. and Malatesta, C. *Boll. Chim. Farm* 1983 Mar; 122(3):137–42.

127. Malatesta P, Bianchi B. and Malatesta C. *Boll. Chim. Farm* 1983 Feb; 122(2):96–103.

128. Ferslew, K.E., Orcutt, R.H. and Hagardorn, A.N. *J. Forensic Sci.* 1986 Apr;31(2): 658–65.

129. Jane, I. and Wheals, B.B. *J. Chromatogr.* 1972 Jul 26;70(1):151–3.

130. Zerba, E.N. and Ruveda, M.A. *J. Chromatogr.* 1972 May 31;68(1):245–7.

131. Sass, S. et al. *Anal. Chem.* 1971 Mar;43(3):462–4.

132. Sreenivasan, V.R. and Boese, R.A. *J. Forensic Sci.* 1970 Jul;15(3):433–42.

133. Ludemann, W.D., Stutz, M.H. and Sass, S. *Anal. Chem.* 1969 Apr;41(4):

679–81.

134. Babakhanian, R.V. et al. *Sud. Med. Ekspert*. 1996 Jan–Mar;39(1):28–9.

135. Ferslew, K.E., Orcut,t R.H. and Hagardorn, A.N. *J. Forensic Sci.* 1986 Apr;31(2):658–65.

136. Fung, T., Jeffery, W. and Beveridge, A.D. *J. Forensic Sci.* 1982 Oct;27(4): 812–21.

137. Leadbeater, L., Sainsbury, G.L. and Utley, D. *Toxicol. Appl. Pharmacol.* 1973 May;25(1):111–6.

138. Cucinell, S.A. et al. *Fed. Proc*. 1971 Jan–Feb;30(1):86–91.

139. Rietveld, E.C. et al. *Arch. Toxicol.* 1983 Oct;54(2):139–44.

140. French, M.C. et al. "The fate of dibenz[b,f]-1,4-oxazepine (CR) in the rat: Part III: The intermediary metabolites." *Xenobiotica.* 1983 Jun;13(6):373–81

141. Furnival, B. et al. "The fate of dibenz[b,f]-1,4-oxazepine (CR) in the rat: Part II: Metabolism in vitro." *Xenobiotica*. 1983 Jun;13(6):361-72.

142. French, M.C. et al. "The fate of dibenz[b,f]-1,4-oxazepine (CR) in the rat, rhesus monkey and guinea-pig: Part I: Metabolism in vivo." *Xenobiotica*. 1983 Jun;13(6):345–59.

143. Doring, G, Zorec-Karlovsek, M. and Berg, S., *Z. Rechtsmed.* 1979 Jul 17;83(2):105–13.

144. Ivanov, A.A. *Sud. Med. Ekspert*. 1998 May–Jun;41(3):27–8.

145. Dautova, Z.A. et al. *Vestn. Oftamol.* 2001 Jan–Feb;117(1):29–30.

146. Schoene, K. et al. *J. of Chromatography A.* Vol. 719, No. 2, pages 401–409.

147. Pitten, F.A. et al. *Sci. Total Environ.* 1999 Feb 9;226(2-3):237–45.

148. http://cns.miis.edu/pubs/week/02110b.htm.

149. Baselt, R.C. *The Disposition of Toxic Drugs and Chemicals in Ma*n, 7th ed. (Foster City, CA: Chemical Toxicology Institute, 2004).

150. http://www.bris.ac.uk/Depts/Chemistry/MOTM/stx/saxi.htm.

151. Wadkins, R.M. et al. *Biosens. Bioelectron.* 1998 Mar 1;13(3–4):407–15.

152. Narang, U. et al. *Biosens. Bioelectron.* 1997;12(9–10):937–45.

153. Gatto-Menking, D.L. et al. *Biosens. Bioelectron.* 1995 Summer;10(6–7): 501–7.

154. O'Brien, T. et al. *Biosens. Bioelectron.* 2000 Jan;14(10–11):815–28.

155. Anderson, G.P. et al. *Biosens. Bioelectron.* 2000 Jan;14(10-11):771–7.

156. Puu, G. *Anal. Chem.* 2001 Jan 1;73(1):72–9.

157. Goldman, E.R. et al. *Anal. Chem.* 2004 Feb 1;76(3):684–8.

158. Ligler, F.S. et al. *Anal. Bioanal. Chem.* 2003 Oct;377(3):469–77.

159. Taitt C.R. et al. *Anal. Chem.* 2002 Dec 1;74(23):6114–20.

160. Taitt C.R. et al. *Microb. Ecol.* 2004 Feb 9.

161. Delehanty, J.B. and Ligler, F.S. *Anal. Chem.* 2002 Nov 1;74(21):5681–7.

162. Despeyroux, D. et al. *Anal. Biochem.* 2000 Mar 1;279(1):23–36.

163. Koja, N., Shibata, T. and Mochida, K. *Toxicon.* 1980;18(5–6):611–8.

164. Griffiths, G.D., Newman, H. and Gee, D.J. *J. Forensic Sci. Soc.* 1986 Sep-Oct;26(5):349–58.

165. Shyu, H.F. et al. *Hybrid Hybridomics.* 2002 Feb;21(1):69–73.

166. Poli, M.A. et al. *Toxicon.* 1994 Nov;32(11):1371–7.

167. Darby, S.M., Miller, M.L. and Allen RO. *J. Forensic Sci.* 2001 Sep;46(5): 1033–42.

168. Groopman, J.D. et al. *Environ. Health Perspect.* 1993 Mar;99:107–13.

169. Nayak, S., Sashidhar, R.B. and Bhat, R.V. *Analyst.* 2001 Feb;126(2):179–83.

170. Weaver, V.M. and Groopman, J.D. *Cancer Epidemiol. Biomarkers Prev.* 1994 Dec;3(8):669–74.

171. Vidyasagar, T. et al. *J. AOAC Int.* 1997 Sep–Oct;80(5):1013–22.

172. Makarananda, K. et al. *J. Toxicol. Sci.* 1998 Jul;23 Suppl 2:155–9.

173. Walton, M. et al. *Chem. Res. Toxicol.* 2001 Jul;14(7):919–26.

174. Alvarez, M.T. et al. *Nat. Toxins.* 1999;7(4):139–45.

175. Sun, G. et al. *Wei Sheng Yan Jiu.* 2001 May;30(3):185–8.

176. Sujatha, N., Suryakala, S. and Rao, B.S. *J. AOAC Int.* 2001 Sep–Oct;84 (5):1465–74.

177. Wang. J.S. et al. *Appl. Environ. Microbiol.* 2001 Jun;67(6):2712–

178. Vidyasagar, T., Sujatha, N. and Sashidhar, R.B. *Food Addit. Contam.* 1997 Jul;14(5):457–67.

179. Vidyasagar, T., Sujatha, N. and Sashidhar, R.B. *Analyst.* 1997 Jun;122 (6):609-13.

180. Kussak, A., Andersson, B. and Andersson, K., *J. Chromatogr. B. Biomed. Appl.* 1995 Oct 20;672(2):253–9.

181. Kussak, A. et al. *Chemosphere.* 1998 Apr;36(8):1841–8.

182. Kussak, A., Andersson, B. and Andersson, K. *J. Chromatogr. B. Biomed. Appl.* 1994 Jun 17;656(2):329–34.

183. Groopman, J.D. and Donahue, K.F. *J. Assoc. Off. Ana.l Chem.* 1988 Sep-Oct;71(5):861–7.

184. Cheng, Z. et al. *Cancer Epidemiol. Biomarkers Prev.* 1997 Jul;6(7):523–9.

185. Korde, A. et al. *J. Agric. Food Chem.* 2003 Feb 12;51(4):843–6.

186. Thirumala-Devi, K. et al. *J. Agric. Food Chem.* 2002 Feb 13;50(4):933–7.

187. Simon, P. et al. *J. Chromatogr. B Biomed. Sci. Appl.* 1998 Aug 7;712(1–2):95–104.

188.. Kussak, A., Andersson, B. and Andersson, K. *J. Chromatogr.* 1993 Jul 2;616(2):235–41.

189. Liu, Z.H. et al. *Biomed. Chromatogr.* 1990 Mar;4(2):83–6.

190. Orti, D.L. et al. *J. Chromatogr.* 1989 Jan 13;462:269–79.

191. Orti, D.L. et al. *J Anal Toxicol.* 1986 Mar–Apr;10(2):41-5

192. Kussak, A. et al. *Rapid Commun. Mass. Spectrom.* 1995;9(13):1234-7.

193. Selim, M.I., Juchems, A.M., Popendorf, W. *Am. Ind. Hyg. Assoc. J.* 1998 Apr;59(4):252–6.

194. Holcomb, M. et al. *J. Chromatogr.* 1992 Oct 30;624(1-2):341–52.

195. Ghosh, S.K. et al. *Am. Ind. Hyg. Assoc. J.* 1997 Aug;58(8):583-6.

196. O'Brien, T. et al. *Biosens. Bioelectron.* 2000 Jan;14(10–11):815–28.

197. Kumar, P. et al. *Biosens. Bioelectron.* 1994;9(1):57–63.

198. Singh, B.R. and Silvia, M.A. *Adv. Ex. Med. Biol.* 1996;391:499–508.

199. Poli, M.A., Rivera, V.R. and Neal, D. *Toxicon.* 2002 Jun;40(6):797–802.

200. Peruski, A.H., Johnson, L.H. 3rd. and Peruski, L.F. Jr. *J. Immuno.l Methods.* 2002 May 1;263(1–2):35–41.

201. Szilagyi M, Rivera VR, Neal D, Merrill GA, Poli MA. *Toxicon.* 2000 Mar;38(3):381–9.

202. Palace, J. et al. *Neurology.* 1998 May;50(5):1463–6.

203. Doellgast, G.J. et al. *J. Clin. Microbiol.* 1997 Mar;35(3):578–8.

204. Doellgast, G.J. et al. *J. Clin. Microbiol.* 1994 Jan;32(1):105–11.

205. Doellgast, G.J. et al. *J. Clin. Microbiol.* 1993 Sep;31(9):2402–9.

206. Szabo, E.A. et al. *J. Appl. Bacteriol.* 1994 Jun;76(6):539–45.

207. Llewellyn, L.E. et al. *Toxicon.* 2002 Oct;40(10):1463–69.

208. Chu, F.S. *Gov't Reports Announcements & Index* (GRA&I), Issue 22, 1988.

209. Chu, F.S. and Fan, T.S. *J. Assoc. Off. Anal. Chem.* 1985 Jan–Feb;68(1):13–6.

210. Usleber, E. et al. *Food Addit. Contam.* 1995 May–Jun;12(3):405–13.

211. Davio, S.R. and Fontelo, P.A. *Anal. Biochem.* 1984 Aug 15;141(1):199–204.

212. Powell, C.L. and Doucette, G.J. *Nat. Toxins.* 1999;7(6):393–400.

213. Mirocha, C.J. et al. *Rapid Commun. Mass Spectrom.* 1992 Feb;6(2):128–34.

214. Mirocha, C.J. et al. *Gov't Reports Announcements & Index* (GRA&I), Issue 09, 1992

215. Stafford, R.G. and Hines, H.B. *J. Chromatogr. B. Biomed. Appl.* 1994 Jul 1;657(1):119–24.

216. Gessner, B.D. et al. *Toxicon.* 1997 May;35(5):711–22.

217. Asp, T.N., Larsen, S. and Aune, T. *Toxicon.* 2004 Mar;43(3):319–27.

218. Garcia, C. et al. *Toxicon.* 2004 Feb;43(2):149–58.

219. Lombaert, G.A. et al. "Mycotoxins in infant cereal foods from the Canadian retail market." *Food Addit. Contam.* 2003 May;20(5):494–504.

220. Meky, F.A. et al. *Food Chem. Toxicol.* 2003 Feb;41(2):265–73.

221. Naseem, S.M., Pace, J.G. and Wannemacher, R.W. Jr. *J. Anal. Toxicol.* 1995 May–Jun;19(3):151–6.

222. Rood, H.D. Jr., Swanson, S.P. and Buck, W.B., *J. Chromatogr.* 1986 Jun 13;378(2):375–83.

223. Dahlem, A.M. et al. *J. Chromatogr.* 1986 May 28;378(1):226–31.

224. Yagen, B., Bialer, M. and Sintov, A. *J. Chromatogr.* 1985 Sep 13;343(1):67–75.

225. Heyndrickx, A., Sookvanichsilp, N. and Van den Heede, M. *Arch. Belg.* 1984;Suppl:143–6.

226. Mirocha, C.J., Pawlosky, R.J. and Chatterjee, K. *Arch. Belg.* 1984; Suppl:210–8.

227. Mirocha, C.J. et al. *J. Assoc. Off. Anal. Chem.* 1983 Nov;66(6):1485–99.

228. Swanson, S.P. et al. *J. Assoc. Off. Anal. Chem.* 1983 Jul;66(4):909–12.

229. Pawlosky, R.J. et al. *J. Assoc. Off. Anal. Chem.* 1989 Sep–Oct;72(5):807–12.

230. Kostianinen, R., Rizzo, A. and Hesso, A. *Arch. Environ. Contam. Toxicol.* 1989 May–Jun;18(3):356–64.

231. Voyksner, R.D., Hagler, W.M. Jr. and Swanson, S.P. *J. Chromatogr.* 1987 May 8;394(1):183–99.

232. Begley, P. et al. *J. Chromatogr.* 1986 Sep 26;367(1):87–101.

233. D'Agostino, P.A., Provost, L.R. and Drover, D.R. *J. Chromatogr.* 1986 Sep 26;367(1):77–86.

234. Black, R.M., Clarke, R.J. and Read, R.W. *J. Chromatogr.* 1986 Sep 26;367(1):103–15.

235. Mirocha, C.J., Pawlosky, R.J. and Abbas, H.K. *Arch. Environ. Contam. Toxicol.* 1989 May–Jun;18(3):349–55.

236. Usleber, E. et al. *Zentralbl. Veterinarmed. B.* 1992 Oct;39(8):617–27.

237. Lee, R.C., Wei, R.D. and Chu, F.S. *J. Assoc. Off. Anal. Chem.* 1989 Mar–Apr;72(2):345–8.

238. Fontelo, P.A. et al. *Appl. Environ. Microbiol.* 1983 Feb;45(2):640–3.

239. Peters, H. et al. *Physiol. Chem.* 1982 Dec;363(12):1437–41.

240. Lee, S. and Chu, F.S. *J. Assoc. Off. Anal. Chem.* 1981 May;64(3):684–8.

241. Schneider, L. et al. *J. Anal. Chem.* 2000 May;367(1):98–100.

242. Teshima, R. et al. *Appl. Environ. Microbiol.* 1990 Mar;56(3):764–8.

243. Ramakrishna N. et al. *J. Assoc. Off. Anal. Chem.* 1990 Jan–Feb;73(1):71–6.

244. Maragos, C.M., Jolley, M.E. and Nasir, M.S. *Food Addit. Contam.* 2002 Apr;19(4):400–7.

245. Maragos, C.M. and Plattner, R.D. *J. Agric. Food Chem.* 2002 Mar 27;50(7):1827–32.

246. Pascale, M., Haidukowski, M. and Visconti, A. *J. Chromatogr. A.* 2003 Mar 14;989(2):257–64.

247. Rupp, H.S. *J AOAC Int.* 2002 Nov-Dec;85(6):1355–9.

248. Lombaert, G.A. *Adv. Exp. Med. Biol.* 2002;504:141–53.

249. Plattner, R.D. and Maragos, C.M. *J AOAC Int.* 2003 Jan–Feb;86(1):61–5.

250. Rodrigues-Fo, E. et al. *Rapid Commun. Mass Spectrom.* 2002;16(19):1827–35.

251. Razzazi-Fazeli, E. et al. *J. Chromatogr. A.* 2002 Aug 30;968(1-2):129–42.

252. Olsson, J. et al. *Int. J. Food. Microbiol.* 2002 Feb 5;72(3):203–14.

253. http://www.epa.gov/nerl/research/2000/pdf_conversions/G2-2.pdf.

254. http://www.fbi.gov/hq/lab/fsc/backissu/april2004/standards/2004_02_standards01.htm.

Chapter 9

The Role of Medical Systems in Responding to Chemical and Biological Terrorism

Michael P. Allswede, D.O.

Synopsis

9.1 Introduction

In the past, medical systems could be reasonably relied on to respond to disasters such as a fires, bombings, or floods through the community response planning process. However, chemical, biological, and radiological terrorism increases the burden on medical systems because recognition of insidious disease or unfamiliar syndromes is needed and rendering care for these victims may place the medical system and its personnel at risk through contamination of the facility. The threat of chemical and biological weapons create situations where crisis and consequence management must occur almost simultaneously. Information collection, analysis, decision-support, needed medications, and rapid surge in treatment capability must occur for the event to be accurately characterized and the victims saved. Chemical and biological events are recognized by the symptoms that they produce in victims. These symptoms must be discriminated from the background of normal disease. Because chemical and biological terrorism starts with ill victims, the medical system is the initial data collector and analyzer for disease recognition. The anthrax events of 2001 and 2002 were initially recognized within the medical system,[1] as was West Nile encephalitis,[2] and Hantavirus pulmonary syndrome.[3] In each of these events, the detection of the disease was made by medical personnel and the initial determination of whether the event was bioterrorism or not was based on medical judgment. With respect to events of terrorism on United States soil, all roads lead to the medical community. Despite these realities, the lead law enforcement agency, Federal Bureau of Investigation, and the overall manager of the event, the Department of Homeland Security, do not have a formal connection to the medical community. This chapter will deal primarily with the function of medical systems, the flow of information, and the decision making structures needed for improved response to chemical and biological threats.

Issues of privacy[4] and national security collide when medical events are converted to criminal investigations and issues of national security. Public health[5] is the designated organization responsible for managing infectious disease threats to the populace. Public health departments, however, are not law enforcement agencies and they do not provide the majority of patient care for ill victims. Epidemic investigation, quarantine, and preventative measures such as prophylaxis and vaccination are the primary mission of most public health departments within the US. Recent events of bioterrorism such as the anthrax events and numerous "white powder" incidents have strained the existing system, often to its limits.[6] Though the FBI is the designated lead federal agency to investigate and determine the criminal aspects of bioterrorism, there exists very little formal connection between the FBI and clinical medicine. The creation of parallel but separate criminal and epidemiological investigations is not a prudent strategy.[7] Rather, integration of epidemiological and criminal investigation with inclusion of the medical community would place the maximum data at the hands of decision-makers.

Should a natural outbreak, chemical spill, chemical weapons attack, or bioterrorism event occur, the key questions are:

- How should an event of chemical or biological terrorism be detected?
- What are the resources needed to contend with the event?
- How should medical systems prepare for terrorism?
- How should an event of chemical or biological terrorism be reported?
- What safeguards are there for privacy?
- How should the event be investigated?
- How can the national security be maintained and improved?

The following chapter will develop these seven questions and suggest a method of rational integration of the medical community in the management of terrorism. Specific recommendations will be made for application and usage by the reader.

9.2 How Should an Event of Chemical or Biological Terrorism Be Detected?

A. Chemical terrorism

Chemical terrorism refers to the use of toxic chemicals to disrupt normal society functions and to sicken or kill victims within the zone of release. Chemical weapon attacks differ from chemical spills by the intent of the terrorist, the use of dissemination devices, and the choice of chemical for maximum impact. There are thousands of chemicals that are toxic to man, but the common "war agents" are

- organophosphate nerve agents like sarin,
- vesicants like mustard,
- chemical asphyxiates like cyanide,
- pulmonary irritants like phosgene, and
- and riot control agents like teargas.

Except for nerve agents, the chemical war agents have distinctive odors, or produce distinctive physiologic signs and symptoms. The discussion of specific chemical weapons will occur in other chapters of this text.

While there are many instances of chemical agents being used during World War I and in various conflicts since, the most instructive example for US preparedness is the use of sarin by the Aum Shinrikyo in 1994 and again in 1995. The sarin attack in Matsumoto in 1994 and in the Tokyo subway in 1995 each created a significant influx of victims prior to accurate information from the scene. Most of the victims were minimally exposed and needed no medical treatment to survive, but some required hospitalizations and aggressive care. Due to a general lack of familiarity with nerve agents, this care was either delayed or insufficiently aggressive until physicians were educated during the ongoing crisis. In addition, up to 23 percent of the hospital staff was contaminated with sarin by the victims and became incapacitated.[8]

Should an organophosphate nerve agent be released into a U.S. city, would the U.S. medical system respond differently? Cholinergic symptoms, such as those produced by sarin, are unusual in the day to day practice of medicine. Without some "just in time" information or references, it is likely that some similar delays would occur. Delays in diagnosis would produce similar delays in protective measures and in decontamination. To be designated as a fully functional emergency department, U.S. medical facilities must possess a decontamination room. The intent of this room is to wash a contaminated victim and to prevent secondary contamination of the medical staff and facility; however the state or readiness of most medical personnel with respect to decontamination and proper use of personal protective equipment is suspect. This decontamination room will typically service a single victim at a time which is sufficient for small volume chemical spills and accidents. The release of a war agent however may produce hundreds or thousands of victims, rendering the single service room insufficient. For these reasons, the medical facilities most accessible to the public would likely become overrun if a chemical weapon was released on a populated venue.

Chemical testing devices do exist to detect various chemical weapons and can be used by staff familiar with the testing devices. The conduct of the test and interpretation of the results is outside the typical scope of practice for most medical facilities and therefore may cause confusion due to the cross reactivity of many common compounds with chemical weapons detection systems. In addition, there is generally an inverse relationship between speed and accuracy in testing materials. While reference laboratory testing may be important for evidentiary purposes, rapid patient symptom recognition and decision-support information geared to the probable agent class is most efficient.

> **Recommendation**. U.S. medical facilities must expand training of emergency personnel to include recognition, protection, decontamination, triage and treatment of chemical weapons syndromes.

B. Biological terrorism

Biological weapons are used to intentionally spread disease causing microbes and toxins. They produce disease that may be nondescript, as in the initial flu-like illness associated with anthrax, or they may cause clearly abnormal disease presentations like the descending paralysis associated with botulinum toxicity. From the medical detection perspective, there are three basic characteristic available to the clinician to differentiate bioterrorism associated disease from background illness. The three characteristics are

- detecting case clusters,
- syndrome recognition, and
- abnormal test results

Detecting a case cluster refers to the observation of a nonspecific disease pattern occurring in a greater than expected frequency among people of a given demographic. Terrorists are associated with victims by ideological disagreements, or by the victim's attendance at a targeted venue. Because clinicians are focused on patient care, not observation of trends, the ability to detect case clusters should be augmented by using some form of syndromic surveillance. Syndromic surveillance can be a simple as reviewing the daily log of patients seen, or as complex as dedicated computer systems.[9]

Syndromic detection strategies are somewhat limited for a number of reasons. Among the more significant limitations of syndromic surveillance are the following; the data monitored is nonspecific, and may be deidentified due to privacy concerns; individuals who are ill, but who do not seek medical attention, or seek alternative treatments are not monitored; natural variations in disease presentation are a challenge as other factors influence disease occurrence such as ill family members and friends, communal living, and mass transit; and lastly, syndromic detection systems only compare the number of ill individuals to relative historical averages, not the total population served. Changes in population will change the number of ill individuals presenting to healthcare facilities. Thus, case cluster detection must also have some form of directed clinical investigations to support or refute the trends in syndromic data. That stated, once a given syndrome is detected, syndromic surveillance processes can greatly enhance the characterization of a infectious outbreak. Case-finding and determination of the scale of the event are key components of response and an electronic syndromic data system can be a significant aid to these tasks.

Disease recognition refers either to definitive case presentations or an unusually severe disease that warrants further work up. The index case of anthrax in 2001 was Bob Stevens of American Media,[10] who presented with unusually severe meningitis that was later proven to be anthrax related. The detection of these cases rests on alert and astute clinicians, with appropriate laboratory backup. Because many bioterrorism diseases are also naturally occurring diseases, the detection of an unusual syndrome should initiate a coordinated epidemiological and law enforcement investigation.[11] The recovery of bioterrorism related microbes from routine culture, or the presentation of unusual test findings is the last method of medical detection. The culture of *Yersinia pestis,* the causative bacteria of plague, from the lungs of a person with pneumonia would be an indicator that the pneumonia may be evidence of bioterrorism. Because plague can also occur naturally in rare cases,[12] bioterrorism must be considered and investigated along with the infectious nature of the disease.

The clinical detection of bioterrorism is clearly imperfect and requires a number of seldom used associations.[13] It should be noted that the role of law enforcement intelligence may be significant in determining the proper response to a worrisome medical anomaly that has yet to be characterized. Knowledge about given targets or likely attack scenarios in association with medical anomalies can be used to guide crisis decisions. Intelligence from law enforcement can potentially identify likely agents, likely target demographics, likely targets and venues of attack, and likely timeframes for an attack to occur. Combining intelligence with clinical indicators is probably the strongest detection strategy for bioterrorism.

Recommendation. The U.S. medical system should develop active interfaces between public health and law enforcement to speed recognition, and improve accuracy of bioterrorism detection.

9.3. What Resources Are Needed to Contend with the Event?

A. Chemical terrorism

One of the greater challenges of a medical facility in responding to a chemical weapon attack is the prevention of contamination. It is likely that the initial victims of a chemical weapon attack will arrive without warning or scene information, and potentially contaminate the medical facility. Thus, medical facilities must be able to respond by limiting access, enforcing decontamination, and surety testing those victims admitted to the facility. By limiting access, a facility may opt to initially deny entry to the contaminated victims until the facility can be configured for decontamination. This response may seem a bit irresponsible, but it may not be. The medical facility has an obligation to its staff and existing patients not to contaminate them. The victims presenting early from a scene are largely those individuals who are minimally exposed and do not need extrication of scene resuscitation. Often, the treatment for minimally exposed chemical casualties is fresh air. Last, if the staff and the facility become contaminated, medical resources are removed and victims are added.

Once properly configured, the medical facility should decontaminate the victims with surety testing. Surety testing refers to the assurance of complete decontamination and the absence of any chemical residue. Gaseous or vapor exposures cause minimal exterior contamination and the individual is most efficiently decontaminated by disrobing. Liquid or solid chemical exposure requires more significant cleansing of the skin surfaces and may be related to more significant exposures. Given the large number of potential victims, significant thought must be given to the ability to engage mass decontamination. Some strategies include; augmentation of hospital capacity by local hazardous material teams, augmentation of hospital capacity by purchasing additional tents or other structures, and making physical changes to the medical facility entrance to ensure no contaminated victim may enter inadvertently. Given the potential deployment of hazardous materials teams during a crisis, it is most wise that the medical facility develop larger volume decontamination capability.

> **Recommendation.** U.S. Medical facilities must improve decontamination facilities to accommodate larger numbers of victims.

Once victims are decontaminated, the next challenge is to triage and deliver medical treatment. An open air gaseous or vapor exposure causes a larger number of minimally exposed victims relative to severely exposed victims due to the dilution of the contaminated air. In contrast, the same amount of contamination within a structure could produce a larger number of severe exposures due to the containment of the contaminated air and its recirculation. A structural contamination can be expected to generate more significant exposures than an open air for this reason, as well as the movement of structure inhabitants and elevators.

Some chemical weapons have specific antidotes such as organophosphate nerve agents and cyanide. Other chemical weapons have no antidotes, such as pulmonary agents, and require only supportive measures. If a hospital stocks antidotal medications for chemical weapons, the volume of medications is probably insufficient to care for a large number of victims because most incidents involving chemical exposure of this sort are small volume industrial or home accidents.

Urban EMS systems now, typically, carry a small amount of antidotes intended for use by the EMS crew in the event of inadvertent exposure. Antidotes for victims are often stockpiled in central locations for ease of inventory control and security. This "stockpile strategy" emphasizes EMS provider care and administrative maintenance but does not maximize victim care. For this reason, a "disseminated strategy" is employed by the US military in which every soldier or sailor carries a potentially lifesaving dosage of medication. This strategy has also been applied to civilian response in Israel with rather minimal health effects.[14] The correct strategy depends on the event with larger events, more frequent events, and more toxic compounds favoring a disseminated strategy.

Regardless of strategy, rapidly available education must also be provided to the treating individual as antidotes are seldom-used medications, or medications used in doses different from their common usage. For these reasons, antidote stockpiles should be accompanied with decision-support material that can be easily disseminated. Figure 9.1 is taken from the RaPiD-T Program.[15] RaPiD-T is the educational and management tool for the city of Pittsburgh EMS and the University of Pittsburgh Medical Center.

Recommendation. Antidotal stockpiles and associated decision-support tools be readily available to medical and EMS systems preparing for chemical terrorism.

Recommendation. Consideration should be given to disseminated antidote strategy with educational material for higher severity and frequency threat areas.

B. Biological terrorism

If one were to believe the media, bioterrorism can occur by releasing smallpox or anthrax in a stadium resulting in thousands or hundreds of thousands of dead and dying.[16] While these scenarios are motivating for certain, there has not been a single instance of that level of attack succeeding.[17] The anthrax events of 2001 for example were a small volume, tightly targeted attack more resembling assassination attempts than a population based attack.[18] Although initially lumped together with al-Qa'eda, the anthrax terrorist actually provided the opportunity to prevent deaths from anthrax by the use of a letter that correctly defined the anthrax pathogen and suggested appropriate antibiotic therapy. The terrorist actually aided the authorities by taking the detection problem away.[19] Twenty-two individuals developed some form of anthrax, five died, but the number of treated individuals is estimated to be 10,000–20,000.[20] Consider for a moment, how much more difficult the fall–winter of 2001 would have been for healthcare systems had the attack been larger or anonymous. Who was exposed? Where were they exposed? Who needs treatment? Which flu is anthrax and which is not? The inability to answer these questions, the disorganization of response, and the resultant panic would have caused significantly more social problems and potentially more deaths.

In responding to bioterrorism, the scale of the attack and the time of detection of the attack are critical components. For example; the mortality of those who acted on the anthrax exposure at the time of the receipt of the letter had a 0-percent death rate from anthrax, but those who waited for a

Organophosphate Nerve Poisons

Recognition: **Vapor** Miosis — **Liquid** Fasciculations, sweating
Protection: Level C minimum
Decontamination: 0.5% hypochlorite
Triage: Based on symptom complex as depicted below

Severity	Vapor-onset in 1–2 minutes	Liquid-onset in several minutes
Mild	miosis, rhinorrhea, dim vision,	local fasciculations, local sweating
Moderate	all above with nausea, vomiting	all above with nausea, vomiting
Severe	convulsions, apnea, death	convulsions, apnea, death

Treatment: Based on triage category as depicted below

Severity	Vapor	Liquid
Mild	observation only	2 mg atropine, 600mg 2-PAM, observation
Moderate	2 mg atropine, 600 mg 2-PAM, observation	2–4 mg atropine, 600–1,200 mg 2-PAM observation
Severe	6 mg atropine, 1,800 mg 2-PAM, 10 mg Diazepam	6 mg atropine, 1,800 mg 2-PAM, 10 mg, Diazepam

The now-infamous sarin gas belongs to the group of super toxic organophosphate compounds, termed "nerve agents." Included in this group are the following compounds: **tabun** (designated GA), **sarin** (designated GB), **soman** (designated GD), and **VX**. The nerve agent compounds are odorless and tasteless, and are readily absorbed through the skin, or by inhalation. They are highly toxic by either route. When inhaled, toxicity is determined by a concentration time product in which the milligram concentration per cubic meter is multiplied by the time of contact. Sarin, for example, has a LCt_{50} of 100 mg-min/m^3. This means that 50-percent mortality is achieved when adult subjects are exposed to 100 mg total exposure. It is important to recognize that the cumulative dose may be achieved by inspiring a low concentration for a longer period of time. It is this feature of nerve agent toxicity that mandates decontamination. In the Tokyo example, a significant number of health personnel were overcome by breathing the vapor contained on victims clothing. Simply disrobing the patients, and setting up a triage post in open air would have alleviated a number of casualties.

Nerve agents are liquids at room temperature and have relatively low vapor pressures. Sarin (GB) is the most volatile at 2 mm Hg, which is similar to water's vapor pressure. The photo to the left demonstrates the physical appearance of common chemical weapons. Note that the compound is an oily brownish liquid. When heated, as in the Matsumoto incident, sarin will come out of solution at a faster rate and produce a highly toxic concentration of agent. The nerve agents are also about four times heavier than air so they collect in low-lying areas. The Tokyo subway attack utilized this property by allowing the unheated vapor to accumulate in the lower reaches of the subway with obvious lethal consequences. The other "G" nerve agents are less volatile than sarin and the agent VX is only considered a contact risk. It is important to note that some of the victims of the subway attack included individuals who attempted to pick up the packets of agent and sustained a subsequent liquid exposure. Liquid exposure presents its own problems in management as the agent VX could be laid down at a location prior to occupation by the intended victims. An understanding of the effect the route of exposure has on the presentation of the clinical toxidrome is critical to the management of the victim.

The toxic effects of nerve agent compounds are achieved through the inhibition of acetylcholinesterase, and the subsequent over-stimulation of the acetylcholine receptor. Muscarinic, nicotinic, and CNS subtypes of receptors are affected. Muscarinic receptors, when stimulated, increase the activity of salivary glands, lacrimal glands, smooth muscle, and pupillary constriction (miosis). The muscarinic syndrome is best remembered by the SLUDGE acronym; S (salivation), L (lacrimation), U (urination), D (diarrhea/diaphoresis), G (general weakness), E (emesis). Of specific concern for medical personnel is the effect upon bronchial smooth muscle and bronchial mucous glands. Nicotinic receptors are found primarily on skeletal muscle as well as certain ganglia, most significantly, the adrenal medulla. Stimulation of nicotinic receptors results in fasciculation and ultimate paralysis of the affected skeletal muscle. The CNS effects of these compounds are sedation, seizure, apnea, and ultimate death.

***Figure 9.1** Selected portion of RaPiD-T manual*

hospital diagnosis had a 70-percent death rate.[21] As America invests in detection technology with better intelligence analysis,[22] biosensors,[23] and syndromic detection,[24] medical interventions will change and survivorship will be increased as bioterrorism is detected earlier. Detection of a bioterrorism attack may occur prior to release (through law enforcement and intelligence services), at the time of release (as in the anthrax cases), at the time of nonspecific symptom occurrence in the exposed population (by a syndromic detection system), at the time of hospital diagnosis of ill individuals, or at the time of deaths or epidemic occurrence. Unfortunately, prior to the events of last fall, detection of unusual disease events occurred only *after* deaths of the intended victims, if at all.[25]

Pre-Release	*Release*	*Symptom Occurrence*	*Illness Occurrence*	*Deaths/Epidemic*
X	X	X	X	X

The time at which disease detection occurs will alter the possible actions of the hospital or healthcare system. Prophylaxis, for example, would be of primary importance early in the timeline, but wane in its effectiveness later in the timeline. The size of a quarantine effort would also markedly change the later on the timeline one detects the bioterrorism event, thus timeline and scale may interact.

A model for quantification of a healthcare system response to bioterrorism should include both scalar effects and timeline of detection. The critical actions and priorities of a hospital or medical system will be primarily effected by these two assessments, as much as pathogen identification. A representative matrix, termed "the Pittsburgh Matrix"[26] after the location of its development, characterizes medical response to bioterrorism by combining these two variables as seen in Figure 9.2

"Current Capacity" would be defined by that number of victims that a hospital or system could absorb without altering normal operations. "Surge Capacity" refers to maximal crisis mode capacity. "Augmented Capacity" refers to capacity derived with external resources, and "Above all Capacity" refers to "battlefield" triage in which maximum good is done for the maximum number.

As a hospital or healthcare system adds resources in terms of better organization and increased capacity, a given numerical scenario will be plotted successively lower on the vertical access. Early recognition and

Above all Capacity					
Augmented Capacity					
Surge Capacity					
Current Capacity					
	Pre Release	Release	Symptom Occurrence	Illness Occurrence	Epidemic

Figure 9.2 *The Pittsburg Matrix*

good early decision-making can move a given scenario from right to left on the horizontal access. Poor decision-making and inadequate planning will move the scenario management to the upper right. Mortality can be expected to increase by moving up and rightward on the matrix.

Specific resources apply well in certain cells and for certain pathogens but not in others. For example, stockpiling oral antibiotics for anthrax is useful in the Release and Symptom Occurrence columns, but loses its effectiveness after severe illness occurs. Likewise, education of physicians to recognize bioterrorism related diseases is only effective after the disease is recognizable in the illness column.

The confusion of fall–winter 2001 can largely be explained by the supposition on the part of most leaders that we were preparing for a "Deaths/Epidemic-Triage of Resources" problem when in fact we were in the "Release-Current Capacity" cell. As a decision support tool, each box can be constructed to contain critical decision and resources identified along with agent specific recommendations.

Hospitals don't take care of matrix cells; they take care of real patients with real infections. Pathogens have a multitude of characteristics that are of medical relevance, but from the planning and response perspective, the three primary concerns are:

Communicability and quarantine needs. This agent characteristic defines quarantine and isolation needs for not only patients but also exposed but asymptomatic individuals. This is a critical characteristic as quarantine will be a difficult civic-medical effort.

Effectiveness of medical treatment. Some bioterrorism diseases are not amenable to treatment, others have unproven treatments, and others have highly effective treatments. The urgency of pharmaceutical intervention and staff can be determined by this analysis. Example: Botulism treatment must be given prior to symptom onset to be effective.

Availability of medical treatment. Certain bioterrorism agents have obscure treatments available only in small amounts. Examples may be antitoxins, heavy metal chelators, or vaccines. The availability of a given treatment may potentially change management strategy from treatment to palliation.

Using a tool like the Pittsburgh Matrix, an accurate assessment of the primary difficulties in managing communicability, effectiveness of treatments, and availability supplies and space can be mapped to matrix cells by the system preparing for the event. By identifying gaps or shortfalls within a cell, improving preparedness on the local level is possible. Armed with these matrices, it is possible for a hospital or medical system to rapidly identify critical needs, estimate casualties, as well as predict future needs as time progresses. By combining mortality expected within each cell, the value in terms of lives saved per dollar spent can be estimated for new detection technologies such as syndromic surveillance technology, or deploying bio-aerosol detectors in various scenarios involving real agents and real events. The value of pre-emptive law enforcement interdiction, a vaccination program, or a new medication can also be evaluated in similar fashion.

Recommendation. Resource planning must be coordinated with an overall understanding of bioterrorism in both timeline of detection and scale of response.

Recommendation. Resource planning for bioterrorism must consist of a "defense in depth" with multiple options and strategies for each stage of the epidemic.

9.4. How Should Medical Systems Prepare for Terrorism?

An old adage in medicine is "The eye does not see what the mind does not know." The purpose of educating the mind is to recognize disease, but most chemical and biological weapons agents are not part of a medical education. There is a need for integrated, sustainable, comprehensive educational process for clinical practitioners in addition to providing them with new resources. Medical facilities must train their personnel on how to use new decontamination systems, access stockpiles of medications, and treat unfamiliar illness. New skills are needed.

Disaster drills have been used in the past to practice mass care, but that care is largely within the normal practice of medicine. While there are a number of good training courses available on chemical and biological weapons, how personnel adapt that knowledge and apply it in practice remains a challenge. Hospitals function like a ship underway, with every person having an assigned job. In times of crisis, additional personnel are added and more work is accomplished. A hospital can not stop its daily work to train for a disaster. When confronted with the need for additional drilling, some hospitals choose to spend money on additional staffing for drill players. While this strategy allows unencumbered drill play, it is expensive and for many hospitals, training a shift at a time is inefficient use of money, time, and personnel. Other hospitals ask for volunteers to avoid the expense of drill pay. While volunteerism is laudable, it only trains those who volunteer for training. This lack of comprehensive approach to training may show the hospital disaster function at its best, but it does not give an accurate picture of how the hospital would function under normal circumstances. Still other hospitals refuse to participate in a disaster drill because they are focused, and paid to do their healthcare jobs, not to treat moulage patients.

No matter what skills may be taught during a disaster drill, they will degrade in time if not used. A key component to responding to high consequence but low frequency events is practice. In the case of caring for victims of hazardous materials events, rendering care in protective gear is an entirely new experience for many. In addition, heat stress, claustrophobia, and attenuation of the senses are just a few challenges of working with personal protective gear. Though blood and body fluid infection control methods are common practice in the U.S., management of airborne pathogens is not. These skills must be reinforced if the hospital is to respond efficiently on the day of the event.

Recommendation. Develop a sustainable educational program focused not only on chemical and biological weapons, but also application of that knowledge to hospital operations.

Recommendation. Develop a sustainable skill acquisition program focused on training unique new skill sets for response to chemical and biological weapons.

A model training program would be sustainable, focused on individual jobs, contain skill acquisition and knowledge acquisition strategies, and have associated knowledge retention tools. Fortunately, most medical practitioners have periodic continuing medical educational (CME) requirements. By adding new skills and knowledge to the ongoing CME process, all can benefit from the training, not just those who participate in the drills. A model of skill acquisition, taken from military training programs is the FAPV (familiarize, acquire, practice and validate) sequence. This is similar to the "crawl, walk, and run" euphemism that often characterizes training efforts.

Familiarization with new knowledge and skills should maximize ease of access for the student. Smaller units of knowledge, testing, and evaluation that one could accomplish during downtime, or on a training day may work better than a larger and more comprehensive program. Distance learning is ideal for this sort of knowledge dissemination. Acquisition of skills requires experiential component. A "training room" experience in which the student wears protective garments, and uses equipment is the goal. An example of a training room experience is the cardiopulmonary resuscitation training in which a mannequin is used to acquire skills. Medical simulation is in its early development but holds significant promise in this area. An opportunity to practice the new knowledge and skills can be created by standard drilling. Validation of response can be assessed in real events, or by using unannounced drills. By developing an educational strategy for new knowledge and skill acquisition and by integrating with existing educational programs, the entire staff performance can not only be improved, it can also be measured.

Recommendation. Integrate new training methods with existing educational programming to create a sustainable and general improvement in personal response to chemical or biological weapons response.

Finally, most U.S. medical facilities are private businesses that employ private citizens for medical jobs. In response to a chemical or biological event, personnel of a medical facility may become alarmed by caring for potentially hazardous patients. Also, should the event alarm the community, one's concerns may be with one's dependents. The choice between professional duty, personal safety, and responsibility to dependents is a difficult one. It is important that some institutional guidance be given to those personnel who would be in that potential position. A family emergency plan is the base document that should be completed by the staff. In addition, some provision for caring for dependents must be made by the institution should a valuable staff member be equally needed at home. In a perfect situation, a sense of duty, purpose, and common bond should be instilled in employees to complete the medical mission despite its challenges. "Psychological immunization" of the workforce by outreach, and motivational programming is needed to mitigate the natural response to crisis.

Recommendation. Medical facilities engage employees in discussions of needs, and develop programs for employee support and motivation.

9.5 How Should an Event of Chemical or Biological Terrorism Be Reported?

Should an anomalous medical event occur and be recognized, the specifics and parameters of the event should be reported to the managing authorities. Specific characteristics of bioterrorism that should be scrutinized:

- **Medical inputs** would include
  - clusters of demographics within ill populations,
  - clusters of nonspecific disease that can be traced to a point of exposure,
  - disease recognition of bioterrorism pathogens, and
  - abnormal laboratory or testing results.

- **Law enforcement inputs** would include
  - likely victims as determined by annunciated threats,
  - likely venues as determined by threat analysis,

- likely timelines as determined by surveillance techniques, and
- likely agents as determined by threat analysis.

- **Public health inputs** would include
  - syndromic detection systems to include active and passive data collection, and
  - the National Laboratory Response System.

As previously stated, the FBI has jurisdiction of the law enforcement investigation, the public health authority has responsibility for the epidemiologic investigation, and the medical system has responsibility to care for the victims. Criminal and epidemiological investigations depend on medical information. There are many impediments to communication including medical privacy concerns, "need to know" thresholds for sharing intelligence, and institutional rivalry. The specific communication can be characterized by Figure 9.3.

Normal disease reporting is best characterized by the normal reporting of specific diseases to the public health authority by clinicians. Most of these reports consist of culture reports or definitive clinical diagnosis of disease submitted by clinicians to local public health authorities. The re-

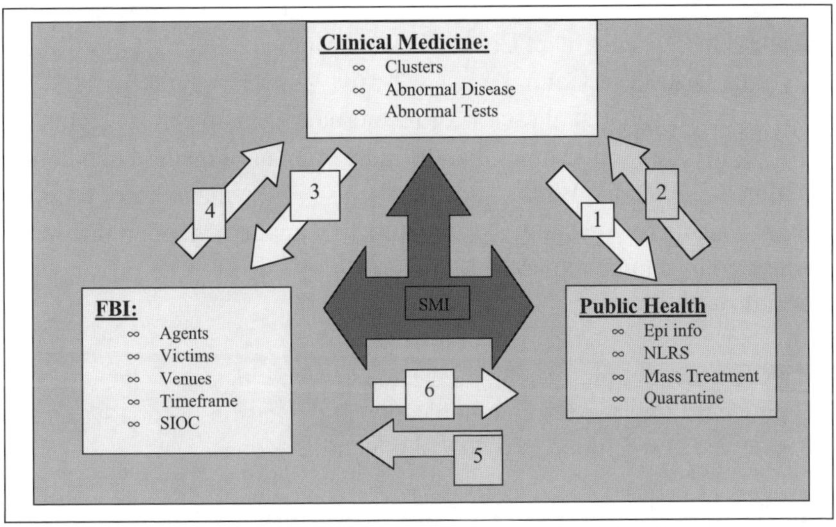

Figure 9.3 *1. Normal disease reporting; 2. public health advisement; 3. law enforcement reporting; 4. law enforcement investigations; 5–6. interagency communication*

porting system is often by the mail and events are recorded by hand. This laborious process is reasonable for nonserious disease or clearly recognizable disease, but may prove disastrously slow in times of infectious disease crisis.[27] Obtaining relevant, timely information has been an identified problem in most emerging diseases, most recently SARS.

Public health advisement in times of crisis has been somewhat problematic as there are multiple public health authorities that must coordinate to send a uniform message. Public health authority is highly irregular across the United States and manifests as city departments of public health, county department of public health, state departments of public health, and various federal agencies to include the CDC, the Surgeon General, and the Office of Emergency Preparedness of the Health and Human Services Department.

Because of the irregular reporting of clinical disease, a certain level of ignorance of bioterrorism detection criteria, and the irregular public health authority, bioterrorism and emerging disease detection and decision-making is not standardized. For example, the agencies and organizations involved in the U.S. Capitol anthrax response included: U.S. Capital Police, Architect of the U.S. Capitol, Sergeant at Arms, U.S. Senate, Office of the Attending Physician of the U.S. Senate, FBI, EPA, CDC, DARPA, HHS, NIOSH, USAMRIID, FEMA, the U.S. Coast Guard, U.S. Marines CBIRF, District of Columbia Department of Health, Office of the Mayor of District of Columbia, U.S. Army, U.S. Navy, and the U.S. Air Force.[28] Further, a casual review of recent bioterrorism and emerging infectious disease events shows that the most often used method of communication is the media. While laudable, the use of the media prior to information sharing by the major stakeholders in management of an infectious disease crisis can be expected to increase confusion, erode privacy, and alarm the public.

Recommendation. The FBI, public health authorities, and clinical medicine must improve the communication and decision-making systems to evaluate and respond to potential infectious events.

9.6 What Safeguards Are There for Privacy?

Reporting of relevant medical information to the FBI is, at present, not governed by any statute or regulation. Instead, there are conflicting regulations that both mandate the reporting of infectious threats to the community, and protect patient privacy.[29] Clinical medicine is restrained in the sharing of clinical data by the Health Insurance Portability and Accountability Act of 1996 (HIPAA). HIPAA was intended to guide medical systems in the routine processing of medical information, not to guide the institution through a bioterrorism crisis response. For example, HIPAA allows the sharing of health information with the FBI under subpoena. To generate a subpoena, the FBI must first generate suspicion that a biocrime has been committed. For this, they must have a reporting structure to receive concerns of the medical community. HIPAA creates a circular logic for the investigation of bio-crimes.

In response to the need for new models of information sharing, the Model State Emergency Health Powers Act[30] (MSEHPA) has created a framework under which information-sharing should be regulated. Specific responsibilities, authority, and constraints must be analyzed for this communication to occur for each of the stakeholders.

- Define **responsibilities** of clinical medicine, public health authorities, and the FBI for use and sharing of data and decision-making.
- Define **authority** of clinical medicine, public health authorities, and FBI for use and sharing of data and decision-making.
- Define **constraints** on clinical medicine, public health authorities, and FBI for use and sharing of medical and intelligence data.

Though not yet in force in the U.S. and opposed by those representing privacy concerns, this analytical construct may prove useful in constructing new legislation to guide and support the sharing of information to determine the nature of infectious disease emergencies, and to guide the roles and responsibilities of the managing authorities. Because of the potential impact of bioterrorism, national executive authority can be expected to be invoked should a significant crisis occur. Thresholds for application of the HIPAA, MSEHPA, and National Command Authority are not well explored and, in practice, will be strongly tied to the context of the event. A suspicious medical anomaly may be treated differently if it occurs at a highly contentious political event such as the United Nations or a political convention.

Just as important as concerns for rapid detection and public safety, are concerns for privacy of the individual. Unregulated reporting of potential bioterrorism in the media "in the public interest" by concerned officials and medical providers has caused examples of privacy violations.

The Council for Excellence in Government has explored the views of the public in this area[31] and found that the public is willing to undergo intrusions of privacy in exchange for safety if the perceived threat is high.

- Sixty-five percent of Americans are satisfied with the government's job protecting civil liberties.
- Only 14 percent of Americans trust the government to use private information appropriately.
- Fifty-six percent of Americans believe that the Patriot Act is good for America.
- Thirty-three percent of Americans believe that the Patriot Act is bad for America.
- Confidence in local emergency responders to provide homeland security is 73 percent.
- Confidence in the FBI to fight terrorism is 49 percent.
- Confidence in the federal government as a whole to provide homeland security is 13 percent.

These various data points indicate that while the federal authorities have funding and strategic direction responsibilities, the local assets are where the public places its trust. For this reason, it is imperative that critical information be obtained, shared, and preserved by the managing FBI, public health authorities, and clinical medicine professionals.

9.7 How Should the Event Be Investigated?

The investigation of chemical and bioterrorism can take two forms. First and best from the perspective of the public interest is pre-event detection. Pre-event detection refers to detection and interdiction of a bioterrorism event prior to the exposure of the target population. Pre-event detection can take the form of surveillance of terrorist cells, "hardening"[32] of target venues, and detecting small medical events that indicate manufacture or acquisition of chemical or biological agents.

Because chemical and biological weapons are toxic or infectious in minute amounts, and because terrorist cells must produce, store, and transport these weapons in clandestine manner under austere conditions, there is potential that small spills, leaks, and inadvertent releases can be detected by monitoring culture results, unusual toxidromes, and perhaps the health of the terrorists themselves.

Like medical reporting of child abuse, spousal abuse, elder abuse, homicidal and suicidal ideation, the reporting of unusual medical events or significant medical events in potential terrorists is in the public interest. The seminal work in this area is detailed in the *Tarasoff* laws[33] in which the physician has a clear and proscribed "duty to warn" the public of imminent danger. While medical findings of abuse or psychiatric cases are well defined and taught to clinicians, and the reporting structures are well-defined and include "whistle-blower" protections to the reporting physician, medical terrorism markers are largely unexplored. Some events that would fall into this category would include

- unexplained blast injury indicating bomb-making,
- unexplained toxidromes of known chemical weapons agents,
- unexplained culture results of known biological weapons agents,
- unexplained findings of radiation illness, and
- unusual cluster of illness in known terrorist cells.

Should a medical terrorism marker occur, it may be unnoticed by an uneducated or overly busy physician. If recognized by a concerned physician, there is no clear reporting mechanism. By following the *Tarasoff*-defined "duty to warn" the reporting individual may have violated HIPAA statutes depending on the eventual finding of the investigation. Finally, it is also a concern that in times of national crisis, physicians may unwittingly report medical information inappropriately in their zeal to guard the public interest during times of attack.

Medical markers of terrorism must also be interpreted correctly by public health authorities and the FBI. It is not clear that either organization has an understanding of how to relate medical findings to syndromic data or intelligence data and how to share in that analysis. Should a concern be elevated due to corroborating threat information and medical or public health data, what is the most prudent course of action? Seemingly drastic responses such a quarantine, or rapid law enforcement interdiction may be lifesaving if employed prior to the spread of disease or execution of a planned attack. Political concerns of these decisions must be weighed not only in their medical context, but also in their political impact. Typically, elected officials are more cautious and require greater surety that a given action is correct if the action will be seen as disruptive to the electorate.

> **Recommendation**. Reporting of medical markers indicating terrorism must be supported by legal statutes and formalized similar to abuse reporting.

The second approach to investigation is reactive, in which an event has occurred to which the medical system must recognize and respond. Reactive investigation is primarily directed at characterizing the event and investigating its public health and criminal potential. Chemical weapons generally exert their symptoms rapidly; therefore the detection issue is less complex as victims emerge from a venue with similar symptoms. Testing for chemical weapons is now available in most hazardous materials teams.

Biological events, particularly discriminating bioterrorism from an emerging disease is more difficult. In past events, there has typically been a significant delay between the detection of a medical anomaly, and the accurate and complete characterization of the event. The New York West Nile outbreak for example took six weeks to fully characterize.[34] The interim time was fraught with confusion and misstatements. Intentional terrorism in which larger numbers of victims are exposed is considerably more difficult to characterize.

Investigations of a bioterrorism event must proceed simultaneously down several avenues. Medical investigations include the laboratory evaluation of the pathogen to include antibiotic resistance, the response of victims to treatment, the development of a "case definition" for unknown diseases, and analysis of virulence features. The medical assets needed to care for the victims must be estimated and recruited. Public health authorities must survey the event to determine the epidemiological cause, and the current size of the event. Victim location is a key for medical asset estimation and public heath authorities have the mandate for this aspect.

Further the movement of national stockpiles, the development of mass treatment guidelines, and reference laboratory capability reside in the various levels of the public health system. The FBI must determine if the medical outbreak could be a crime and if so, collect sufficient evidence to identify and apprehend the perpetrators and guide national command authority. Potentially this investigation may lead to national command authority action and result in military action.

The longer an event remains undetected, or under appreciated, the more difficult will be the eventual investigation and response. Speed and accuracy are essential for all investigations, but thresholds for the determination of event character and potential decisions are not well defined. A few sample questions would be:

- How is disease determined to be bioterrorism or an emerging disease?
- If two or more diseases are occurring in a population, are how are they both managed?
- Can medical facilities, which are largely private businesses, be compelled to care for hazardous infectious patients by public health authority?
- Can physicians, who are private citizens, be compelled to care for hazardous infections patients by the public health authority?
- Can private citizens be compelled to receive medical care against their wishes by public health authority?
- Who will manage civic unrest if infectious disease is threatening a community?
- Who determines who must be quarantined or treated, where they will be quarantined or treated, and what shall be the proper use of force for those resisting detention or treatment?

Forced quarantine has in the past resulted in civil unrest.[35] Quarantine has been inappropriately applied and has resulted in deaths.[36] Though we have yet to encounter bioterrorism challenges of this nature, imagine for a moment the anthrax events of 2001 and 2002 without the annunciated threat letter. If the anthrax terrorist used the spores to contaminate a mall, or airport, or stadium, these decisions may have confronted us and the resultant lack of organization[37] may have been disastrous.

Recommendation. Create structures to share information and decision-making must be developed to include public health, the FBI, local medical leaders, and political leadership to coordinate key decisions and assessments of potential terrorist events.

9.8 How Can the National Security Be Maintained and Improved?

The Japanese word for "crisis" is composed of two pictograms read vertically, one for "danger," the other for "opportunity." This poignant combination of meanings is particularly applicable in describing the current United States' preparation for bioterrorism. We all agree that we face a new danger in the potential of bioterrorism within our borders in the hands of terrorists. However, bioterrorism for all its great potential has only been responsible for five deaths in the last year. Bioterrorism represents our current national crisis, but we have been afforded the opportunity to prepare the great resources of this nation prior to a more adept application of bioterrorism.

A key feature of our preparedness efforts must be to better understand and characterize the specific responsibilities and duties of the key stakeholders. No single entity holds the solution to terrorism challenges, but together, medical, public health, and law enforcement entities can combine to create a "defense in depth." Defense in depth refers to specific strategies employed by specific entities or organizations to mitigate specific threats. Roughly separated, the stages of defense and their attendant strategies are summarized by the following.

- **Pre-event detection and mitigation**. The FBI and intelligence agencies must be augmented in their detection mission by appropriate sharing of medical indicators of terrorism and public health surveillance for maximum effectiveness for pre-event interdiction.
- **Release detection and venue protection**. Technology based detection systems and facility hardening should be deployed at high value venues by facility and municipal safety officers.
- **Symptomatic recognition strategy**. Public health surveillance of nonspecific disease trends must be coordinated with directed medical investigations to determine at the earliest possible moment the presence of an unusual disease or syndrome. These findings must be

corroborated to intelligence services and coordinated management plans developed between political leaders, the FBI, public health, and clinical medical leadership.

- **Disease recognition strategy**. Training physicians to recognize unusual diseases or toxidromes must be supported and needed antidotes and medications stockpiled in accessible locations for maximal utility and lifesaving. Critical decisions involving mass treatment and control of the population must be coordinated with public health authorities, law enforcement and political leadership.

To manage this defense in depth strategy, a focused flexible system of local management is optimal. The components of such a system are surveillance, monitoring, reporting, synthesis, analysis, and response. Due to the highly technical nature of each component, it is not efficient to train every physician, medical facility, or public health official to a high degree of competence. It is however necessary to train a smaller group or team to respond to these challenges.[38] This team would respond to local threat changes and national threat levels by deploying different threat-based strategies for detection and response. Should a concerning finding occur, corroboration and analysis would be initially performed by this group and reported to the stakeholder communities. Strategy and decision-making would then ensue and incorporate local, state and federal partners as indicated. Response would be coordinated in similar manner. Early detection, systematic preparations, and a defense in depth strategy are the key needs in developing a better system to respond to chemical and biological terrorism.

Recommendation. Adopt a systematic approach to preparedness that is focused on increasing local competence in detection, evaluation and response to terrorist threats.

9.9 Conclusion

If terrorism could be reasonably relied on to produce a few victims per year, as bad as that would be, terrorism management would not be a priority. However, chemical and biological terrorism has the capability to overwhelm our resources and alter the course of this nation and potentially the world. Taking well reasoned steps toward preparedness is the responsibility of medical systems and providers. Strengthening local medial systems will create better detection and response capability. Local action will make the nation safer, one community at a time.

In the development of a competent, flexible, system of making informed decisions to manage bioterrorism, the medical systems must understand its role in the recognition of these threats, the protection of its staff and patients, the need for nontraditional operations like decontamination, and finally train and guide its staff in the management of chemical and biological weapons events. This challenge takes resources and committed leadership, but is also requires the ability to characterize the new challenges and to create new organizational structure.

Similar to the intelligence community, information sharing under HIPAA has largely been governed by a "need to know" rationale. "Need to know" refers to the general lack of information sharing unless it is determined that an individual has a need for that information. As this nation prepares for terrorist threats, information sharing will become a key for good decision-making. A "need to share" paradigm should be adopted in which key bioterrorism or chemical terrorism related information must be shared under proper controls. Shared information and decision making are in the best interest of the nation.

Endnotes

1. Larry M. Bush et al. "Index case of fatal inhalational anthrax due to bioterrorism in the United States," *NEJM*, November 29, 2001.

2. NYC encephalitis outbreak of 1999.

3. Forty-two deaths of suspicious pneumonia in Four Corners region of Southwest 1994.

4. Health Insurance Portability and Accountability Act (HIPAA).

5. Public health refers to municipal, county, state, and federal agencies.

6. Bioterrorism: Public Health Response to Anthrax Incidents of 2001; GAO-04-152, Washington DC, Oct 15, 2003.

7. Bioterrorism, note 6.

8. Tetsu Okumura et al. "Lessons learned from the Tokyo subway sarin attack." *Prehosp. Disast. Med.* 15(3):s30 (2000).

9. **Syndromic detection** refers to the science of collecting and analyzing data to determine anomalous disease patterns. Examples would include the computer-based Real-Time Outbreak Detection System (RODS), the system in place during the Salt Lake City Winter Olympics http://www.health.pitt.edu/rods/ or clinical systems like standard public health sentinel physician networks.

10. Bush, note 1.

11. D.A. Henderson, T.V. Inglesby and T. O'Toole. "Bioterrorism: Guidelines for medical and public health management," *JAMA & Archives Journals*, 2002.

12. Plague occurs in fewer than ten cases per year in the U.S.

13. Committee on Assuring the Health of the Public in the 21st Century, Institute of Medicine, *The Future of the Public's Health in the 21st Century* (Washington. DC: National Academy Press, 2003).

14. Yona Amitai et al. "Atropine poisoning in children during the Persian Gulf Crisis: A national survey in Israel," *JAMA* 268(5) (1992).

15. Michael Allswede, Joe Suyama and Walt Stoy, Center for Emergency Medicine, University of Pittsburgh. *RaPiD-T Program* (Prentice-Hall-Brady; publication pending).

16. Example: "Dark Winter" exercise June 2001.

17. Example: In 1992, the Aum Shinrikyo released anthrax aerosol in downtown Tokyo for three days with no human deaths.

18. Limited dissemination, tightly targeted releases directed at famous people.

19. The letters contained an accurate description of the pathogen and suggested antibiotics that were also correct.

20. Henderson, note 12.

21. David Heyman. *Lessons from the Anthrax Attacks: Implications for U.S. Bioterrorism Response: A Report on a National Forum on Biodefense,* Center for Strategic Studies, DTRA01-02-C-0013 (Defense Threat Reduction Agency, 2002).

22. Refers to current intelligence pooling initiatives.

23. Refers to detection of pathogenic biological aerosols.

24. Refers to detection of latent illness in population by data mining and analysis.

25. Examples: Sin nombre virus 1992, and West Nile outbreak 2000.

26. Pittsburgh Matrix Project, Michael Allswede, Lucy Savitz, Agency for Healthcare Resources and Quality; Bioterrorism Toolbox Presentations, San Diego CA, Atlanta GA, 2003 and 2004.

27. Heyman, note 21.

28. Heyman, note 21.

29. Amy Fairchild and Ronald Bayer. "Ethics and the conduct of public health surveillance." *Science*, January 30, 2004, p. 631.

30. Center for Law and the Public's Health at Georgetown and Johns Hopkins Universities. *The Model State Emergency Health Powers Act, Prepared for the Centers for Disease Control and Prevention, to Assist National Governors Association, National Conference of State Legislatures, Association of State and Territorial Health Officials, and the National Association of County and City Health Officials* (December 2001). Available online at http://www.publichealthlaw.net/.

31. Council for Excellence in Government. "From the Home Front to the Front Lines: America Speaks out about Homeland Security." (Washington, DC: Council for Excellence in Government, 2004). Available at http://www.excelgov.org/displaycontent.asp?keyword=prhHomePage.

32. **Hardening** is a term borrowed from the cold war in which the target venue is made more difficult to attack by making its heating ventilation and air conditioning systems more difficult to contaminate, creating better surveillance systems, or by placing early warning monitors in vulnerable locations.

33. Tarasoff v. Regents of the University of California, 17 Cal.3d 425, 1976.

34. D. Nash et al. (1999 West Nile Outbreak Response Working Group). "The outbreak of West Nile virus infection in the New York City area in 1999." *N. Engl. J. Med.* 344(24):1807–14 (2001)

35. W. Eidson. "Confusion, controversy, and quarantine: The Muncie smallpox epidemic of 1893." *Indiana Magazine of History*, 86 (1990).

36. H. Markel. "Knocking out the cholera: Cholera, class, and quarantines in New York City, 1892." *Bull. Hist. Med.* 69 (1995).

37. Heyman, note 21.

38. Gerald Joyce et al. *Biodetection Architectures*, JASON JSR-02-330 (McLean, VA: Mitre Corporation, 2003). Available on line at http://www.fas.org/sgp/news/secrecy/2004/01/012104.html.

Chapter 10

Public Health Aspects and Preventive Measures

Bruce W. Dixon, M.D.

Synopsis

10.1 Introduction

Public health has a key role in biological and chemical terrorism response and works closely with law enforcement agencies and emergency response agencies at the local, state, and federal levels. Public health is an over-arching term that includes not only government agencies but private individuals and institutions whose unifying purpose in the event of a terrorist attack is to contain, control, to educate people at risk or perceived to be at risk, and to educate people who have fears of being affected by such an event. These activities are a part of the core functions of public health as defined by the Institute of Medicine, and include assessment and assurance functions as well as policy development to maximize safety by reducing hazards. Public health's role in responding to biological and chemical terrorism is part of a larger role as a support agency in disaster response, whether naturally occurring or man made. It may include issues beyond the scope of this chapter, such as building collapse, possibly from structural deficiency; natural disaster, such as a fire, or a man-made disaster such as a bomb; and may include radiological accidents such as occurred at Three Mile Island, near Harrisburg, Pennsylvania, and more recently at Chernobyl in the Ukraine. Although beyond the scope of this chapter, it is important to recognize that combinations of terrorist events may occur so that biological or chemical weapons disseminated by a bomb could result in building collapse and radiation release as well. The initial response must look at the latter two situations in order to assure the safety of first responders. Building integrity and lack of radiation threat must be rapidly ascertained and assured before the assessment of biological or chemical risk begins. It is only within the last decade that attention has been paid to the potential for biological or chemical terrorism so concepts for identification, response, and public health intervention are in their infancy and are constantly changing. For purposes of defining public health response, it is convenient to think of public health activities in two broad categories; those activities that occur prior to any terrorist event and which are ongoing as part of the overall mission of public health, and those specific activities that would occur post-terrorist event which are targeted specifically to that event.

10.2 Pre-Event Activities

Pre-event activities on the part of public health that relate to biological or chemical terrorism fall in three general categories (1) surveillance, (2) laboratory capabilities, and (3) education and training. All three activities are core functions of public health at the local, state, and federal level and have a long and distinguished history. However, the threat of terrorism has caused a rethinking of all of these activities and further clarification and definition of their role.

A. Surveillance

Traditional infectious disease surveillance has been a public health activity since at least the eighteenth century and has been responsible for major breakthroughs in disease recognition and intervention. Throughout much of its history, however, disease surveillance has been a passive process. Physicians and, more recently, hospitals, laboratories, and infection-control nurses have reported definitive diagnoses of disease to a health authority that, by virtue of its legal mandate, has then taken some action to control, stop the spread, and eventually eliminate the infectious disease process. Regardless of the circumstances—whether the control of cholera in nineteenth-century England by eliminating contamination of the city well by sewage or, more recently, the limitation of cases of paralytic polio by vaccination or the elimination of smallpox from the globe by vaccination—the principles have remained the same. Traditional surveillance has been called into question, however, by the threat of terrorism. For many years, this system has been a passive one that depended on voluntary reporting of disease states. Today, that process is being supplanted by active surveillance systems that go out and search for disease by a variety of mechanisms, with the goal of reducing the time between occurrence and recognition of illness. The scope of individuals involved in active surveillance has been increased as well, so that nurses, pharmacists, laboratory directors and technicians, and other health care-related personnel are actively surveyed for potential biological disease. The process is labor intensive, however, and requires personal interactions to achieve reporting of a significant number of conditions of interest. The surveyor must establish personal communications with the reporting entity and survey them regularly and repetitively.

As a result, there are growing initiatives to create automated surveillance systems. Electronic surveillance systems capable of managing large and redundant amounts of data are being developed, especially at the federal and state levels. The National Electronic Disease Surveillance System (NEDSS), presently under development and deployment by the Centers for Disease Control, is one such system designed to facilitate surveillance. There have been various state revisions to this system to accommodate special interests and needs, but the overall intent is to have a variety of healthcare professionals enter data suggestive of, or confirmatory of, an infectious disease or other condition and to allow public health practitioners wide access to that data so that they can associate disparate bits of information and begin to see patterns of disease occurrence and spread. Such a system allows a local jurisdiction to see patterns of spread within their own area of concern, allows a larger entity, such as a state, to see patterns of spread between jurisdictions, and has the potential for a government agency such as the CDC to see potential spread on a much wider area involving multiple states or territories. Most present-day surveillance (whether active or passive) has been disease specific and has depended on either laboratory or clinical confirmation before reporting occurs. In order to be better prepared to respond to a biological event, it is necessary to shorten the time that elapses between the event and its detection, and for that reason, syndromic reporting of illness becomes desirable. Since most biological terrorist agents, and indeed, most chemical terrorist agents, will result in a fairly limited number of clinical manifestations, looking at clinical syndromes of respiratory disease, gastrointestinal disease, neurologic disease, and dermatologic conditions should result in the detection of virtually all chemical and biological terrorist agents. By their training, physicians and other health professionals have been accustomed to think in terms of clearly defined disease entities; retraining to think in terms of broad clinical presentations has proven to be difficult to achieve. In addition, most of the potential biological or chemical agents that would be considered terrorist threats result in rare diseases. As a result, health professionals do not recognize them or may ascribe them to some more common illness and miss the opportunity for early intervention. One researcher, in 2000, showed photographs of smallpox to physicians involved in family practice, internal medicine, and infectious disease. The infectious disease specialists suggested smallpox to a greater degree than did the internists or family practitioners. But the overall identification rate was poor and resulted in a positive diagnosis far less than 50 percent of the time. Indeed, the tendency of health practitioners to ascribe a rare event to a common occurrence is common behavior. For instance, in the early cases of anthrax which occurred in 2001, which were subsequently shown to be spread by the mail service, the index case was thought to have been acquired by natural means in central Florida, although the septic form of that illness had not been seen there for at least two decades. All efforts of disease surveillance have been largely concentrated thus far on hospitals and large, freestanding clinics. The reality is, however, when looking for unusual disease, that it will probably show up in an individual physician's office; thus the need for continuing education of the practice community and the continued need to reassure physicians that they do not need to have a specific diagnosis in order to report an infectious disease. Indeed, simply recognizing that a patient seems to have an unusual illness should be sufficient cause to report and then allow others to help with the diagnosis and solution. Frequently, practitioners and other health professionals will raise the issue of confidentiality in failing to report a potential infectious disease. Every state has reporting laws that give public health broad authority to receive and protect such reported disease information. HIPAA requirements recently enacted by the Department of Health and Human Services have a major exception for public health reporting which is not confined to an illness for which there is a specific reporting provision or statute. Because of the uncertainties and inexact nature of disease surveillance, even with active surveillance, a variety of surrogate reporting systems have been developed or are in development. The United States Postal Service has recently deployed a biological detection system (BDS) in thirteen facilities, that depends on scanning mail in stamping machines and sampling the surrounding air at frequent intervals with PCR (polymerase chain reaction) for anthrax. Although conceivably, this automated process could be expanded to other pathogens, the specific antigen must be loaded into the BDS and so its applicability for unusual disease or unrecognized disease is quite limited. The University of Pittsburgh has embarked on a project known as "RODS" (reactive outbreak and disease surveillance) that depends on a variety of direct and surrogate indicators of health conditions including emergency room visits, pharmaceutical purchases, absences from schools and other workplaces. The difficulty with RODS is that it is unlikely to pick up a single occurrence of a rare disease and, although it may pick up large concentrations of individuals who may be afflicted with one or another syndromic conditions, it is not specific enough to distinguish naturally occurring illness from unusual and perhaps, terrorist-related illness. Further refinement may reveal that there is some use, however, for this data mining process. In addition to these human health surveillance efforts, a variety of environmental efforts have recently been deployed. Funded by the Environmental Protection Agency, several cities have a bioshield project that samples the air at a variety of sites and rapidly performs an analysis, in most instances, by PCR for pathogens. While there is some theoretic likelihood for success with such a system, the small amount of air sampled, the limited geographic area from which a sample is obtained, and the need to compare it with known pathogen standards make it unlikely that it will have a significant impact on detecting biological agents that may be generally released into the environment. Similarly, although issues around food safety have been raised and the Rajneesh cult in Oregon placed salmonella in foodstuffs, routine surveillance is not likely to pick up any food contamination.

B. Laboratory capabilities

As a result of the inexact nature of surveillance, laboratory identification of organisms of particular concern for bioterrorism has remained the standard. While the reporting system from laboratories has generally been quite good, there is an obvious time delay between obtaining an environmental specimen or a specimen from a potential victim of bioterrorism, having it processed in the laboratory, and obtaining a result. There is, in addition, a dynamic tension between law enforcement and public health, as far as laboratory determinations are concerned. Although the FBI has been designated as the primary response agency for acts of bioterrorism, its focus is largely criminal prosecution, where the interest of public health is to rapidly ascertain whether or not a pathological agent is present and to intervene. While a laboratory which processes specimens from a variety of medical providers may occasionally find an organism suggestive of bioterrorism, specimens obtained from a suspected site of terrorism must be handled in such a way that a chain of custody is maintained to be useful for prosecution. For that reason, laboratories processing specimens from a suspected terrorist scene, in general, are laboratories under the control of government, either at the local, state, or federal level who can use and attest to the chain of custody. Such laboratories must be close enough to the site of potential terrorism that long delays in transportation do not hinder the rapid identification of a pathogen by the laboratory. For instance, in many parts of the country, a public health laboratory is several hours' distance, even by plane, from the site and although today, the technology exists to identify an organism in as short a time as forty minutes, the long delays in getting the specimen to the laboratory make the rapid identification of lesser value. To deal with these concerns, several laboratories, including those of state and local health departments and CDC, have been certified as parts of the Laboratory Response Network, to allow for specimens to be rapidly identified using newer antigens and techniques and to be sent on to other more specialized facilities for diagnostic confirmation. Laboratories processing such specimens should at the very minimum, meet the qualifications of Biosafety Level III, as promulgated by the Centers for Disease Control, to allow the identification of pathogens with safety for the laboratory technicians. When used for bioterrorism, many of the organisms will be weaponized—that is, in sufficient size that it results in a greater infectivity than would occur in nature. Laboratory safety is therefore of paramount concern. Similarly, within the laboratory network, there needs to be sufficient redundancy so that if the capabilities of one laboratory are exceeded or are rendered inoperable, other laboratories are able to rapidly provide the capabilities necessary. More specialized laboratories able to perform genetic fingerprinting are part of the network so that one can associate infections disassociated in time or space with a common source. Determination of chemical agents, like bacteriological agents, requires specialized laboratory equipment and specialized safety measures for staff. Many of the potential chemical agents, including a variety of neurotoxins, represent gases that must be collected safely and analyzed either by mass spectroscopy or infrared chromatography in equipment that doesn't expose the laboratory technicians to undue risk. Because of the unique nature of chemical agents and their rapid onset, many emergency response units have been equipped with portable gas chromatography-mass spectroscopy units to identify the agent, at least preliminarily, in the field.

C. Training

Public health training is another pre-event function important to the overall bioterrorism effort. Continued training of health professionals and related staff is vital to transmit not only new knowledge, but to refresh principles of disease surveillance and response among health practitioners who have had relatively little training during their formal education. Since it is likely, should an event occur, that people with specialized skills would be needed to care for injured or affected individuals, collaboration and sharing of resources is once again important. The Medical Reserve Corps grants, funded by the Department of Health and Human Services, have allowed jurisdictions to recruit a variety of health practitioners, including physicians, nurses, and pharmacists to assist should a terrorist event occur. Training of those individuals in not only disease recognition but also triage and dispensation of medications, including vaccines and technical knowledge, is imperative. It is felt to be prudent that a small number of individuals who represent this level of health practitioners should be immunized against common pathogens for which vaccines exist so that they can be used as immediate responders or to help vaccinate other individuals. Vaccines for smallpox have been deployed by the federal government with questionable success. Small groups of people appear to be available in most regions of the country with sufficient protection either from former or revaccination to allow them to be first responders if a smallpox outbreak does occur. Similarly, although there is controversy around the use and potential side effects from anthrax vaccine, a small but diverse group of people have been immunized for anthrax and could serve as first responders from a public health point of view. Specialized knowledge continues to advance and it is important that ongoing training and education be available. For consistency, many jurisdictions have adopted Internet-based training so that the training is not only comprehensive, but allows one to receive training at their own pace and with similar content. This becomes more important if some sort of a mass hazardous event occurs which will require people to come to an area to assist not only with public health, but also with patient care.

The Metropolitan Medical Response System has been a preparedness system initially deployed in many of the larger cities throughout the United States and gradually expanded to cities and regions of more moderate size. This is a planning effort to ensure that those jurisdictions most at risk for some type of man-made or natural disaster have begun the planning process to ensure there is coordination between healthcare providers, local and state health systems, and emergency management personnel and systems.

10.3 Post-Event Activities

There have been relatively few events that have tested the post-event response to large scale public health emergencies. The radiation emergencies at Three Mile Island and Chernobyl were several years ago and the capacity to detect and respond has improved significantly since those two events. A sarin gas release in a Japanese subway is often cited as an example of a chemical release and the release of methylisocyanate at Bhopal, India, also provided experience with the release of a chemical agent. Again, both events occurred long enough ago that significant improvement in knowledge has occurred since then. More recently, the dissemination of anthrax in multiple areas by U.S. mail has provided an opportunity to study response to a biological agent in which person-to-person spread and secondary cases does not occur. While there has been no purposeful release of an agent in which person-to-person spread occurs, there are clearly naturally occurring examples which can be used as models of such an event. These range from such conditions as pulmonary tuberculosis to the more-recently described, severe acute respiratory syndrome (SARS) and the latter served as an excellent model for post-event planning. The areas of interest and concern for public health in a post-event situation again can conveniently be grouped in a series of initiatives:

- surveillance and epidemiology
- communication
- interaction with hospitals and health professionals to accomplish treatment and risk reduction
- deployment of medical materials, including vaccines and medications to both treat affected individuals and prophylactically treat individuals at risk
- removal of individuals from areas of risk
- segregation of individuals known to be affected or at risk to reduce further spread
- mental health issues
- other considerations

A. Surveillance

Surveillance in a post-event situation is somewhat distinct from pre-event surveillance in that a known agent has been recognized and the emphasis shifts from detection of an unusual event to detection of individuals who exhibit the symptom complexes characteristic of the agent known to have been released. Epidemiologic investigation begun by questioning individuals who have the symptoms becomes extremely important in identifying other individuals who may either be incubating disease or who may have been put at risk. This activity must be coordinated since individuals have a tendency to travel large distances in a relatively short period of time and multiple sites may be infected simultaneously or in succession by a noxious agent. It is necessary that surveillance activities be available twenty-four hours daily, seven days a week, to not only receive information but to respond in a rapid fashion. Complementing an active surveillance system, it is necessary to have a responsive laboratory, which is equipped with the latest technologies for infectious diseases and to a lesser degree, chemical identification. A level-A hospital laboratory or other freestanding laboratories should have agreements in place to forward specimens to a laboratory of level-B or C capability and ideally, one that is a member of the Laboratory Response Network which can handle not only hazardous pathogens but do so in a way that preserves chain of custody for potential future legal prosecution. As previously noted, it is necessary that those laboratories, in the Laboratory Response Network, have surge capacity so that, in the event they become overwhelmed by specimen acceptance, they can have additional resources available for the quick turnaround of results. Efforts are presently underway to facilitate electronic data reporting and sharing. The laboratory component of the National Electronic Disease Surveillance System (NEDSS) has been made operational to a variable degree in many states.

B. Communication

A unified command and an incident command system is critical to any emergency response. While public health is a key component, many of the direct response functions are the responsibility of a local or regional emergency management agency and the close working between those two entities as well as the private healthcare system is key to any emergency response. In order to facilitate coordination, it is necessary that communication devices be available which are compatible and optimally redundant means of communication be available. Ideally, a senior public health official is part of the incident command and emergency operation center to receive information from the field and to help formulate a cohesive plan for response. While it has been common for various groups such as police, fire, emergency management, and public health to deploy radio systems, in many instances the frequencies have not been compatible and such lack of consistency has led to fragmentation of effort, on occasion with serious or fatal consequence. Cell phone and land line phones are other means of communication and are useful for communication with agencies at a distance from an event that may not be reachable by radio transmission. Electronic computer-based communication with partners at both state and federal levels provides additional redundancy for the transmission of information. The Centers for Disease Control has recently deployed a Health Alert Network; this electronic form of data exchange is being used regularly to disseminate information of health importance with the goal of having people become comfortable enough with its use that it could be rapidly switched over in an emergency situation to disseminate important information to health providers and field personnel. In addition to communication between various health practitioners, health providers, and responders, communication with the public and at-risk communities becomes extremely important. It is necessary that this be done in a coordinated way, to avoid misinformation, and be presented by someone with known credibility. The goal should be to identify individuals who have been at risk, as well as to avoid panic among a larger number of individuals who have no actual risk but who may, because of lack of information, unnecessarily clog the healthcare delivery system or jam roadways by trying to avoid an area, thus making it difficult for responders to reach an area of concern. Such actions put more people at risk. By properly informing the public about potential health events, the electronic and print media are important allies and participants. The electronic media has the advantage of being able to rapidly transmit information and radio networks, in particular, have demonstrated their abilities to remain active in a wide variety of environmental conditions. The print media, although a somewhat slower avenue to disseminate information, has the advantage of covering facts in much greater detail and providing a written document to which people can repetitively refer for instructions. In some cities, local telephone companies have made use of supplements to their telephone directories to have generic information about emergency response. This, again, is an important avenue to reduce panic. It is clear that, in almost every incidence of both naturally occurring and man-made disaster, panic is the single biggest event. Clearly, a prime goal of terrorist activity is to produce panic and fears of the unknown as evidenced by the large number of people collecting dust and powders for analysis during the recent anthrax events.

C. Interaction with hospitals and health professionals to accomplish treatment and risk reduction

Hospitals and other acute-care facilities play an obvious central role in any public health response to natural or man-made disasters. Not only are the most seriously ill patients hospitalized, but hospital emergency rooms are apt to be jammed with self-referred individuals either because of risk or perceived risk. The ability to communicate that risk and delay the concerns of those individuals who are not at risk has a direct relationship to the number of people seeking emergency room evaluation. Good communication keeps a hospital emergency room from being unnecessarily congested. Central to any mass casualty event is field triage and, depending on the circumstances, it may be carried out by paramedics and other emergency response personnel, by nurses, in some instances by physicians and, in situations of extreme emergency, by other allied health practitioners. Surveillance information obtained soon after an event is of extreme importance to the triage personnel because they themselves may be exposed as part of this activity to either a biological or chemical agent. In order to err on the side of caution until the exact nature of an event is known, it is prudent in most instances that those individuals use protective garments and, occasionally, self-contained breathing apparatus. Triage needs to occur in proximity to the location of an event, particularly when there are multiple victims. But also, it needs to be far enough away to reduce the risk of further injury. There needs to be a close interaction with law enforcement personnel to ensure that the boundaries of a triage area are not violated and that casual onlookers do not have ready access to the area. It is anticipated in those areas, particularly those that have a Medical Reserve Corps, that people from the Corps would serve as the triage staff. It makes no sense that skilled and tertiary care physicians are asked to leave their hospital in order to accomplish field triage when there is a greater need for them to care for the most seriously ill patients who are apt to be transported to their institution for care. Similarly, as part of the triage activities, those tertiary-care hospitals close to an event would probably become the hospitals for the most critically ill patients. Those with less severe needs but requiring evaluation would be taken to institutions at greater distances. In the event of a large-scale disaster with multiple victims, if the capacities of a Reserve Corps were exhausted, triage individuals would need to come from contiguous jurisdictions and surrounding institutions that did not have the critical need for inpatient staffing. Depending on the nature of the event, it may be necessary for individuals to be decontaminated either in the field or on arrival at the hospital emergency room. Many large hospitals have established decontamination facilities and procedures in the event that decontamination is necessary. Decontamination, in some instances, may be as simple as removing clothing and showering, but may be complicated if exposure to vesicant agents or inhalational toxins has occurred. Should an infectious agent be implicated, particularly one that is spread person-to-person, such as smallpox, it is prudent that appropriately immunized staff be available to care for that individual and minimize risk to the caregivers. Similarly, many hospitals have either built negative-pressure emergency rooms or have been retrofitted with negative air pressure, at least in portions of the emergency room, and installed air handling systems which separate the emergency room from the main hospital system to reduce the potential spread of infectious agents to the at-large hospital population. Included in hospital contingency plans are schema to identify the least seriously ill patients and discharge them to provide beds for victims of a widespread catastrophe. Elective procedures, from radiology to surgery, would be curtailed so that such facilities would be at the ready. Mortuary facilities need to be established off site to tend to those who have died at a scene, and in the hospital to care for victims that expire in the hospital, and to allow for the rapid examination of remains to further define causative agents under the direction of the appropriate coroner or medical examiner. Depending on the nature and size of the event, and if the ordinary means of postmortem holding are exhausted, this may require the use of refrigerated trucks or warehouses or in the event of an extreme emergency, the use of large facilities, such as an airport hangar with the need to bring in refrigeration equipment. Depending on the nature of the contagion, the medical examiner may order cremation of the remains to control and reduce the contagion. Such issues are discussed in greater detail in other chapters.

D. Deployment of medical materials

Many regions have accumulated local stockpiles of emergency medications, vaccines, and equipment to use in the event of a natural or man-made emergency. These range from such measures as equipping firemen, paramedics, emergency medical technicians and other first responders with self-contained breathing apparatus and protective clothing to equipping paramedics and field personnel with agents such as atropine or 2-PAM (pralidoxime) to treat cholinesterase inhibitor poisonings. Most hospitals have at least small quantities of ciprofloxicin available to treat individuals who may have been exposed to anthrax or to begin prophylactic treatment of individuals who may be at risk. Larger public health agencies may have additional supplies of ciprofloxicin and in many instances, have small quantities of smallpox vaccine to begin immunization of healthcare workers and individuals at risk, should smallpox exposure occur. Although large numbers of healthcare workers did not volunteer to receive smallpox immunization, most areas have a small contingent of people who are appropriately immunized who could begin both epidemiologic investigation and treatment. It is reassuring to note that many individuals who previously had been immunized for smallpox and were re-immunized had an accelerated reaction, which would suggest that they have some residual immunity from the previous immunization. Based on the nature and size of a disaster, it may be necessary to mobilize the Strategic National Stockpile of pharmaceuticals and equipment, which are maintained at sites throughout the United States. The mobilization of the SNS is on request of a governor, after consultation with the Secretary of Health and occurs at a statewide level. Multiple sites for acceptance of the SNS have been determined and the supplies, along with a minimal staff of expert consultants, can be made available within forty-eight hours of request. The dissemination of materials from the accepting site is, however, a local responsibility and requires appropriate numbers of pharmacists, pharmacy technicians, and couriers at the acceptance site to break down packaging and disseminate the materials to hospitals or predetermined community sites, for instance, for the administration of vaccines or medications. Such sites, in general, would be staffed with public health workers supplemented by nurses and physicians from the Medical Reserve Corps. Clerical staff and security staff needs to be obtained from the local workforce. Most areas have planned and practiced to be able to provide medications including immunizations to the entire population of an affected area within 100 hours using multiple sites.

E. Segregation of individuals known to be affected or at risk to reduce further spread

A general evacuation of an area affected by some type of disaster may be necessary because of continued hazard or the potential for further damage. In general, individuals affected by such an evacuation tend to be well or minimally affected by the initial event and would be temporarily housed in shelters such as schools, auditoria, or a combination of private and public facilities, including those already equipped for domiciliary care such as hotels and motels and those that can be converted with minimal effort to house individuals. The large numbers of people cohabiting leads to the potential spread of common infectious diseases such as respiratory illnesses as well as psychological unrest due to the sudden change of environment. At-risk individuals, such as the elderly, may be disproportionately impacted by any evacuation exercise and public health has a role to ensure that the mental anguish is minimized, that the unrelated infectious diseases are evaluated and treated as necessary to reduce spread, and that ongoing medical conditions present in the individuals so evacuated such as hypertension, diabetes, and other common but chronic illnesses are cared for, particularly when medications may not be readily available. Individuals on dialysis or respirators may pose special challenges as may prisoners. A second and more important public health initiative is the segregation of individuals known to be at risk or minimally affected with a potentially infectious condition in order to reduce spread. The isolation of people with person-to-person spread infectious diseases in either hospitals or at home has been a long-standing public health practice and has been widely used in the past to reduce the spread of infectious disease; it has become less common as potent antimicrobials have been developed so that the periods of infectivity of disease have become much shorter. There are still, however, times when such isolation is necessary. A good example is tuberculosis, where it is commonplace to restrict the movement of an individual with infectious disease until they are rendered noninfectious. More recently, it was the practice to restrict individuals with sudden acute respiratory syndrome (SARS) to their home during their period of infectivity. This endeavor proved effective when used to reduce person-to-person spread of that illness. The authority to restrict peoples' movement is well established by law and although the exact conditions of that restriction vary from region to region, in some instances requiring review in a timely fashion with the courts, the authority of public health to do so is a well established principle in all areas. Federal legislation has been enacted to allow for the emergency isolation of individuals and those areas with weak statutory authority have adopted that federal regulation and others have used it as a model to improve their existing regulatory authority. One of the goals of the federal regulation and always one of the goals of public health is to balance the individual's needs against the needs of society to protect itself and the federal regulation allows for the rapid isolation of individuals if, on review, it is found to be necessary. Such isolation or quarantine may extend to a forced isolation either in a home or institution equipped to restrict the movement of an individual and may require close coordination with law enforcement to ensure that the terms of that isolation are being met.

F. Mental health issues

Some of the mental health issues resulting from a disaster have been mentioned above and are more fully described in other chapters. However, since mental health programs in many jurisdictions are a part of the public health system and in others are closely aligned with public health, the public health system has a major role in providing mental health services. Those services must be in place not only for the workers, who in many instances are exposed to conditions and situations with which they are not familiar, or are not comfortable and that have at times resulted in long-term posttraumatic stress syndromes, but also include mental health services for victims who may be displaced from their usual domicile, are rendered unemployed, are unable to locate close family members and loved ones, or who may be overwhelmed by the enormity of the situation. Just as in every other area of public health, sharing of responsibilities is important. Many times, pastoral care is a useful adjunct included in pre-established mental health teams.

G. Other considerations

The public health system has operated on a principle, in general, that events confined to a single jurisdiction are handled by that jurisdiction so long as they are able. If more than one jurisdiction is involved, then there is a sharing of responsibility with the next highest level, which may be either a state or a region. The federal government has teams in place to assist in instances of severe disaster and although they have tremendous expertise, mobilizing them takes a reasonable amount of time and often, they are not familiar with local conditions that must be considered. Teams such as National Disaster Medical Assistance Team (NDMATS), Veterinary Medical Assistance Teams (VMATS), and Mortician Teams (DMORTS) are available for consultation and help in a large disaster. Other skills and other agencies may be involved, depending on the unique nature of a particular incident. In the case of a zoonotic illness, teams of veterinarians may be mobilized to help with investigation and control. Food safety public health experts, including members of the FDA and

Department of Agriculture, may be useful in the event of a food-borne illness. The unique nature of every public-health-related disaster requires constant re-evaluation of the circumstances, consultation with individuals who can share expertise, and a scaling up or scaling down of interventions and resources as the situation evolves.

Chapter 11

The Role of the Medical Examiner and Coroner in the Investigation of Terrorism

Michael M. Baden, M.D.

Medical examiners, coroners and forensic pathologists are at the forefront of the war on terrorism. It is they who have statutory authority to investigate the victims of suspicious and violent deaths which include deaths from explosions, in aircraft crashes and from exposure to toxic gases or microbiologic agents. It is they who investigate deaths on planes or boats entering the country. It is they who must contribute to the determination as to whether any of those deaths are related to terrorism. And it is only after the entire investigation is completed that a conclusion can be made as to whether or not the deaths were the result of a terrorist act.

An autopsy is a powerful investigative tool. A complete autopsy should be performed whenever there is the possibility that a death is terrorism-related so that information can be obtained not only as to the identity of the decedent and as to the cause of death, but also so that evidence of any explosive device, any chemical agent, or any micro-organism, that may have entered the body can be identified, retrieved and documented. Photographs should be taken to document all injuries and patterns of injury. X-rays should be taken to assist in identifying any possible bomb device fragments in the body, as well as to assist in the identification process. Toxicologic analyses should test for chemicals that might be present. Microbiologic studies should look for appropriate bacteria, viruses or other microorganisms. Further, the medical examiner can provide expertise at the scene of death in identifying, documenting and recovering bodies and body parts and in assuring that no evidence is lost in the process of moving the remains to the morgue. If the staff can't perform these tasks, arrangements should be made with others to assist as appropriate—there must be no pride of jurisdiction. Someone should be available from the medical examiner or coroner's office to speak to families on a twenty-four-hour basis every day during the investigation to provide information and to comfort them and to receive information from them as to dental records, medical history and scars and tattoos that might assist in the identification process.

Accurate and prompt identification of bodies is the most important contribution that a medical examiner provides to the family of the deceased. Direct visual identification, fingerprints, dental analysis, DNA technologies and comparison to prior x-rays of any of the 206 bones in the body should all be employed as necessary. Clothing, wallets and purses, and jewelry permit presumptive identification, which should be confirmed. Most terrorist attacks around the world and in this country have involved explosions, often with after-coming fires, which can make identification difficult. The following cases illustrate the New York experience in investigating possible terrorist incidents.

Case 1. Identification was a major concern when a liquid natural gas container explosion occurred in Staten Island, New York in 1973. Forty-three men from Italy between twenty and forty years of age died after an explosion in the very large cement container they were working in with a subsequent fire that burned for many hours before the bodies could be removed. The skin of all of the workers was severely charred which precluded direct visual or fingerprint identification. However, the teeth remained intact which permitted rapid identification of all decedents. (Figures 11.1 and 11.2) Subsequent investigation determined that the explosion was accidental.

Case 2. When TWA flight 800 exploded in 1996 about 13,000 feet above the Long Island Sound in Suffolk County, New York shortly after takeoff from JFK Airport, all 220 people on board died. Initial reports stressed the likelihood of a terrorist bomb. Complete autopsies of all recovered victims and body parts with total body photographs and x-rays, fingerprinting, examination of all clothing and DNA analysis of unidentified remains, resulted in the identification of every one of the victims and permitted the comparison of injury patterns with seat assignments, and the recovery of all foreign objects from the bodies. None of the thousands of objects removed from the bodies proved to be from an explosive device. The injury patterns did not suggest an explosion of a bomb on the airplane. The full investigation concluded that the plane exploded accidentally from ignition of vapors in the empty middle fuel tank and not as the result of terrorism.

The great majority of the bodies were recovered intact because the terminal velocity of a freely falling human body, even from more than 13,000 feet high, reaches only 120 miles per hour on impact, sufficient to cause extensive and immediate lethal internal injuries but not sufficient to tear the skin and cause the body to fragment (Figure 11.3).

Unfortunately, New York City officials kept the families of the victims housed together at one hotel at John F. Kennedy Airport, more than sixty miles from the Suffolk County Medical Examiner's Office where the bodies were examined. It is important in a mass disaster for families to be able to directly view their loved ones and to see progress being made as other families identify theirs. That families were unable to go to the Medical Examiner's Office to identify loved ones quickly caused great dissatisfaction among many families that was passionately and frequently expressed to the throngs of media at the hotel. To this day, many victims' families remain upset at what they feel was insensitive treatment by city and county officials that caused delays in their ability to view and identify loved ones.

The most common form of terrorist attacks worldwide and in this country has been by means of explosive devices in public places, in symbolic places or in vehicles. Explosives are an inexpensive, low-tech means of quickly getting attention and terrorizing a population.

Case 3. In 1972, a bomb exploded outside historic Fraunces Tavern on Wall Street in New York City, where General George Washington said good-bye to his troops. Four men lunching at the nearest table were killed by shrapnel injuries from flying debris - forks, glass, nails and wood. (Figures 11.4 and 11.5) This homemade device was the type used by the FALN, a Puerto Rican nationalist group.

Case 4. A bomb exploded in a car in Upstate New York near the Canadian border in 1998, causing death and extensive injury to the only occupant. Autopsy examination and x-rays demonstrated radio-opaque shrapnel that had blown upward into the right upper and lower extremities, which showed what their positions were when the explosion occurred: right hand on the turned ignition key and right foot on the depressed gas pedal. Among the many metal objects removed from the body and given to Bureau of Alcohol, Tobacco and Firearms' investigators present, one, and only one, proved to be part of a bomb device of the type that had been used in Canada in a motorcycle gang war in Montreal in which fifty people had been killed. (Figures 11.6 and 11.7).

Case 5. An explosion at LaGuardia Airport in 1976 killed eleven people standing in line in front of the TWA check-in desk. The deaths resulted from a plastic explosive device, placed in a metal luggage locker by Croatian nationalists, that caused metal fragments and other materials in the locker to act as secondary missiles. (Figures 11.8, 11.9 and 11.10) It was not determined whether the explosion was intended to occur at the time or place that it did.

Case 6. In 1993, a car bomb exploded in the basement garage at the World Trade Center killing six people. It was the investigation by police who recovered parts of the vehicle at the scene, that contained the bomb that was critical in leading to the identification and successful prosecution of the Islamic terrorist who had parked the car and of some of his associates.

Case 7. On September 11, 2001, two commercial airplanes were used as suicidal explosive weapons by terrorists and were flown into the two World Trade Center Towers in New York City. The resultant jet fuel fire caused the buildings to collapse. Officially, 2,749 people were killed. The bodies of those who jumped, many from more than ninety stories high, were intact when they struck the ground (Figure 11.11) but most bodies were then fragmented when struck by after-coming, falling building debris.

A decision was made to clear the scene as rapidly as possible and not to treat it with the care that a crime scene requires. This decision may have proved to be politically correct and greatly enhanced national morale and pride. However, it severely compromised forensic investigations, particularly the ability to search for bodies and body parts, identify all of the terrorists, and determine if a bomb device was used. The scene was not examined by crime scene investigators nor by staff medical examiners from other jurisdictions who responded to the emergency. Rather, firemen were given the responsibility to look for bodies and body remnants. Large front-loader type machines removed unexamined steel girders and debris commingled with body parts, sometimes even with unrecognized intact bodies, and placed them into trucks, some of which illegally drove to metal recovery and dump sites in New Jersey. The site was cleared ahead of schedule to the nation's great approval, but evidence was lost and 40 percent of the bodies still remain unidentified at this time.

Biochemical weapons have limited effectiveness outdoors because of dilution by air and dispersal by air currents but can be effective indoors and in closed areas such as subway systems. Anthrax is a bacteria that does not spread from person to person and caused only five deaths when sent through the mails shortly after 9/11. However, its presence caused enormous terror in this country, far greater than its ability to cause infections. Smallpox, a virus that spreads from person to person and has a mortality rate of about 30 percent of those infected, would be a much more potent biologic weapon than anthrax.

There have been no significant terrorist chemical incidents in this country and, most fortunately, no nuclear agents have been used. Should there be a biologic, chemical or nuclear attack, special precautions and autopsy facilities previously planned for would be necessary.

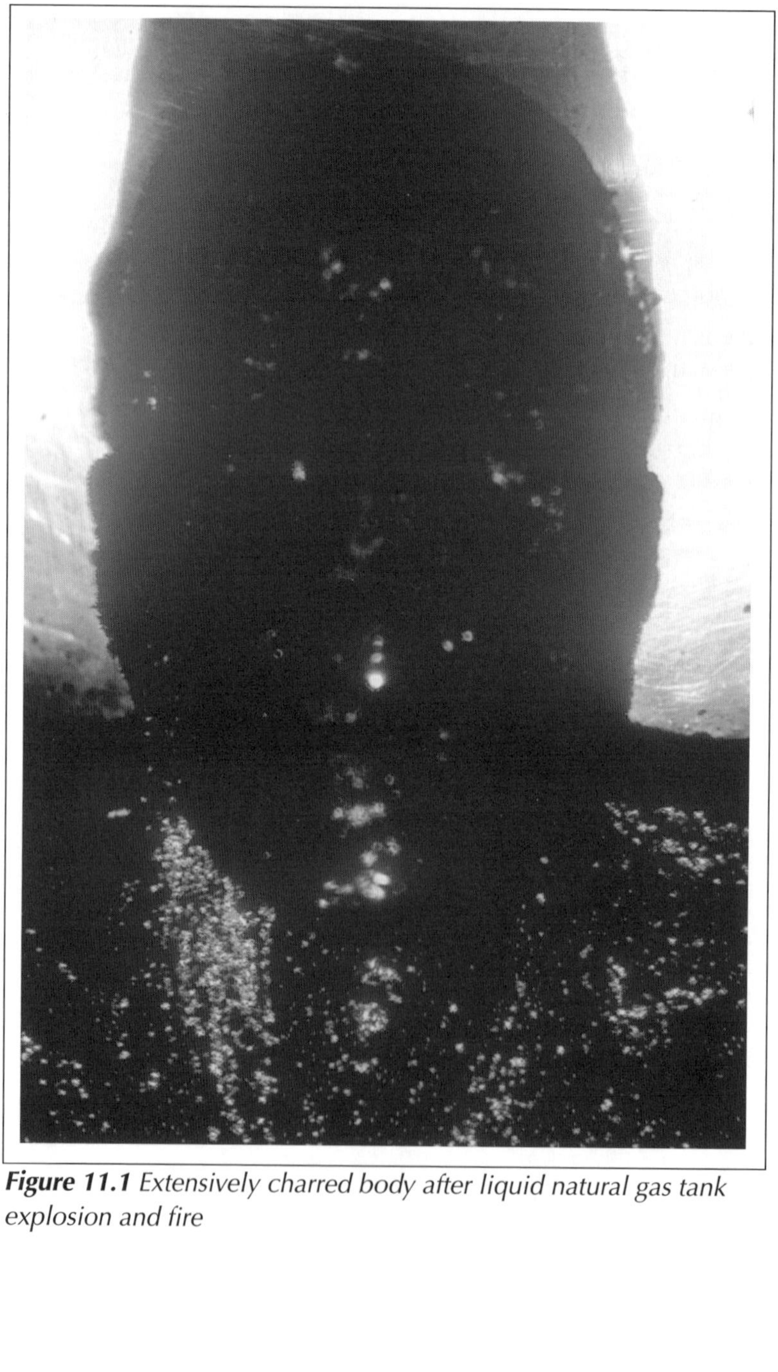

Figure 11.1 *Extensively charred body after liquid natural gas tank explosion and fire*

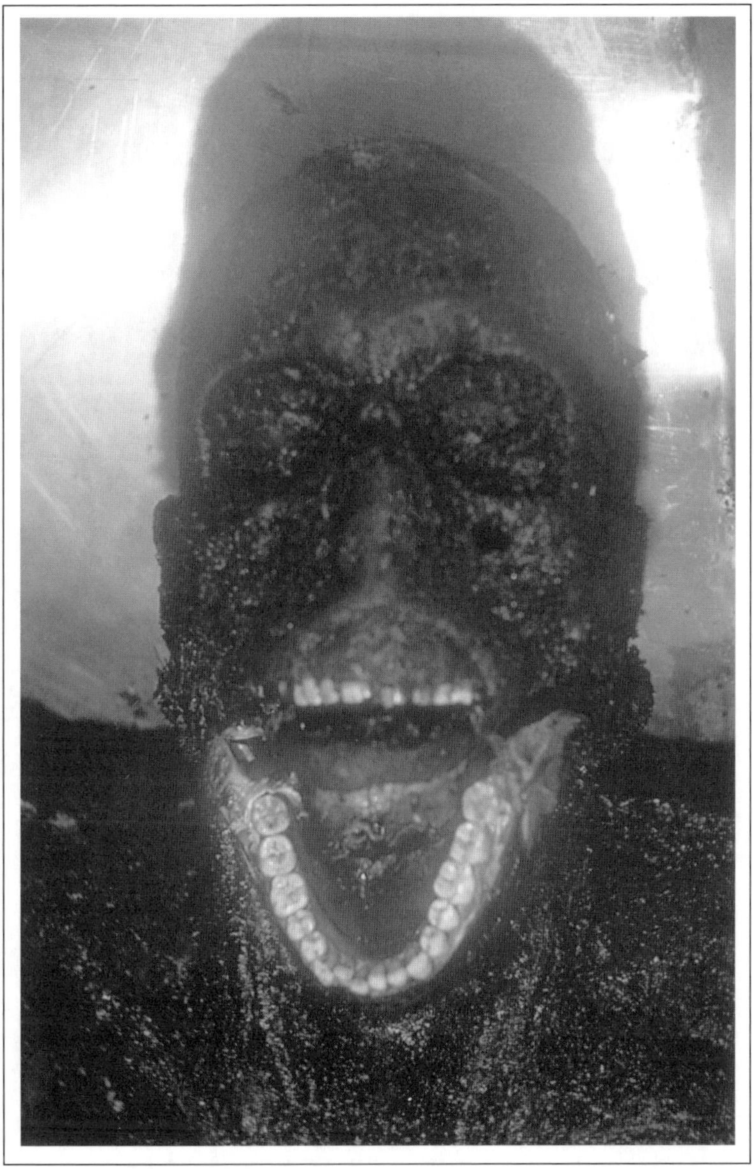

Figure 11.2 *Same body showing teeth still intact and suitable for identification purposes*

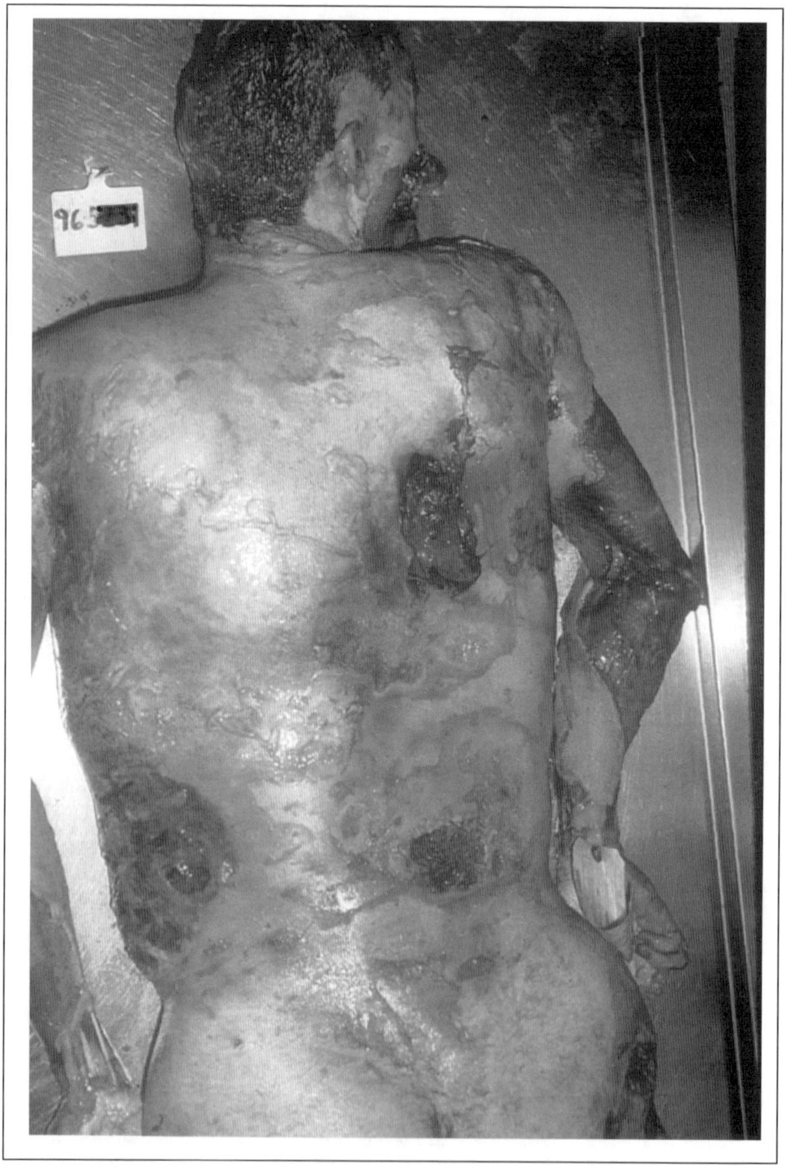

Figure 11.3 *TWA 800 explosion. The body fell 13,000 feet and remained 100 feet underwater for two weeks before recovery. Note that the coldness of the water prevented bacterial growth and decomposition but there is loss of soft tissues from fish and other animal activity.*

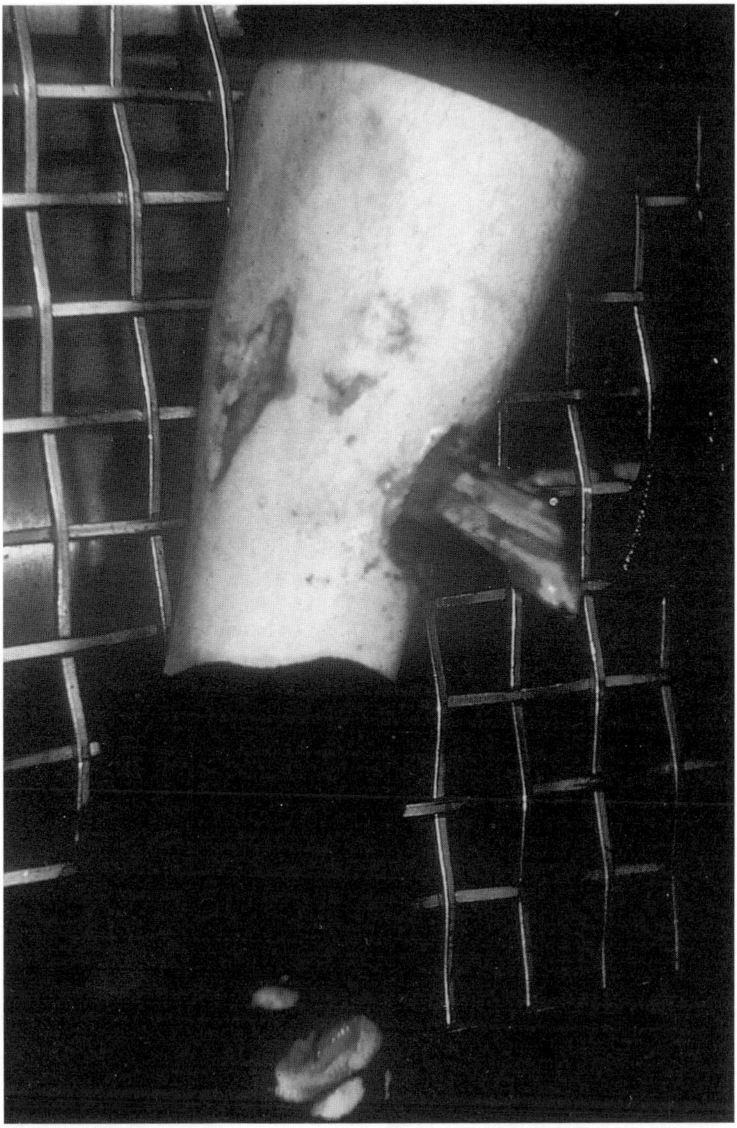

Figure 11.4 *Fraunces Tavern explosion: secondary debris missiles in lower extremity*

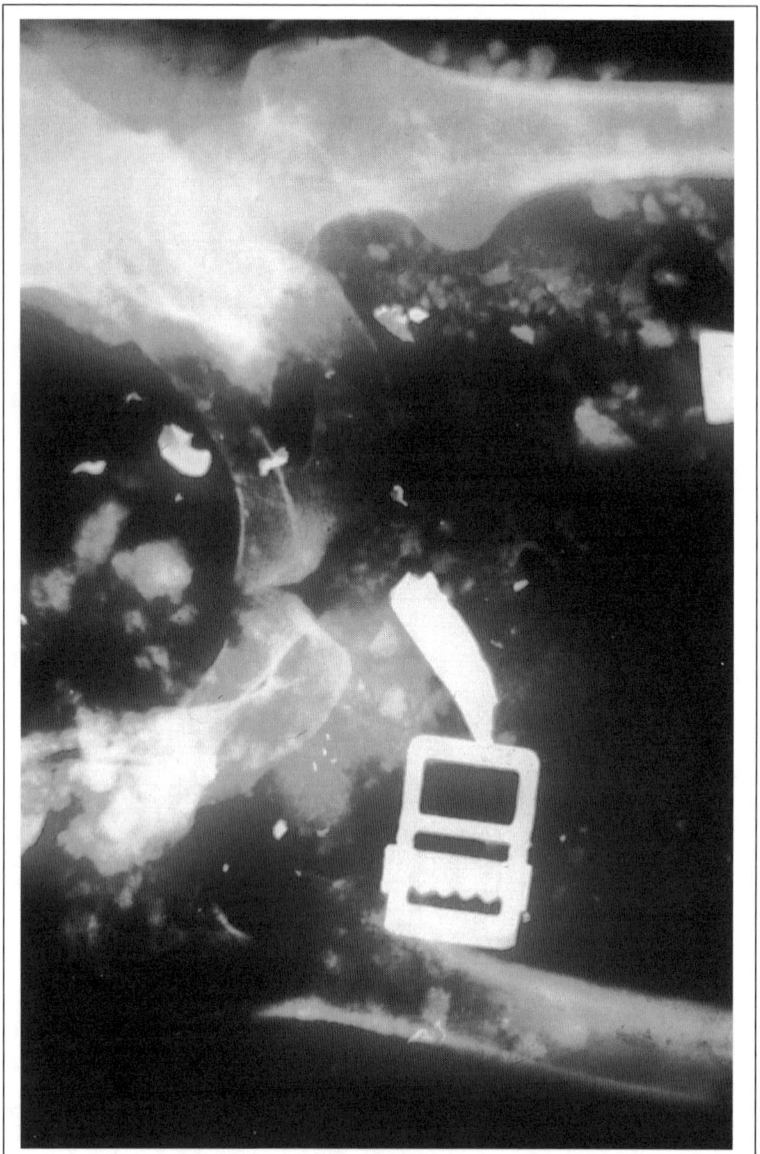

Figure 11.5 *Fraunces Tavern explosion: X-ray of pelvis showing secondary shrapnel that entered body*

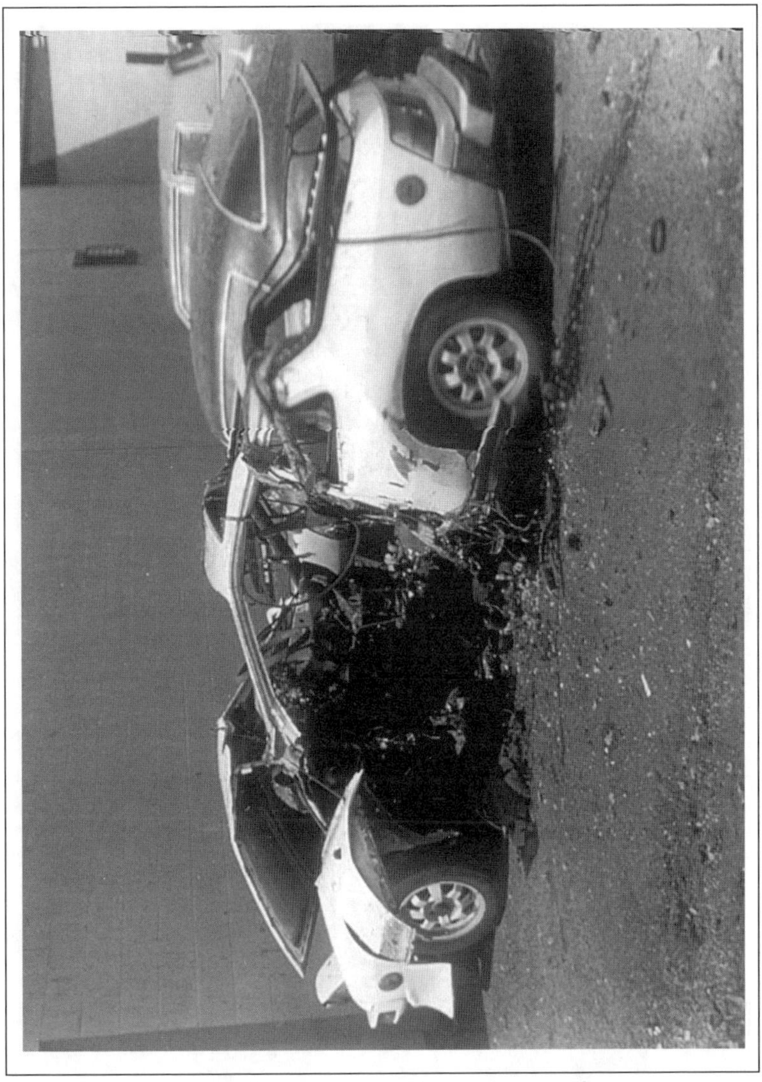

Figure 11.6 *Car bombing: explosive device was under car*

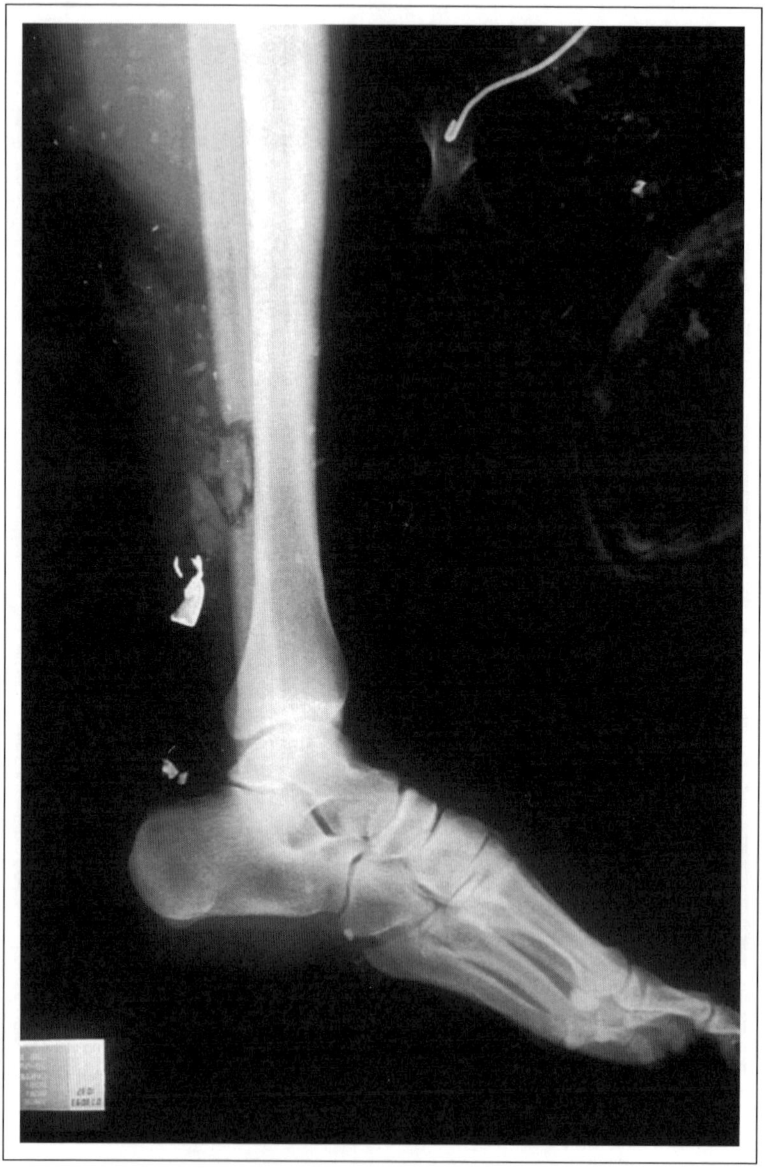

Figure 11.7 *X-ray of right leg shows metal fragments from bomb device that were blown into the body*

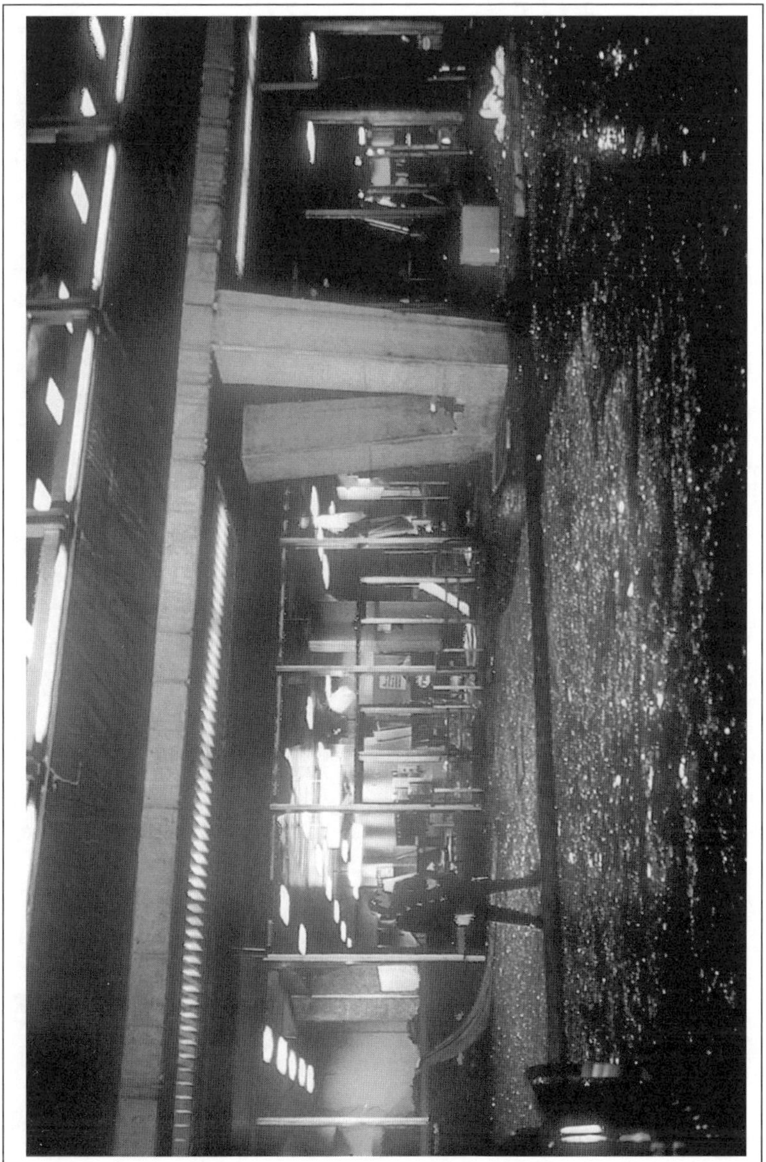

Figure 11.8 *Bomb explosion at LaGuardia Airport: plastic explosive left in metal locker at TWA terminal*

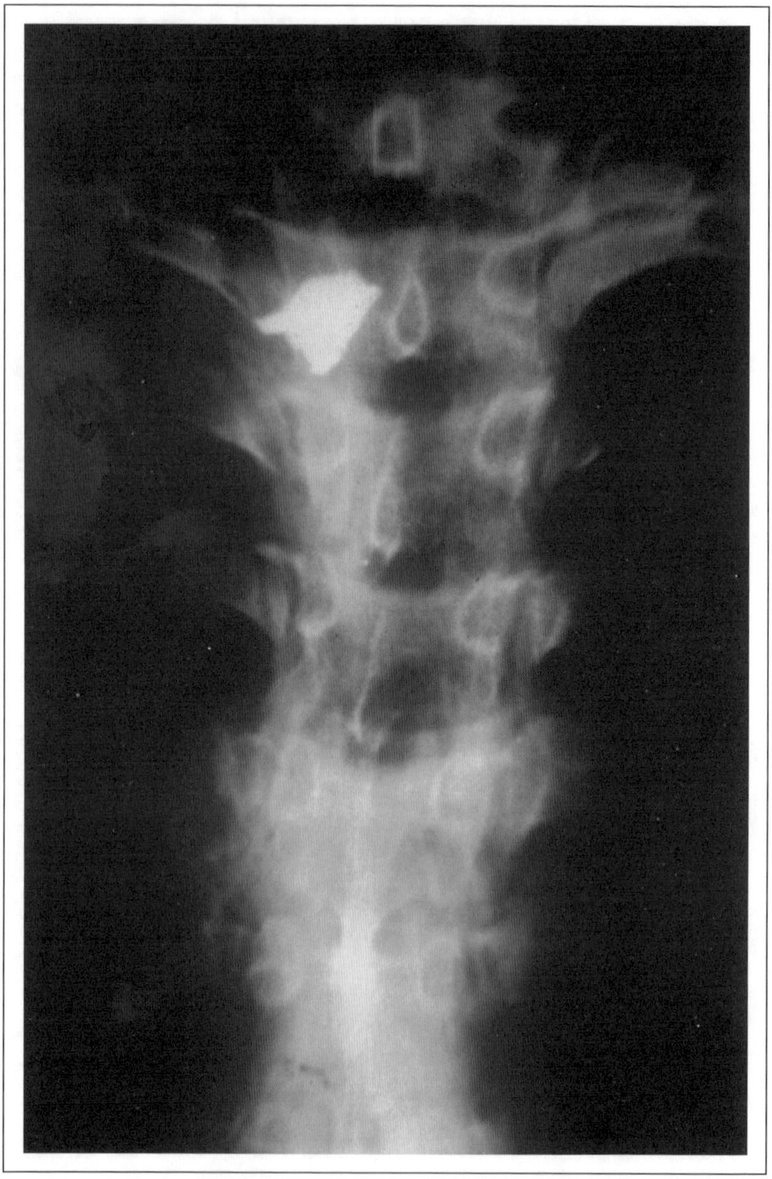

Figure 11.9 *Bomb explosion at LaGuardia Airport: X-ray showing metal fragment from locker that acted as secondary missile and fatally severed the right carotid artery*

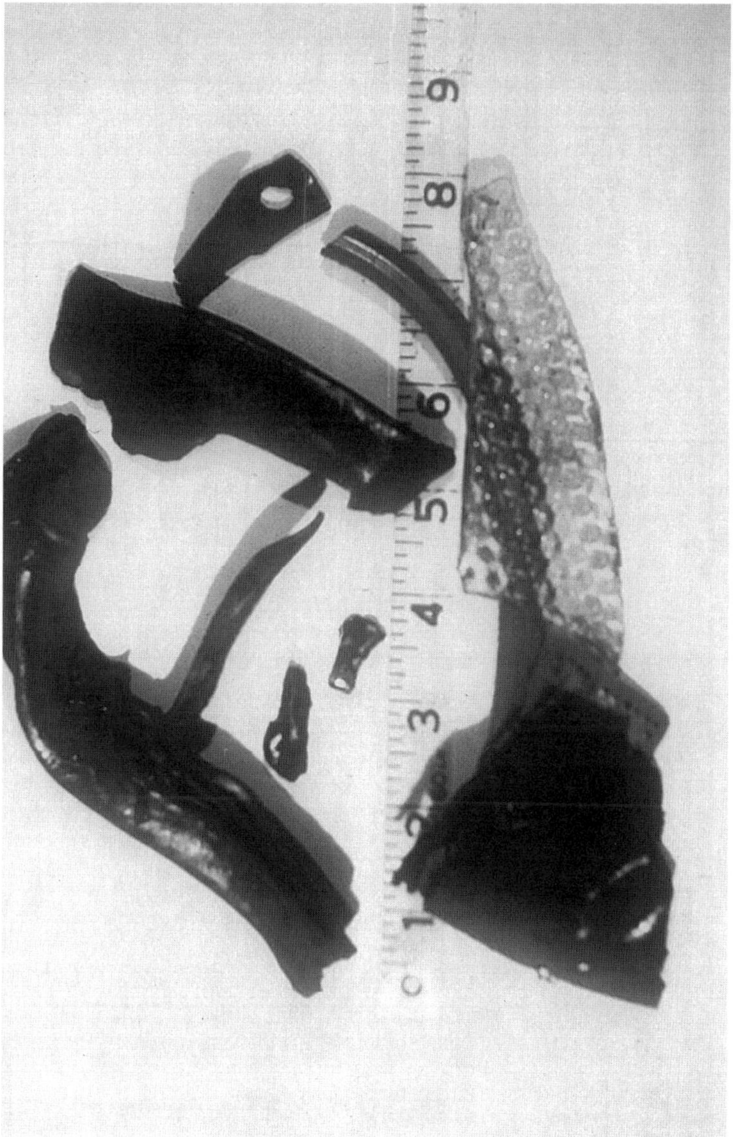

Figure 11.10 *Bomb explosion at LaGuardia Airport: lethal objects removed from decedents*

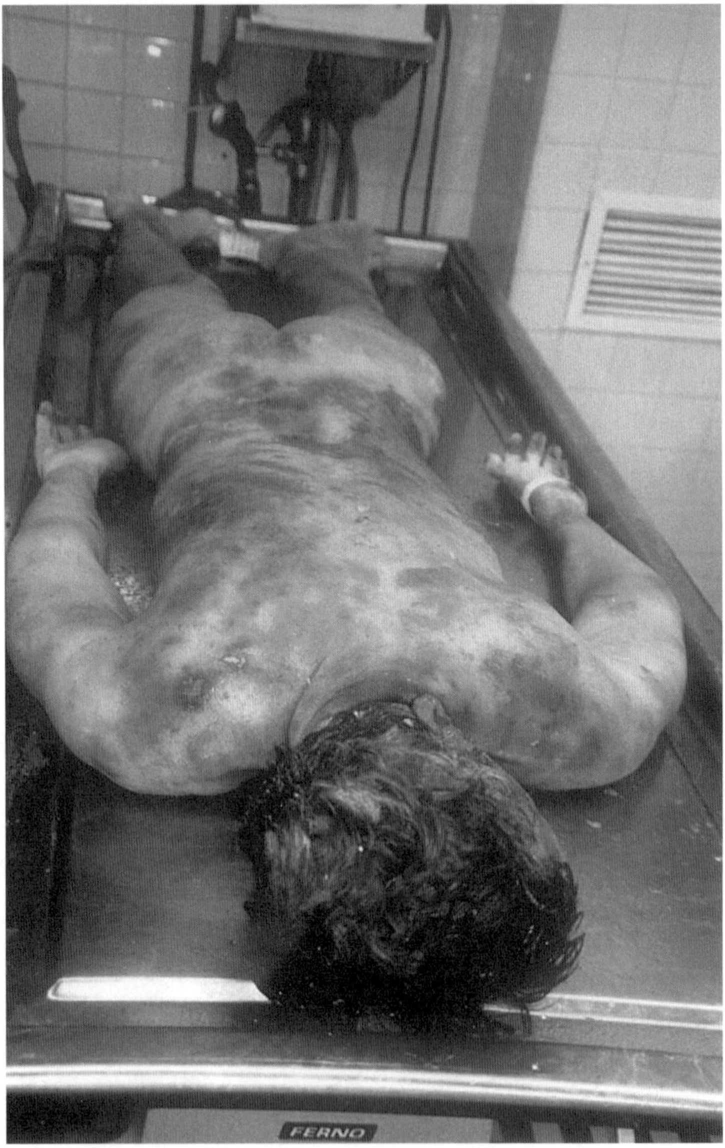

Figure 11.11 *Victim of World Trade Center collapse fell from 85th floor. Body intact but with extensive internal injuries.*

Chapter 12

Medical Examiners, Coroners, and Biologic Terrorism: A Guidebook for Surveillance and Case Management

Kurt B. Nolte, M.D.,[1,2*] Randy L. Hanzlick, M.D.,[2,3*] Daniel C. Payne, Ph.D.,[4] Andrew T. Kroger, M.D.,[5] William R. Oliver, M.D.,[6*] Andrew M. Baker, M.D.,[7*] Dennis E. McGowan,[3*] Joyce L. DeJong, D.O.,[8*] Michael R. Bell, M.D.,[7] Jeannette Guarner, M.D.,[9] Wun-Ju Shieh, M.D., Ph.D.,[9] and Sherif R. Zaki, M.D., Ph.D.[9]

The material in this report originated in the Epidemiology Program Office, Stephen B. Thacker, M.D., M.Sc., Director; the Division of Public Health Surveillance and Informatics, Richard Hopkins, M.D., M.S.P.H., Acting Director; the National Center for Infectious Diseases, James M. Hughes, M.D., Director; and the Division of Viral and Rickettsial Diseases, James LeDuc, Ph.D., Sc.D., Director.

Summary

Medical examiners and coroners (ME/Cs) are essential public health partners for terrorism preparedness and response. These medicolegal investigators support both public health and public safety functions and investigate deaths that are sudden, suspicious, violent, unattended, and unexplained. Medicolegal autopsies are essential for making organism-specific diagnoses in deaths caused by biologic terrorism. This report has been created to (1) help public health officials understand the role of ME/Cs in biologic terrorism surveillance and response efforts and (2) provide ME/Cs with the detailed information required to build capacity for bio-

---

Reprinted with permission from *Morbidity and Mortality Weekly Report*, June 11, 2004.

logic terrorism preparedness in a public health context. This report provides background information regarding biologic terrorism, possible biologic agents, and the consequent clinicopathologic diseases, autopsy procedures, and diagnostic tests as well as a description of biosafety risks and standards for autopsy precautions. ME/Cs' vital role in terrorism surveillance requires consistent standards for collecting, analyzing, and disseminating data. Familiarity with the operational, jurisdictional, and evidentiary concerns involving biologic terrorism-related death investigation is critical to both ME/Cs and public health authorities. Managing terrorism-associated fatalities can be expensive and can overwhelm the existing capacity of ME/Cs. This report describes federal resources for funding and reimbursement for ME/C preparedness and response activities and the limited support capacity of the federal Disaster Mortuary Operational Response Team. Standards for communication are critical in responding to any emergency situation. This report, which is a joint collaboration between CDC and the National Association of Medical Examiners (NAME), describes the relationship between ME/Cs and public health departments, emergency management agencies, emergency operations centers, and the Incident Command System.

Introduction

Terrorist events in recent years have heightened awareness of the risk of terrorist acts involving unconventional agents, including biologic and chemical weapons. The need for terrorism preparedness and planning for response at multiple levels is now recognized, including planning and response by medical examiners, coroners (ME/Cs), and the medicolegal death-investigation system.

Federal, state, and local agencies have developed plans to detect and respond to terrorism by using a multidisciplinary approach that requires active participation of health-care providers, law enforcement, and public health and safety staff. Because ME/Cs have expertise in disease surveillance, diagnosis, deceased body handling, and evidence collection, they serve a vital role in terrorism preparedness and response. ME/Cs should ensure that their role in surveillance for unusual deaths—and response to known terrorist events—is a critical part of the multidisciplinary response team. Terrorism-related drills and practical exercises conducted by public health, law enforcement, and public safety agencies should include training on postmortem operations and services.

This report, prepared as a joint effort between the National Association of Medical Examiners (NAME) and CDC, is a first step in providing specific guidance to ME/C death investigators and public health officials. This report can help bridge gaps that exist in local terrorism preparedness and response planning. By discussing the substantial contributions of ME/Cs, this report can also serve as a foundation for identifying the needs of medicolegal death-investigation systems and for addressing those needs through adequate training and funding.

This report provides guidance, identifies support services and resources, and discusses the roles and responsibilities of ME/Cs and affiliated personnel in recognizing and responding to potential biologic terrorism events. Certain questions being asked by ME/Cs and their public health partners are answered in this report, including the following:

- What are the likely biologic agents to be encountered?
- What are the expected case fatality rates and time courses for the different agents?
- What types of ongoing surveillance are needed to detect potential biologic terrorism-associated incidents?
- What protective equipment and procedures are needed to ensure the safety of death investigation and forensic pathology personnel?
- What are the appropriate facilities in which to perform postmortem examinations in cases of suspected biologic terrorism?
- What are the best methods for ensuring biosafety during the mortuary process?
- How will hospitals, emergency personnel, health departments, and ME/Cs effectively communicate during a suspected or known incident?
- How will local ME/C systems interact with the Federal Bureau of Investigation (FBI) and other investigative agencies?
- What is the minimum extent of examination that will be required? For example, will a complete autopsy be required in every suspected case to support the criminal justice process?

- What pathology-specific tests are available; which ones are the best to use to make an accurate diagnosis; and which ones are the best for making a rapid diagnosis?
- Which laboratories are best suited to perform the necessary postmortem testing?
- What role does public health law play in determining disposition of bodies?
- What legal authority do public health agencies have in making decisions during potential biologic terrorism events?
- What federal resources are available to assist ME/Cs?

Background

Medicolegal death investigators

CDC has identified medicolegal death investigators (i.e., ME/Cs) as essential partners in terrorism preparedness and response.[1] This report is designed to assist ME/Cs and their public health partners in developing appropriate capacity for recognizing and responding to deaths that are potentially a consequence of biologic terrorism.

The organization of medicolegal death investigative systems within the United States varies by state.[2] As ME/Cs and public health and public safety departments prepare to respond to terrorism-associated events, each state should consider how its medicolegal death investigation system is organized. These systems can be medical examiner-based (twenty-one states and the District of Columbia), coroner-based (ten states), or both (nineteen states) (Figure 12.1). Typically, coroners are elected lay persons who use medical personnel to assist in death investigation and autopsy performance. Medical examiners are usually appointed physicians and pathologists who have received special training in death investigation and forensic pathology.

Medicolegal death investigation systems can be either centralized (i.e., investigations emanate from one state-level office) or decentralized (i.e., investigations are conducted in more than one regional-, county-, or city-based office). A total of twenty-three states plus the District of Columbia have centralized systems; twenty-seven states are decentralized. States with medical examiner systems might have a state-based medical examiner office, and also have county-level autonomous medical exam-

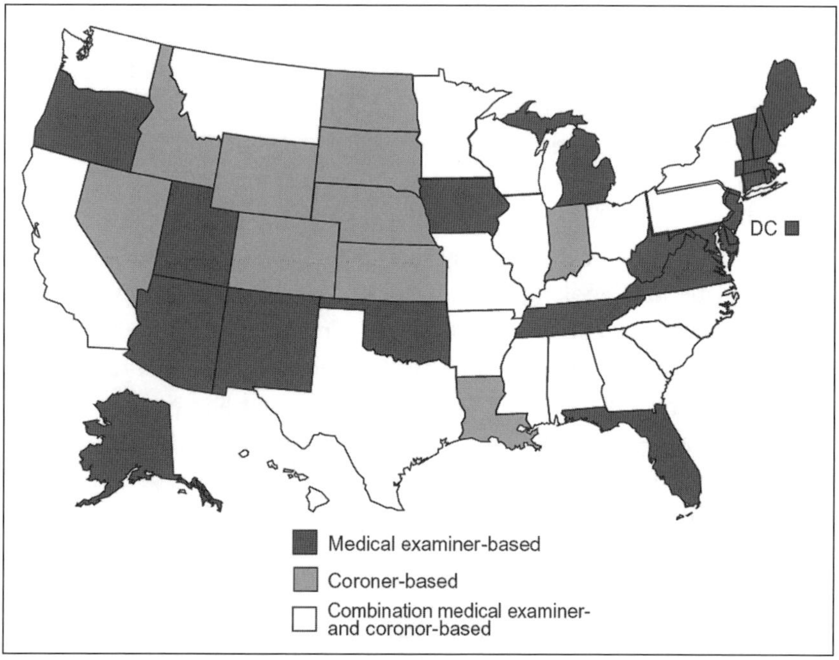

Figure 12.1 *Medicolegal death investigative systems in the United States*

iner offices that perform their own autopsies and manage their own data and administrative systems.

ME/C offices can also vary in their organizational position within the government. ME/C offices might be a component of the public health department or the public safety department, or be independent of other government agencies. All types of medicolegal death investigation systems should be considered when determining the roles, responsibilities, and participation of ME/Cs in a jurisdiction's terrorism preparedness and response plans.

Biologic terrorism

Biologic terrorism is defined as "the use or threatened use of biologic agents against a person, group, or larger population to create fear or illnesses for purposes of intimidation, gaining an advantage, interruption of normal activities, or ideologic activities. The resultant reaction is dependent on the actual event and the population involved and can vary from a minimal effect to disruption of ongoing activities and emotional reaction, illness, or death."[3] In the United States in 1984, an outbreak of terrorism-related Salmonella dysentery caused 715 persons to become ill, but no fatalities resulted.[4] In 2001, the intentional distribution of anthrax spores through the U.S. Postal Service resulted in five deaths from inhalational anthrax.[5–8] MEs were critical members of the response team during the anthrax outbreak, performing autopsies on each fatality to confirm the cause of death as anthrax and to identify the manner of death as homicide.

ME/Cs have state statutory authority to investigate deaths that are sudden, suspicious, violent, unattended, or unexplained;[9] therefore, these investigators have a role in recognizing and reporting fatal outbreaks, including those that are possibly terrorism-related, and a role in responding to a known terrorist event.[10–12] Deaths of persons at home or away from health-care facilities fall under the jurisdiction and surveillance of medicolegal death investigators,[13] who often identify infectious diseases that are not terrorism-related. For example, in 1993, MEs recognized an outbreak of hantavirus pulmonary syndrome, a disease with symptoms that can mimic terrorism-related illnesses.[14] Deaths of patients in hospitals can also fall under medicolegal jurisdiction if the patient dies precipitously before an accurate diagnosis is made or if a public health concern exists.[10] Fatalities caused by known terrorist events are homicides and therefore fall under the statutory jurisdiction of ME/Cs.

Risk assessment for potential biologic terrorism is an uncertain process. Hypothetical terrorism scenarios can involve a limited number of cases or millions of cases, with proportionate numbers of fatalities. For example, in 2002, the Dark Winter smallpox exercise included in the scenario 3 million fourth-generation cases of smallpox and approximately 1 million deaths.[15] In 2000, the TOPOFF (Top Officials) plague exercise included in the scenario 2,000 fatalities in a one-week period.[16] Given such possibilities if a biologic terrorist event occurred, ME/Cs should proactively identify appropriate resources and links to the public health, emergency response, healthcare, and law enforcement communities. With appropriate resources and links, ME/Cs can assist with surveillance for infectious disease deaths possibly caused by terrorism and provide confirmatory diagnoses and evidence in deaths clearly linked to terrorism. Conversely, public health agencies should recognize ME/Cs as a vital part of the public health system and keep them informed of infectious disease outbreaks occurring in their jurisdictions so that they are better able to recognize related fatalities. Additionally, public health agencies should provide ME/Cs with appropriate resources to enhance their surveillance and response capacities for terrorism.

An ME/C's principal diagnostic tool is the autopsy. This procedure enables pathologists to identify the dead, observe the condition of the body, and reach conclusions regarding the cause and manner of death. Autopsies are valuable in diagnosing unrecognized infections, evaluating therapy, understanding the pathogenesis and route of infection for uncommon or emerging infections, and developing evidence for subsequent legal proceedings.[10,17] In 1979, an anthrax outbreak occurred that was associated with an unintentional release of spores from a bioweapons factory in the Soviet city of Sverdlovsk; pathologists used autopsies to identify the cause of death as anthrax and the route of infection as inhalation.[18] In a 1945 smallpox outbreak, autopsy pathologists, rather than clinicians, were the physicians who recognized the sentinel case.[19]

Probable Biologic Terrorism Agents, Diseases, and Diagnostic Tests

Agent categories

In this report, the list of potential biologic terrorism agents has been prioritized on the basis of the risk to national security (Box 12.1).[1] Biologic agents are classified as high-risk, or Category A, because they can (1) be easily disseminated or transmitted person to person; (2) cause high mortality, with potential for major public health impact; (3) might cause public panic and social disruption; or (4) require special action for public health preparedness. The second highest priority, or Category B, agents include those that (1) are moderately easy to disseminate; (2) cause moderate morbidity and low mortality; or (3) require enhanced disease surveillance. The third highest priority, or Category C, agents include emerging pathogens that can be engineered for future mass dissemination because of (1) availability; (2) ease of production and dissemination; or (3) potential for high morbidity and mortality and major health impact.

Recognizing pathologic features of different biologic agents is important, as demonstrated by the inhalational and cutaneous anthrax cases that occurred in the United States during 2001[5,8,20–23] The autopsy of the index patient was performed to determine how the person had acquired anthrax (cutaneous, gastrointestinal, or inhalational). After inhalational anthrax

Box 12.1
Classification of Biologic Terrorism Agents

Category A Agents

- Variola major (smallpox)
- *Bacillus anthracis* (anthrax)
- *Yersinia pestis* (plague)
- *Clostridium botulinum* toxin (botulism)
- *Francisella tularensis* (tularemia)
- Hemorrhagic fever viruses, including
  - Filoviruses including Ebola and Marburg hemorrhagic fever
  - Arenaviruses, including Lassa (Lassa fever) and Junin (Argentine hemorrhagic fever) and related viruses

Category B Agents

- *Coxiella burnetii* (Q fever)
- *Brucella* species (brucellosis)
- *Burkholderia mallei* (glanders)
- Alphaviruses including Venezuelan encephalomyelitis and eastern and western equine encephalomyelitis viruses
- Ricin toxin from *Ricinus communis* (castor beans)
- Epsilon toxin of *Clostridium perfringens*
- *Staphylococcus* enterotoxin B
- Food- and waterborne pathogens
  - *Salmonella* species
  - *Shigella dysenteriae*
  - *Escherichia coli* O157:H7
  - *Vibrio cholerae*
  - *Cryptosporidium parvum*

Category C Agents

- Nipah virus
- Hantaviruses
- Tickborne hemorrhagic fever viruses
- Tickborne encephalitis viruses
- Yellow fever virus
- Multidrug-resistant *Mycobacterium tuberculosis*

was diagnosed, public health officials were able to better define potential sources of the airborne *Bacillus anthracis* spores.

Diagnostic tests

If possible, given the constraints of case volume and biosafety concerns, complete autopsies with histologic sampling of multiple organs should be performed in deaths potentially caused by infections with biologic terrorism agents. Autopsy diagnostic procedures for the Category A agents include microscopic examination, combined with the collection of specimens for additional tests that will aid in determining a definitive organism-specific diagnosis. Blood, cerebrospinal fluid, and tissue samples or swabs should be placed in transport media that will allow bacterial and viral isolation. Serum should be collected for serologic and biologic assays. Tissue samples should be frozen for polymerase chain reaction (PCR). Tissue samples should also be placed in electron microscopy fixative (glutaraldehyde). Microscopic examination of formalin-fixed, paraffin-embedded tissues stained with hematoxylin and eosin (H&E) is essential to characterizing the patterns of tissue damage defining a syndrome and establishes a list of possible microorganisms in the differential diagnosis. To enhance surveillance for these conditions, a matrix of potential pathology-based syndromes has been developed to guide autopsy pathologists in recognizing potential cases.[24] Special stains (e.g., tissue Gram and silver impregnation stains [Steiner's or Warthin-Starry]), can be helpful in identifying bacterial agents. Additionally, specific immunohistochemical (IHC) and direct fluorescent assays (DFA) for the Category A terrorism agents have been developed and are available at CDC.† These tests can be performed on formalin-fixed tissues. Clinical and pathologic characteristics of the Category A agents and corresponding diagnostic methods are summarized in this report (Tables 12.1 and 12.2).

Anthrax

Agent: *Bacillus anthracis*

Pathologic findings. Anthrax has three pathologic forms. **Cutaneous anthrax** is characterized by an eschar that forms where the bacteria entered the skin (Figure 12.2). Microscopically, the epidermis has necrosis and crusts, whereas the dermis demonstrates necrosis, edema, hemorrhage, perivascular inflammation, and vasculitis. The lymph nodes that drain the skin site eventually become enlarged, necrotic, and hemorrhagic. **Gastrointestinal anthrax** is distinguishable by hemorrhagic ulcers in the terminal ileum and caecum accompanied by mesenteric hemorrhagic lymphadenitis and peritonitis. **Inhalational anthrax** is characterized by hemorrhagic mediastinal lymphadenitis (Figure 12.3) accompanied by pleural effusions. Histologically, lymph nodes have abundant edema, hemorrhage, and necrosis with limited inflammatory infiltrate (Figure 12.4).[18,25–29] As any of the three anthrax forms progresses, the bacteria can spread to abdominal organs, producing petechial hemorrhages, and to the central nervous system, producing hemorrhagic meningitis (i.e., cardinal's cap) (Figure 12.5).

Diagnostic specimens. Performing a complete autopsy with histologic sampling of multiple organs will help determine the distribution of bacilli and the portal of entry. The specimens that harbor the highest number of *B. anthracis* organisms vary by the pathologic form of anthrax. For example, diagnosis of cutaneous anthrax requires skin samples from the center and periphery of the eschar, whereas for inhalational anthrax, pleural fluid cell blocks, pleura tissue, and mediastinal lymph nodes have the highest amounts of bacilli and antigens.

Diagnostic tests. If the patient has not received antibiotics, bacilli can be observed in tissues with H&E, Gram, and silver impregnation stains

Table 12.1
Selected Epidemiologic Characteristics of Illnesses Caused by Category A Biologic Agents*

Disease	Incubation period	Duration of illness	Case fatality rates
Inhalational anthrax	1–6 days	3–5 days	Untreated, 100% Treated, 45%
Botulism	6 hr–10 days	24–72 hrs	Outbreak-associated, first patient, 25% Subsequent patients, 4% Overall, 5%–10%
Tularemia	1–21 days	2 weeks	Untreated, 33% Treated, <4%
Pneumonic plague	2–3 days	1–6 days	Untreated, 40%–70% Treated, 5%
Smallpox	7–17 days	4 weeks	Overall, 20%–50%
Viral hemorrhagic fevers	4–21 days	7–16 days	Overall, 53%–88%

* Source: CDC. Bioterrorism: Agent Summary. Atlanta, GA: US Department of Health and Human Services, CDC, 2001.

Table 12.2
Primary Pathologic Features and Differential Diagnoses of Illnesses Caused by Category A Biologic Agents

Agent/disease	Primary pathologic features	Differential diagnosis
Smallpox virus (variola major)	Multiloculated vesicles, ballooning degeneration of epithelial cells, intracytoplasmic inclusions (Guarnieri bodies)	Chicken pox, monkeypox, parapox, tanapox, herpes simplex, secondary syphilis
Bacillus anthracis (anthrax)	Inhalational anthrax—hemorrhagic mediastinitis, hemorrhagic lymphadenitis, hemorrhagic pleural effusion	Inhalational anthrax—community acquired pneumonia, pneumonic tularemia or plague, hantavirus pulmonary syndrome, bacterial/fungal/tuberculous mediastinitis or meningitis, fulminate mediastinal tumors, aortic dissection
	Cutaneous anthrax—hemorrhage, edema, necrosis, perivascular infiltrate, vasculitis	Cutaneous anthrax—rickettsialpox, spider bite, ecthyma gangrenosum, ulceroglandular tularemia
	Gastrointestinal anthrax—hemorrhagic enteritis, hemorrhagic lymphadenitis, mucosal ulcers with necrosis in the terminal ileum and cecum, peritonitis	
	CNS involvement—hemorrhagic meningitis	
	Bubonic plague—acute lymphadenitis with surrounding edema	Bubonic plague—tularemia, other bacterial adenitis
	Pneumonic plague—severe, confluent, hemorrhagic, and necrotizing bronchopneumonia, often with fibrinous pleuritis	Pneumonic plague—inhalational anthrax, community acquired pneumonia, pneumonic tularemia, hantavirus pulmonary syndrome
	Septicemic plague—generalized lymphadenitis, foci of necrosis in lymph nodes and other reticuloendothelial organs, disseminated intravascular coagulation (DIC) with widespread hemorrhages and thrombi	Septicemic plague—other bacterial sepsis
	CNS involvement—meningitis	Plague meningitis—other bacterial or fungal meningitis
Yersinia pestis (plague)	Ulceroglandular tularemia—skin ulcer with associated suppurative necrotizing lymphadenitis	Ulceroglandular tularemia—cutaneous anthrax, rickettsialpox, spider bite, ecthyma gangrenosum
	Glandular tularemia—suppurative necrotizing lymphadenitis without associated skin ulcer	Glandular tularemia—pyogenic bacterial infections, cat-scratch disease, syphilis, chancroid, lymphogranuloma venereum, tuberculosis, nontuberculous mycobacterial infection, toxoplasmosis,sporotrichosis, rat-bite fever, anthrax, plague
Francisella tularensis (tularemia)	Oculoglandular tularemia—eyelid edema, acute conjunctivitis and edema, small conjunctival ulcers, regional lymphadenitis	Oculoglandular tularemia—pyogenic bacterial infections, adenoviral infection, syphilis, cat-scratch, disease, herpes simplex virus infection
	Pharyngeal tularemia—exudative pharyngitis or tonsillitis with ulceration, pharyngeal membrane formation, regional lymphadenitis	Pharyngeal tularemia—streptococcal pharyngitis, infectious mononucleosis, adenoviral infection, diphtheria
	Typhoidal tularemia—systemic involvement, DIC, focal necrosis of major organs	Typhoidal tularemia—typhoid fever, brucellosis, Q fever, disseminated bacterial, mycobacterial or fungal infection, rickettsioses, malaria
	Pneumonic tularemia—acute inflammation, diffuse alveolar damage	Pneumonic tularemia—community-acquired pneumonia, pneumonic plague, hantavirus pulmonary syndrome
Viral hemorrhagic fevers	Filoviruses (Ebola and Marburg)—massive hepatocellular necrosis, filamentous inclusions in hepatocytes, extensive necrosis in other major organs, diffuse alveolar damage	Other systemic infections caused by viral, bacterial, or rickettsial agents
	Arenaviruses (Lassa, Junin, Machupo, Guanarito) —massive hepatic necrosis, diffuse alveolar damage	

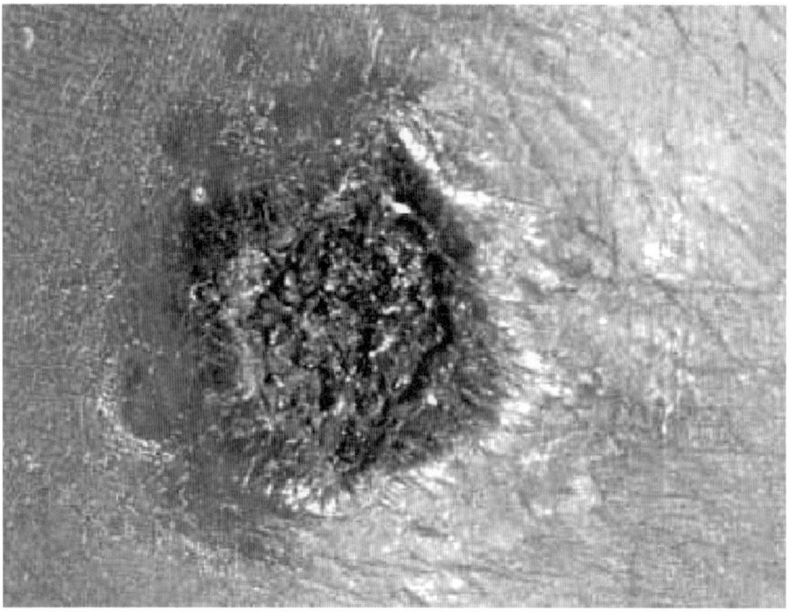

Figure 12.2 *Cutaneous anthrax—eschar lesion. Public Health Image Library, CDC*

and IHC assays (Figures 12.6 and 12.7). However, after antibiotic treatment has been instituted, only silver stains and IHC assays will highlight the bacilli. IHC assays for *B. anthracis* can demonstrate bacilli, bacillary fragments, and granular bacterial fragments in formalin-fixed tissues, even after ten days of antibiotic treatment. Although a DFA test is available for *B. anthracis*, it is not used on formalin-fixed tissues.

Plague

Agent: *Yersinia pestis*

Pathologic findings. Similar to anthrax, the clinicopathologic manifestations of plague are classified on the basis of the portal of entry of *Y. pestis*. Bubonic plague refers to an acute lymphadenitis that occurs after the bacteria have penetrated the skin (Figure 12.8). Usually, skin lesions are inconspicuous or have a small vesicle or pustule that might not be evident at the time the infected lymph node (bubo) appears. Histologically, the bubo exhibits edema, hemorrhage, necrosis, and a ground-glass amphophilic material that represents masses of bacilli. Primary pneumonic

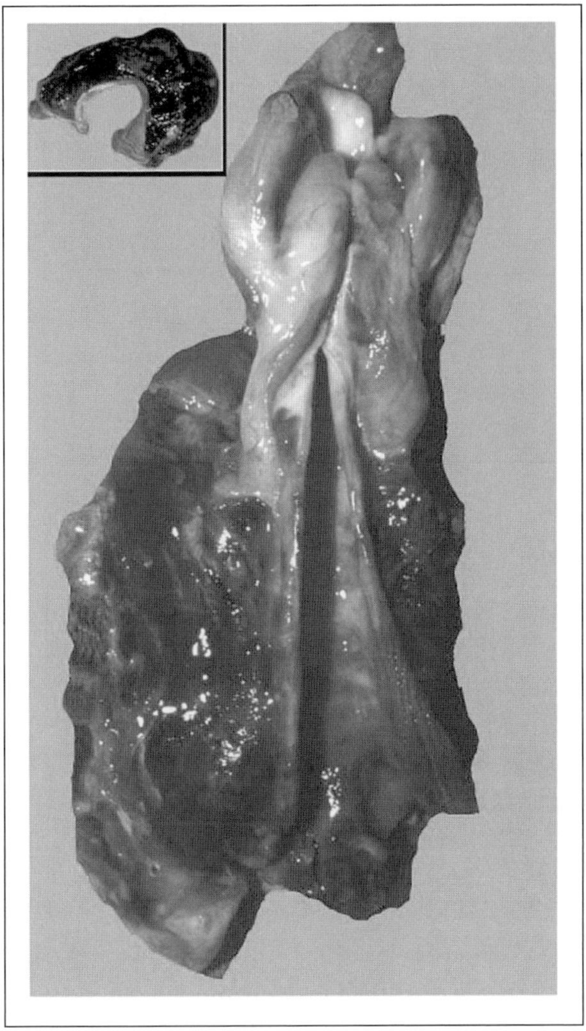

Figure 12.3 *Inhalational anthrax—hemorrhagic mediastinal lymphadenitis surrounding trachea; inset, cross-section of trachea surrounded by hemorrhagic soft tissue and lymph nodes. Reprinted courtesy of New York City Office of the Chief Medical Examiner.*

plague refers to the infection caused by inhalation of airborne bacteria, producing intra-alveolar edema accompanied by varying amounts of acute inflammatory infiltrate and abundant bacteria. Primary septicemic plague occurs when *Y. pestis* enters through the oropharyngeal route. In septicemic plague, the cervical lymph nodes draining the infected region

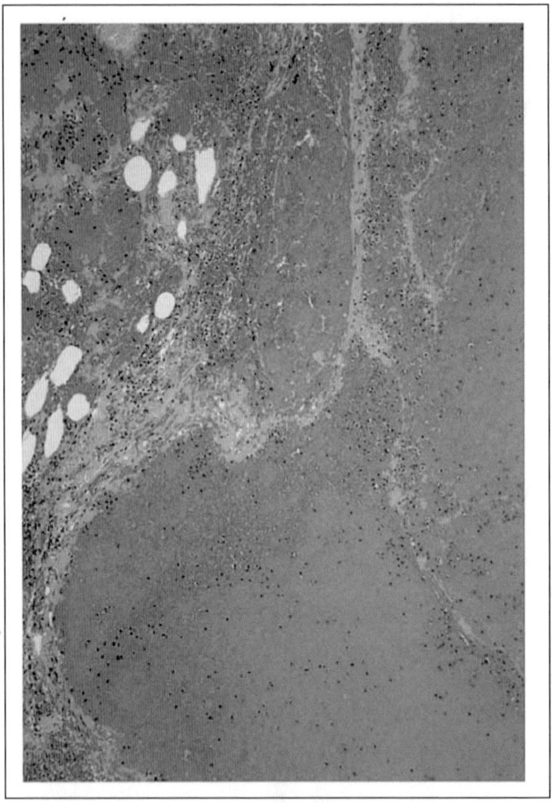

Figure 12.4 *Inhalational anthrax—histologic section of mediastinal lymph node with hemorrhage, necrosis, and sparse inflammatory cell infiltrate (hematoxylin and eosin stain). Infectious Disease Pathology Activity, CDC*

will display the previously described pathologic features. As the disease progresses, bacteria are distributed widely throughout the body, and findings consistent with shock and disseminated intravascular coagulation are observed. Septicemic plague with bacterial seeding of the lungs results in secondary pneumonic plague (Figure 12.9A, left).[30–35]

Diagnostic specimens. Performing a complete autopsy with histologic sampling of multiple organs will help determine the distribution of bacteria and the portal of entry. Enlarged, soft, hemorrhagic lymph nodes should be sampled and tested for *Y. pestis*. The lungs should be sampled to determine whether a primary or secondary infection existed.[30]

Diagnostic tests. *Y. pestis* can be visualized in formalin-fixed tissues by using H&E, Gram, silver impregnation, and Giemsa stains; however,

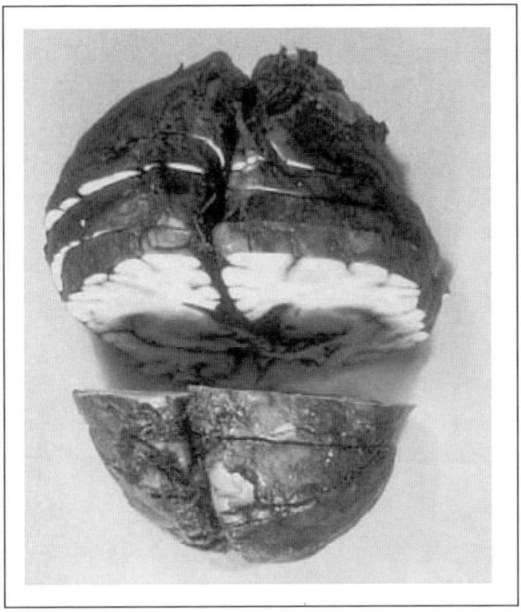

Figure 12.5 *Anthrax—hemorrhagic meningitis. Public Health Image Library, CDC*

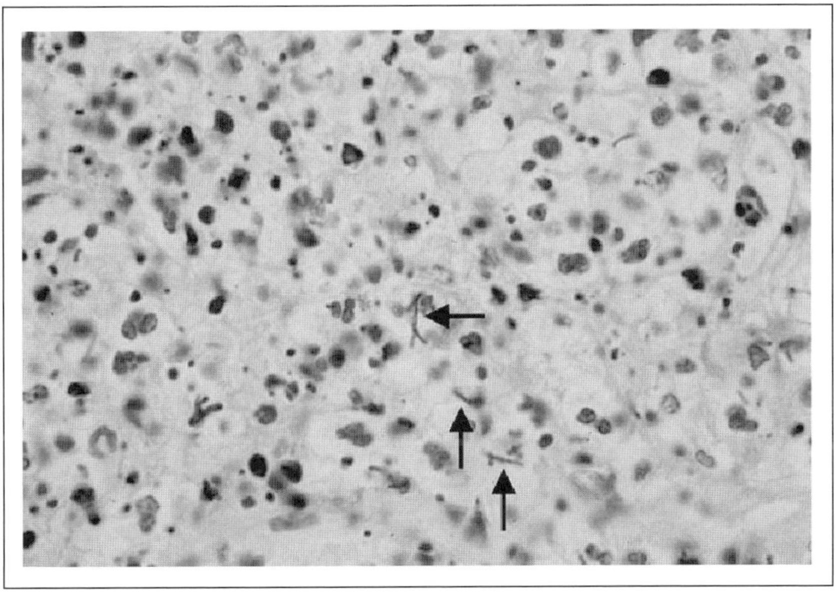

Figure 12.6 *Anthrax—*Bacillus anthracis *rods in mediastinal lymph node (Gram stain). Infectious Disease Pathology Activity, CDC*

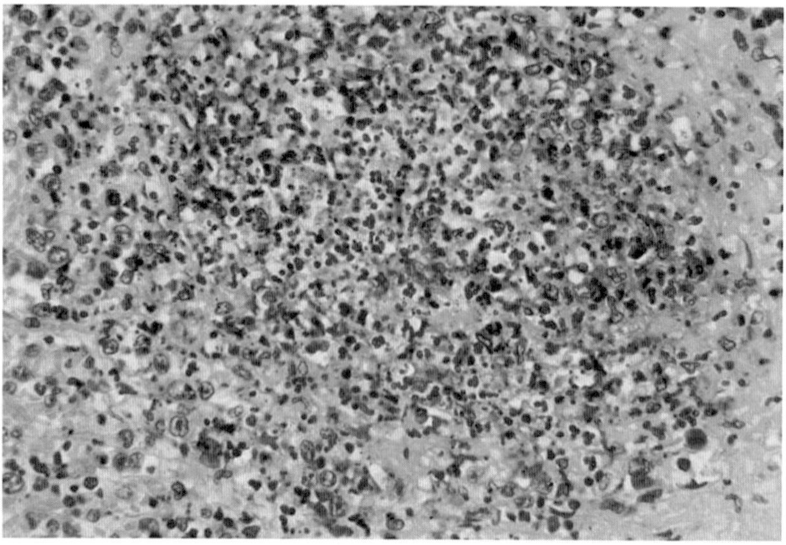

Figure 12.7 *Anthrax—*Bacillus anthracis *rods, bacillary fragments and granular bacterial fragments in spleen(immunohistochemistry). Infectious Disease Pathology Activity, CDC*

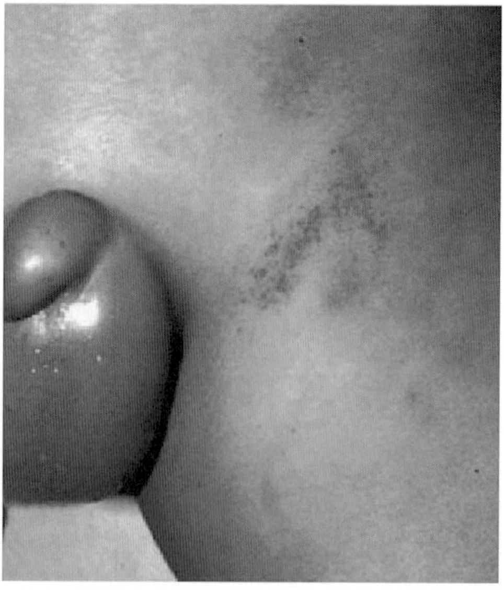

Figure 12.8 *Bubonic plague—lymphadenitis. New Mexico Office of the Medical Investigator*

specific identification of the bacilli in tissues can only be performed by using IHC or DFA (Figure 12.9B, right).

Tularemia

Agent: *Francisella tularensis*

Pathologic findings. Tularemia can also have multiple clinicopathologic forms, depending on the portal of entry, including ulceroglandular, oculoglandular, glandular, pharyngeal, typhoidal, and pneumonic. In all forms, the primary draining lymph nodes demonstrate necrotizing lymphadenitis surrounded by a neutrophilic and granulomatous inflammatory infiltrate. In the ulceroglandular form, a skin ulcer or eschar with corresponding lymph node involvement is present, but skin lesions are absent in the glandular form. In the oculoglandular form, the eye exhibits conjunctivitis with ulcers and soft-tissue edema. The pharyngeal form is characterized by pharyngitis or tonsillitis with ulceration. The lungs in pneu-

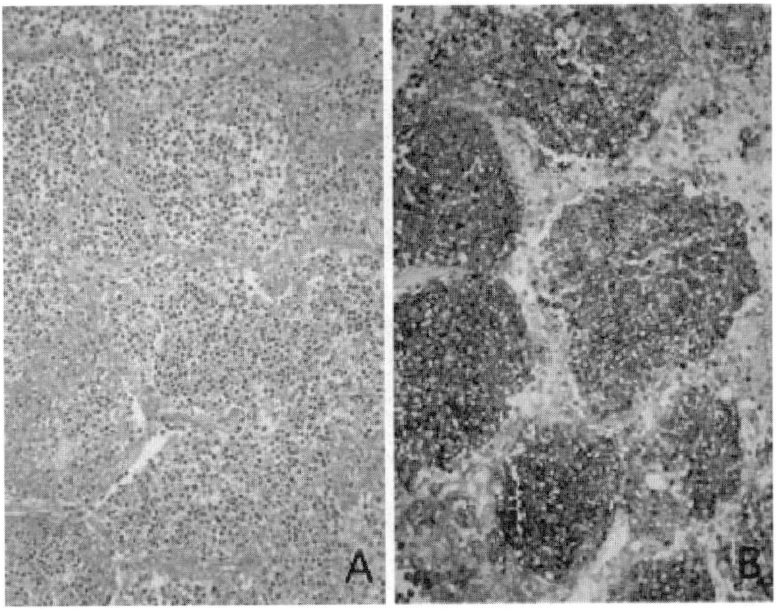

Figure 12.9 *Secondary pneumonic plague—Histologic sections of lung with (A, left) neutrophilic infiltrate in space (hematoxylin and eosin stain) and (B, right) pestis bacteria (immunohistochemistry). Infectious Disease Pathology Activity, CDC*

monic tularemia exhibit abundant fibrinous necrosis accompanied by varying amounts of mixed inflammatory infiltrate (Figure 12.10A, left). Typhoidal tularemia refers to systemic involvement with focal areas of necrosis in the major organs and disseminated intravascular coagulation, but lacks a group of primary draining lymph nodes.[36–40] In cases of tularemia sepsis, organisms can be seen with blood smears (Figure 12.11).

Diagnostic specimens. Performing a complete autopsy with histologic sampling of multiple organs will help determine the distribution of bacteria and the portal of entry. Enlarged, necrotic lymph nodes should be sampled and tested for *F. tularensis*. Culture swabs from the potential portals of entry (e.g., skin, conjunctiva, or throat) can be useful.

Diagnostic tests. The microorganisms are difficult to demonstrate with special stains; however, IHC and DFA have been successfully used in formalin-fixed tissues to demonstrate the bacteria (Figure 12.10B, right).

Botulism

Agent: Absorption of *Clostridium botulinum* toxin

Pathologic findings. *C. botulinum* elaborates a potent, preformed neurotoxin. The most important diagnostic feature of botulism is the clinical history because the histopathologic changes are nonspecific (e.g., central nervous system hyperemia and microthrombosis of small vessels).[41]

Diagnostic specimens. When botulism is suspected because of a symmetrical, descending pattern of weakness and paralysis of cranial nerves, limbs, and trunk, the pathologist should obtain tissue for anaerobic cultures from the suspect entry sites (i.e., wound, gastrointestinal tract, or respiratory tract) and serum for botulinum toxin mouse bioassay.

Diagnostic tests. Microbiologic culture and botulinum toxin mouse bioassay with serum are necessary.

Smallpox

Agent: Variola virus (Orthopoxvirus)

Pathologic findings. Smallpox is an acute, highly contagious illness caused by a member of the *Poxviridae* family. *Variola major* refers to the form with a higher mortality rate, and variola minor or alastrim is a milder

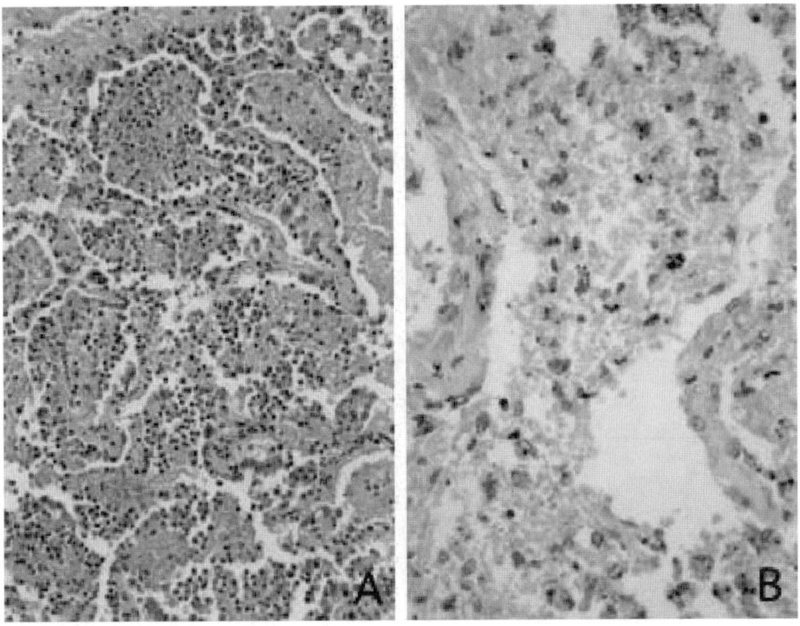

Figure 12.10 *Primary pneumonic tularemia—histologic sections of lung with (A, left) neutrophilic infiltrate in alveolar space (hematoxylin and eosin stain) and (B, right)* Francisella tularensis *bacteria (immunohistochemistry). Infectious Disease Pathology Activity, CDC.*

form. The lesions develop at approximately the same time and rate, starting in the palms and soles and spreading centrally; they first appear as macules and papules, and then progress to vesicles and umbilicated pustules (Figure 12.12), followed by scabs and crusts, and end as pitted scars. Occasionally, a hemorrhagic and uniformly fatal form occurs. This form has extensive bleeding into the skin and gastrointestinal tract and can be grossly taken for meningococcemia, acute leukemia, or a drug reaction.[42] Microscopically, the skin exhibits multiloculated, intraepidermal vesicles; ballooning degeneration of epithelial cells; intracytoplasmic, paranuclear, and eosinophilic viral inclusions (i.e., Guarnieri bodies) (Figure 12.13); and occasionally intranuclear viral changes. Secondary infections (e.g., bronchitis, pneumonia, and encephalitis) can complicate the clinical appearance.[43–48]

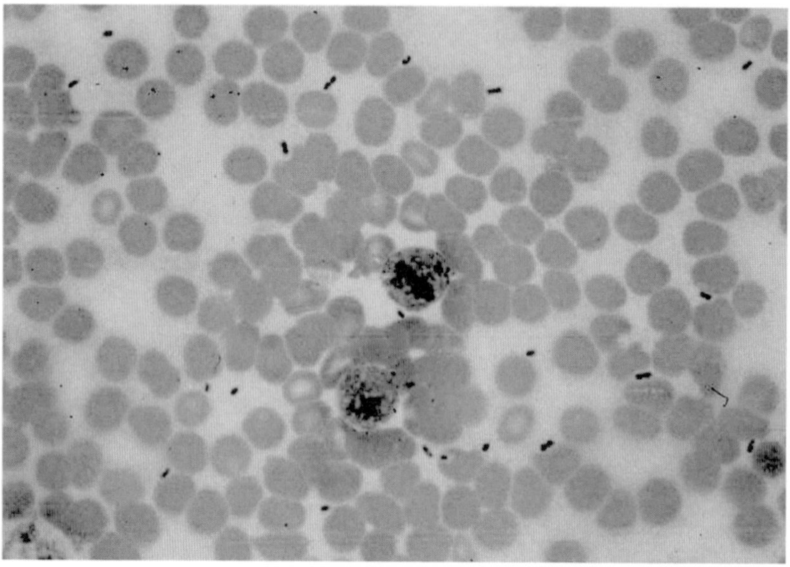

Figure 12.11 *Tularemia—blood smear demonstrating* Francisella tularensis *bacteria (Giemsa stain). Infectious Disease Pathology Activity, CDC.*

Diagnostic specimens. Cutaneous lesions are the most important sample for smallpox. Samples should include fluid from vesicles to be studied by electron microscopy, and skin samples fixed in formalin for histopathology and immunohistochemistry. Performing a complete autopsy with histologic sampling of multiple organs will help determine the extent and distribution of the virus, as well as the occurrence of secondary infections.

Diagnostic tests. Electron microscopic studies of vesicle fluid or skin samples can identify characteristic viral particles (Figure 12.14). IHC studies have demonstrated the virus in the epithelial cells and in the subjacent fibroconnective tissue.

Viral Hemorrhagic Fevers

Agents: Multiple

Viruses that can cause hemorrhagic fevers belong to different families, including Filoviridae (Ebola, Marburg viruses), Flaviviridae (yellow fever, dengue viruses), Bunyaviridae (Rift Valley fever, Crimean Congo,

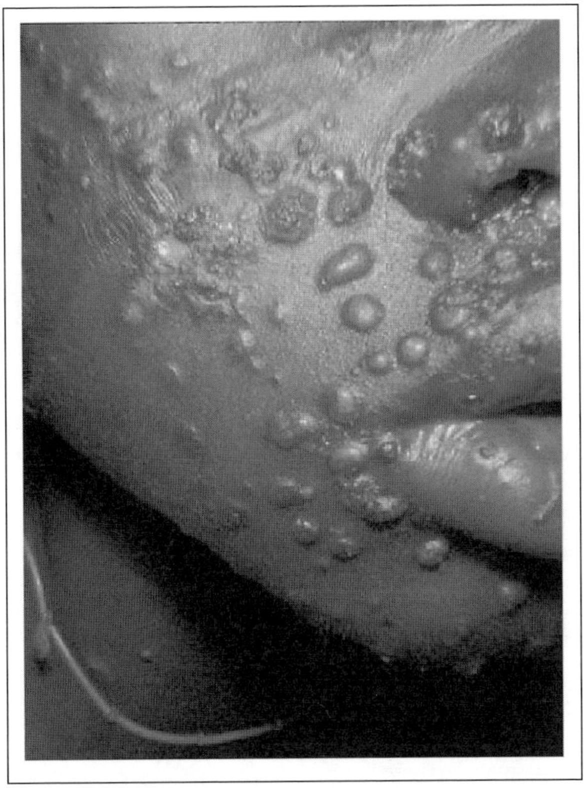

Figure 12.12 *Smallpox—cutaneous papules and vesicles. Public Health Image Library, CDC.*

Hantaan, Sin Nombre viruses), and Arenaviridae (Junin, Machupo, Guanarito, Lassa viruses).

Pathologic findings. The term viral hemorrhagic fever is reserved for febrile illnesses associated with abnormal vascular regulation and vascular damage. Common pathologic findings at autopsy include petechial hemorrhages and ecchymoses of skin, mucous membranes, and internal organs. Although systemic hemorrhages occur in the majority of viral hemorrhagic fevers, certain agents infect specific cells and thus histopathologic features can differ among agents. Necrosis of liver and lymphoid tissues, as well as diffuse alveolar damage, occur in the majority of viral hemorrhagic fevers, but can be more prominent for certain infections (e.g., midzonal hepatocellular necrosis is prominent in yellow fever, but not in dengue). Viral inclusions can be visualized in hepatocytes with

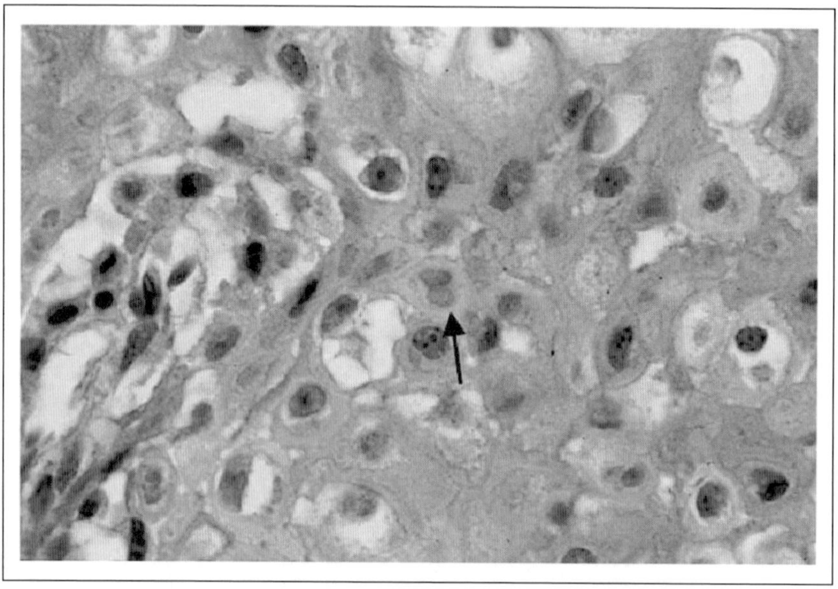

Figure 12.13 *Smallpox—histologic section of skin with intraepidermal vesicles and ballooning degeneration of epithelial cells with viral inclusions (Guarnieri bodies [arrow]) (hematoxylin and eosin stain). Infectious Disease Pathology Activity, CDC.*

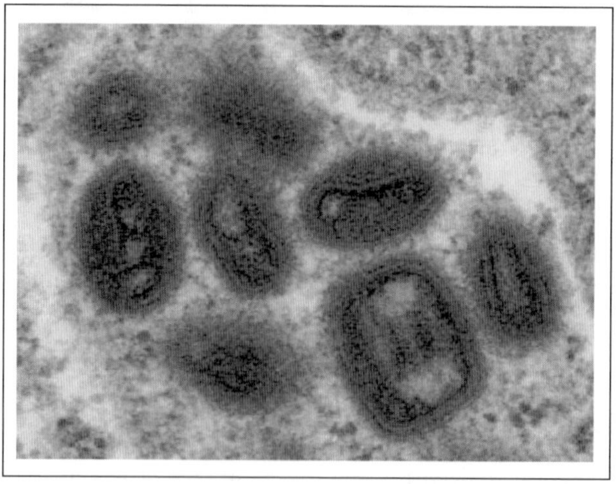

Figure 12.14 *Intracellular mature variola virus particles grown in cell culture. Note: The barbell-shaped inner core and two lateral bodies are surrounded by an outer membrane. One brick-shaped particle is also illustrated (thin section electron microscopy). Infectious Disease Pathology Activity, CDC.*

Ebola or Marburg infections by using light and electron microscopy (Figure 12.15).[49–54]

Diagnostic specimens. Performing a complete autopsy with histologic sampling of multiple organs can determine the extent of the disease and help identify the specific virus. After a specific etiologic agent has been isolated or identified from an index case, targeted sampling of additional cases with similar symptoms can decrease the exposure of autopsy personnel to these hazardous agents and still yield diagnostic material. For example, during outbreaks of Ebola hemorrhagic fever in Africa, using IHC on skin punch biopsy samples was sufficient to provide a diagnosis in a substantial number of fatalities and minimized the risk to the medical personnel who obtained the specimens.[49]

Diagnostic tests. Serum and skin samples can be tested by using PCR, immunohistochemistry, and electron microscopy (Figure 12.16). Additionally, serum can be inoculated into experimental animals or culture cells for viral isolation.

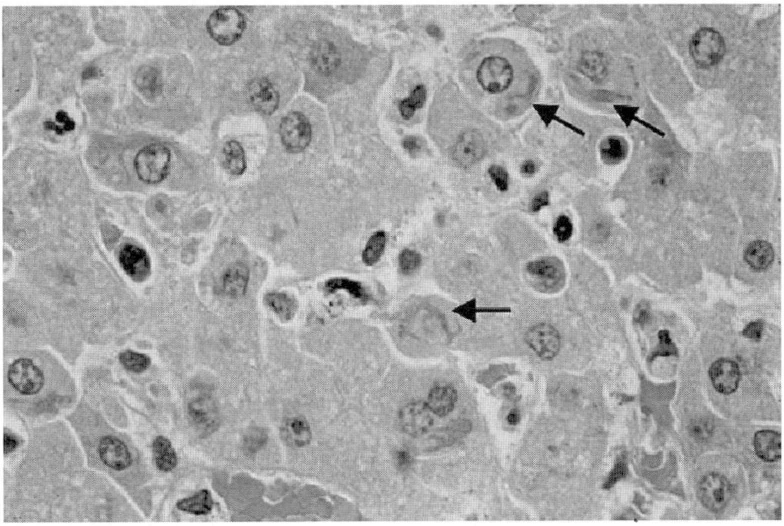

Figure 12.15 *Ebola hemorrhagic fever—necrotic hepatocytes with filamentous intracytoplasmic inclusions (arrows) (hematoxylin and eosin stain). Infectious Disease Pathology Activity, CDC.*

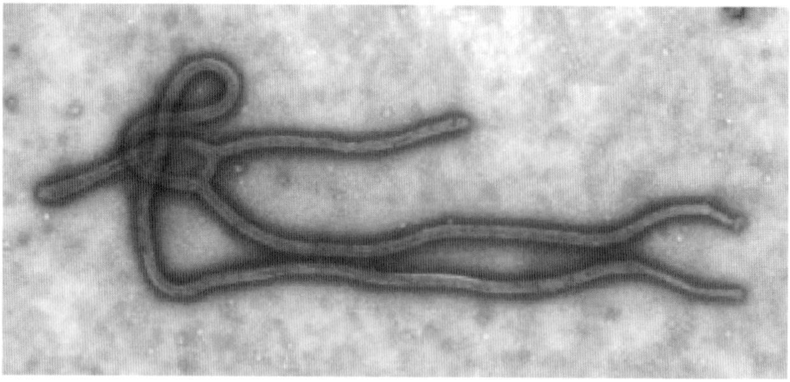

Figure 12.16 *Ultrastructural appearance of Ebola virus (electron microscopy negative stain). Infectious Disease Pathology Activity, CDC.*

Laboratory Response Network

CDC, in collaboration with the Association of Public Health Laboratories (APHL), the FBI, and other federal agencies, has developed the Laboratory Response Network (LRN) as a multilevel system of linked local, state, and federal public health laboratories as well as veterinary, food, and environmental laboratory partners.[55–57] The primary components of LRN are the state public health laboratories representing each of the fifty states. Within certain states, laboratories are located in different counties and more populated cities. In addition, federal laboratories within LRN include CDC, the Food and Drug Administration (FDA), the Environmental Protection Agency (EPA), the U.S. Army Medical Research Institute of Infectious Diseases (USAMRIID), and other Department of Defense laboratories.

Each laboratory has been assigned a designation (Table 12.3), predicated on their diagnostic capability, ranging from sentinel status (i.e., Level A for presumptive-level screening) through national laboratory status (i.e., Level D for genetic subtyping and confirmatory testing).[55–57] Hospital clinical laboratories are designated as sentinel laboratories (Level A); they have a rapid rule out and forward mission when handling presumptive clinical cases. County, city, and state public health laboratories are designated as confirmatory reference facilities (Level B, core, or Level C, advanced), depending on their degree of containment capacity and technical proficiency in performing agent-specific confirmatory

Table 12.3
Selected Characteristics and Capabilities by Functional Level of the Laboratory Response Network for Terrorism

Laboratory Level	Biosafety Level (BSL)	Capabilities	Testing Resource
D	BSL-4	• Probe for universal agents • Perform all Level A– C tests • Validate new assays • Detect genetic recombinants • Provide specialized reagents • Bank isolates • Molecular typing • Negative stain electron microscopy for smallpox virus	CDC; U.S. Army Medical Research Institute of Infectious Diseases
C	BSL-3	• Nucleic acid amplification assays • Molecular typing • Toxicity testing • Provide surge capacity	Selected state public health laboratories
B	BSL-3 Recommended or BSL-2 facilities with BSL-3 practices	• Rule in specific agents • Isolate and identify • Forward specimens to higher level laboratories • Process environmental samples • Perform confirmatory testing • Antimicrobial susceptibility testing	Selected state and county public health laboratories and other veterinary, environmental, and food testing laboratories
A	BSL-2	• Antimicrobial susceptibility testing • Rule out specific agents • Early detection of presumptive cases • Forward specimens to higher level laboratories	Clinical and other sentinel laboratories

analyses and rapid presumptive testing by PCR for nucleic acid amplification and time-resolved fluorescence for antigen detection. The Level D designation is reserved for CDC and USAMRIID laboratories. No regional laboratories exist; the network functions by channeling the specimens through the designated levels to a pathogen-specific conclusion.

ME/Cs should submit specimens from suspected biologic terrorism-related cases to the state public health laboratory through the local or county laboratory that serves their jurisdiction, unless their standard reporting protocol makes them a direct client of the state laboratory. These primary laboratories conduct the tests that fall within the scope of their ability and refer specimens to the state laboratory for more advanced tests. The state laboratory processes and refers specimens in a similar manner to other state laboratories or CDC (Figure 12.17). Contact information for all state diagnostic laboratories is included in this report (Appendix 12.A). The point of contact for ME/Cs should remain the laboratory where the specimens were first submitted, unless they are directed to contact a reference laboratory (e.g., a state laboratory) to track the progress of the testing. Before the need for LRN services arises, ME/Cs should establish con-

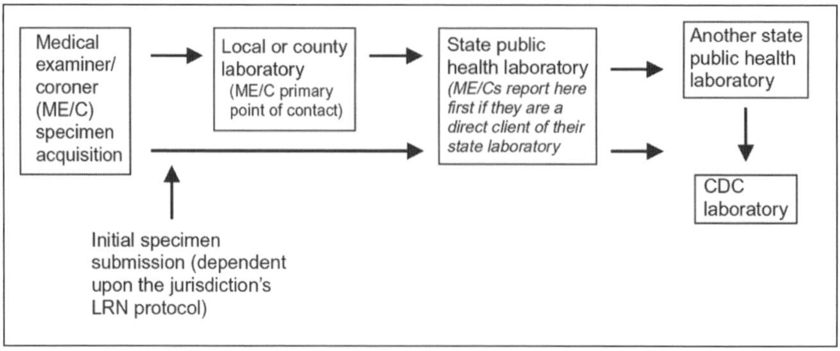

Figure 12.17 *Process for submitting specimens containing suspected Category A, B, or C* biologic agents (except smallpox virus) for testing within the Laboratory Response Network (LRN) * Note: Dependent upon the LRN-designated capacity (Level A, sentinel; Level B, core; Level C, advanced), laboratory confirmation might occur on-site or require referral to the next higher-level laboratory for confirmatory testing or correct biocontainment.*

tact with the public health laboratory serving their jurisdiction and determine how the laboratory services can be best accessed when needed. Such a relationship might require a memorandum-of-understanding, which should be prepared and agreed to in advance.

All specimens that are to be tested for potential biologic terrorism pathogens are handled through the same reporting and submission process except specimens potentially containing smallpox virus. Because smallpox virus should only be handled in a Biosafety Level 4 facility, the specimen should be transported to CDC.[57] If ME/Cs suspect this agent, they should notify their state public health department, which can test for other agents that cause a vesiculopustular rash (i.e., varicella zoster, vaccinia, and monkeypox viruses) and either further test or refer the specimen for rapid presumptive screening for smallpox virus by PCR. The same laboratories will be able to coordinate submission of the specimen to CDC as needed for pathogen confirmation. In advance, ME/Cs should establish contact with the state health department representative who would coordinate smallpox specimen submission. In their surveillance capacity and concurrent with specimen submission, ME/Cs should notify the epidemiologic investigation unit in their local or state health department of the suspected smallpox-infected decedent.

Biosafety Concerns

Autopsy risks

Biosafety is critical for autopsy personnel who might handle human remains contaminated with biologic terrorism agents. Tularemia, viral hemorrhagic fevers, smallpox, glanders, and Q fever have been transmitted to persons performing autopsies (i.e., prosectors); certain infections have been fatal.[49,58–70] Infections can be transmitted at autopsies by percutaneous inoculation (i.e., injury), splashes to unprotected mucosa, and inhalation of infectious aerosols.[71] All of the Category A pathogens are potentially transmissible to autopsy personnel, although the degree of risk varies considerably among these organisms.

Additionally, autopsies of persons who die as the result of terrorism-related infections might expose autopsy personnel to residual surface contamination with infectious material. For example, botulinum toxin has the potential to be inhaled by autopsy personnel if it is present on the body surface at the time of examination.[72] Heavy surface contamination of the body is unlikely because of the incubation period for the majority of infectious agents and the likelihood that a victim will have bathed and changed clothes after exposure and before becoming symptomatic and dying.[73] However, if such residual material (e.g., powder) is present, examination and specimen collection should be undertaken by using appropriate biosafety procedures to protect autopsy and analytic laboratory personnel from possible exposure to more concentrated infectious material.

Because human remains infected with unidentified biologic terrorism pathogens might arrive at autopsy without warning, basic protective measures described in this report should be maintained for all contact with potentially infectious materials.[74,75] In addition to these measures, certain high-risk activities (e.g., use of oscillating saw) are known to increase the potential for worker exposure and should be performed with added safety precautions.

Autopsy precautions

Existing guidelines for biosafety and infection control for patient care are designed to prevent transmission of infections from living patients to care providers, or from laboratory specimens to laboratory technicians.[76,77] Although certain biosafety and infection-control guidelines are applicable to the handling of human remains, inherent differences exist in transmission mechanisms and intensity of potential exposures during autopsies that require specific consideration.[71]

As with any contact involving broken skin or body fluids when caring for live patients, certain precautions must be applied to all contact with human remains, regardless of known or suspected infectivity. Even if a pathogen of concern has been ruled out, other unsuspected agents might be present. Thus, all human autopsies must be performed in an appropriate autopsy room with adequate air exchange by personnel wearing appropriate personal protective equipment (PPE).[71] All autopsy facilities should have written biosafety policies and procedures; autopsy personnel should receive training in these policies and procedures, and the annual occurrence of training should be documented.

Standard Precautions are the combination of PPE and procedures used to reduce transmission of all pathogens from moist body substances to personnel or patients.[77] These precautions are driven by the nature of an interaction (e.g., possibility of splashing or potential of soiling garments) rather than the nature of a pathogen. In addition, transmission-based precautions are applied for known or suspected pathogens. Precautions include the following:

- **airborne precautions**. Used for pathogens that remain suspended in the air in the form of droplet nuclei and that can transmit infection if inhaled;
- **droplet precautions**. Used for pathogens that are transmitted by large droplets traveling 3–6 feet (e.g., from sneezes or coughs) and are no longer transmitted after they fall to the ground; and
- **contact precautions**. Used for pathogens that might be transmitted by contamination of environmental surfaces and equipment.

All autopsies involve exposure to blood, a risk of being splashed or splattered, and a risk of percutaneous injury.[71] The propensity of postmortem procedures to cause gross soiling of the immediate environment also requires use of effective containment strategies. All autopsies generate aerosols; furthermore, postmortem procedures that require using devices (e.g., oscillating saws) that generate fine aerosols can create airborne particles that contain infectious pathogens not normally transmitted by the airborne route.[71,78–81]

PPE

For autopsies, standard precautions can be summarized as using a surgical scrub suit, surgical cap, impervious gown or apron with full sleeve coverage, a form of eye protection (e.g., goggles or face shield), shoe covers, and double surgical gloves with an interposed layer of cut-proof synthetic mesh.[71] Surgical masks protect the nose and mouth from splashes of body fluids (i.e., droplets > 5 μm); they do not provide protection from airborne pathogens.[82,83] Because of the fine aerosols generated at autopsy, prosectors should at a minimum wear N-95 respirators for all autopsies, regardless of suspected or known pathogens.[84] However, because of the efficient generation of high concentration aerosols by mechanical devices in the autopsy setting, powered air-purifying respirators (PAPRs) equipped with N-95 or high-efficiency particulate air (HEPA) filters should be considered.[85–87] Autopsy personnel who cannot wear N-95 respirators because of facial hair or other fit limitations should wear PAPRs.

Autopsy procedures

Standard safety practices to prevent injury from sharp items should be followed at all times.[77] These include never recapping, bending, or cutting needles, and ensuring that appropriate puncture-resistant sharps disposal containers are available. These containers should be placed as close as possible to where sharp items are used to minimize the distance a sharp item is carried. Filled sharps disposal containers should be discarded and replaced regularly and never overfilled.[77]

Protective outer garments should be removed when leaving the immediate autopsy area and discarded in appropriate laundry or waste receptacles, either in an antechamber to the autopsy suite or immediately inside the entrance if an antechamber is unavailable. Handwashing is requisite upon glove removal.[77]

Engineering strategies and facility design concerns

Air-handling systems for autopsy suites should ensure both adequate air exchanges per hour and correct directionality and exhaust of airflow. Autopsy suites should have a minimum of twelve air exchanges/hour and should be at a negative pressure relative to adjacent passageways and office spaces.[84] Air should never be returned to the building interior, but should be exhausted outdoors, away from areas of human traffic or gathering spaces (e.g., air should be directed off the roof) and away from other air intake systems.[88,89] For autopsies, local airflow control (i.e., laminar flow systems) can be used to direct aerosols away from personnel; however, this safety feature does not eliminate the need for appropriate PPE.

Clean sinks and safety equipment should be positioned so that they do not require unnecessary travel to reach during routine work and are readily available in the event of an emergency. Work surfaces should have integral waste-containment and drainage features that minimize spills of body fluids and wastewater.

Biosafety cabinets should be available for handling and examination of smaller infectious specimens; however, the majority of available cabinets are not designed to contain a whole body.[76,90] Oscillating saws are available with vacuum shrouds to reduce the amount of particulate and droplet aerosols generated.[80] These devices should be used whenever possible to decrease the risk of dispersing aerosols that might lead to occupationally acquired infection.

Vaccination and postexposure prophylaxis

Vaccines are available that convey protection against certain diseases considered to be potentially terrorism-associated, including anthrax, plague, and tularemia.[76] However, these vaccines are not recommended for unexposed autopsy workers at low risk. Consistent application of standard safety practices should obviate the need for vaccination for *B. anthracis* and *Y. pestis*. In 2003, the U.S. Department of Health and Human Services (DHHS) initiated a program to administer vaccinia (smallpox) vaccine to first responders and medical personnel. In this context, persons who might be called on to assess remains or specimens from patients with smallpox should be included among this group (Box 12.2).[91]

The administration of prophylactic antibiotics to autopsy workers exposed to potentially lethal bacterial pathogens is sometimes appropriate. For example, autopsy personnel exposed to *Y. pestis* aerosols should consider receiving such treatment regardless of vaccination status.[92] Similarly, because tularemia can result from infection with a limited number of organisms, an exposure to *F. tularensis* should also prompt consideration of antimicrobial prophylaxis. However, decisions to use antimicrobial postexposure prophylaxis should be made in consultation with infectious disease and occupational health specialists, with consideration made of

Box 12.2
Smallpox Immunization Considerations for Medicolegal Death Investigators*

Because the distribution of the smallpox vaccine to the civilian U.S. population was discontinued in 1983,° essentially all U.S. residents having contact with a smallpox case are at increased risk for infection. Although probably susceptible to smallpox, with appropriate precautions, medicolegal death investigators can reduce their risk of smallpox infection if they must examine or autopsy a decedent suspected to be infected with smallpox. Three risk-reduction activities during the postmortem period might be considered, (1) voluntary vaccination after the occurrence of smallpox has been confirmed in the community; (2) modification of autopsy procedures to limit the possible aerosolization of smallpox virus; and (3) exclusion of embalming procedures (see text). In the event of mass fatalities resulting from a smallpox outbreak, CDC recommends that health departments consider planning for vaccinating mortuary personnel and their families. This recommendation is relevant for medical examiners, coroners, and other forensic death investigators who have a high likelihood of handling smallpox-infected decedents during a mass fatality event.

In considering vaccination plans, attention should be given to the risk of adverse effects from smallpox vaccination as well as to its potential benefits. During a smallpox-associated mass fatality event, the federal government might propose that vaccinia inoculations be offered on a voluntary basis to appropriate personnel. Vaccinia inoculations have been effective in preventing smallpox infection but also pose certain risks for causing adverse reactions in the vaccinee and, less frequently, for spreading the vaccinia virus to other close contacts. Because of the increased risk of adverse effects, the Advisory Committee on Immunization Practices (ACIP) recommends that the following persons not receive vaccinia inoculation:

- persons with immunosuppressive conditions;
- those receiving immunosuppressive medical treatments or pharmaceutical regimens;

- those with eczema or who have a close contact having eczema;
- anyone who is allergic to the vaccine or any of its components;
- women who are breastfeeding;
- anyone aged < 12 months; and
- pregnant women or women expecting to become pregnant within four weeks.[1]

ACIP recommends that persons be excluded from the pre-event smallpox vaccination program who haveknown underlying heart disease, with or without symptoms, or who have more than three known major cardiac risk factors (i.e., hypertension, diabetes, hypercholesterolemia, heart disease at age fifty years in a first-degree relative, and smoking).[**] Persons at increased risk for adverse reactions to the vaccine should be counseled regarding the potential risks before being vaccinated.

[*] **Source:** Adapted from Payne DC. Smallpox considerations for forensic professionals. *National Association of Medical Examiners (NAME) News* 2003;11(1):2.

[°] **Source:** CDC. Smallpox vaccine no longer available for civiliansÑ United States. *MMWR* 1983;32:387.

Source: CDC. Smallpox response plan, smallpox vaccination clinic guide. Annex 3–38. Atlanta, GA: U.S. Department of Health and Human Services, CDC, 2002. Available at http://www.bt.cdc.gov/ agent/smallpox/response-plan/files/annex-3.pdf.

[1] **Source:** CDC. Recommendations for using smallpox vaccine in a preevent vaccination program: supplemental recommendations of the Advisory Committee on Immunization Practices (ACIP) and the Healthcare Infection Control Practices Advisory Committee (HICPAC). *MMWR* 2003;52(No. RR-7):1–16. Available at http:// www.cdc.gov/mmwr/preview/mmwrhtml/rr5207a1.htm.

[**] **Source:** CDC. Supplemental recommendations on adverse events following smallpox vaccine in the pre-event vaccination program: recommendations of the Advisory Committee on Immunization Practices [Notice to readers]. *MMWR* 2003;52:282–4. Available at http://www.cdc.gov/mmwr/preview/mmwrhtml/mm5213a5.htm.

vaccination status, nature of exposure, and safety and efficacy of prophylaxis.

Decontamination of body-surface contaminants

If human remains with heavy, residual surface contamination (i.e., visible) must be assessed, they should be cleansed before being brought to the autopsy facility and after appropriate samples have been collected in the field. Surface cleaning should be performed with an appropriate cleaning solution (e.g., 0.5% hypochlorite solution or phenolic disinfectant) used according to manufacturer's instructions. If the number of remains requiring autopsy is limited (i.e., one or two), cleaning of heavily contaminated remains can be undertaken in an autopsy facility that has the infrastructure, capacity, and hazardous materials (HAZMAT)-trained personnel to perform the cleaning safely. Heavily contaminated remains should not be brought to facilities where patient care is performed. Both personnel carrying contaminated remains and personnel occupying areas through which remains are being carried should wear PPE. HAZMAT personnel should perform large-scale decontamination outdoors in a controlled setting. To ensure mutual understanding of the roles and responsibilities of HAZMAT and death-investigation personnel in situations with contaminated remains, ME/Cs should develop response protocols with HAZMAT personnel before such an event occurs.

Waste handling

Liquid waste (e.g., body fluids) can be flushed or washed down ordinary sanitary drains without special procedures. Pretreatment of liquid waste is not required and might damage sewage treatment systems. If substantial volumes are expected, the local wastewater treatment personnel should be consulted in advance. Solid waste should be appropriately contained in biohazard or sharps containers and incinerated in a medical waste incinerator.[73,75]

Storage and disposition of corpses

The majority of potential biologic terrorism agents (*B. anthracis*, *Y. pestis*, or botulinum toxin) are unlikely to be transmitted to personnel engaged in the nonautopsy handling of a contaminated cadaver. However, such agents as the hemorrhagic fever viruses and smallpox virus can be transmitted in this manner. Therefore, standard precautions[77] should be followed while handling all cadavers before and after autopsy.

When bodies are bagged at the scene of death, surface decontamination of the corpse-containing body bags is required before transport. Bodies can be transported and stored (refrigerated) in impermeable bags (double-bagging is preferable), after wiping visible soiling on outer bag surfaces with 0.5% hypochlorite solution. Storage areas should be negatively pressured with 9–12 air exchanges/hour.

The risks of occupational exposure to biologic terrorism agents while embalming outweigh its advantages; therefore, bodies infected with these agents should not be embalmed. Bodies infected with such agents as *Y. pestis* or *F. tularensis* can be directly buried without embalming. However, such agents as *B. anthracis* produce spores that can be long-lasting and, in such cases, cremation is the preferred disposition method. Similarly, bodies contaminated with highly infectious agents (e.g., smallpox and hemorrhagic fever viruses) should be cremated without embalming. If cremation is not an option, the body should be properly secured in a sealed container (e.g., a Zigler case or other hermetically sealed casket) to reduce the potential risk of pathogen transmission. However, sealed containers still have the potential to leak or lose integrity, especially if they are dropped or are transported to a different altitude.[93]

ME/Cs should work with local emergency management agencies, funeral directors, and the state and local health departments to determine, in advance, the local capacity (bodies per day) of existing crematoriums, and soil and water table characteristics that might affect interment. For planning purposes, a thorough cremation produces approximately 3–6 pounds of ash and fragments. ME/Cs should also work with local emergency management agencies to identify sources and costs of special equipment (e.g., air curtain incinerators, which are capable of high-volume cremation) and the newer plasma incinerators, which are faster and more efficient than previous incineration methods. The costs of such equipment and the time required to obtain them on request should be included in state and local terrorism preparedness plans.

ME/C's Role in Biologic Terrorism Surveillance

ME/Cs should be a key component of population-based surveillance for biologic terrorism. They see fatalities among persons who have not been examined initially by other physicians, emergency departments, or hospitals. In addition, persons who have been seen first by other healthcare providers might die precipitously, without a confirmed diagnosis, and therefore fall under medicolegal jurisdiction. Autopsies are a critical component of surveillance for fatal infectious diseases, because they provide organism-specific diagnoses and clarify the route of exposure.[94] With biologic terrorism-related fatalities, organisms identified in autopsy tissues can be characterized by strain to assist in the process of criminal attribution.

Models for ME surveillance for biologic terrorism mortality include sharing of daily case dockets with public health authorities (e.g., King County, Washington, and an active symptom-driven case acquisition and pathology syndrome-based public health reporting system developed in New Mexico[24]). Different areas of responsibility exist for ME/Cs regarding their role in effective surveillance for possible terrorism events. The following steps should be taken in local jurisdictions to enable ME/Cs to implement biologic terrorism surveillance:

- Death-investigation laws should be changed to enable ME/Cs to assume jurisdiction and investigate deaths that might constitute a public health threat, including those threats that are probably communicable.
- Any unexplained deaths possibly involving an infectious cause or biologic agent should be investigated to make etiology (organism)-specific diagnoses.[94]
- Uniform standards for surveillance should be used. For example, the Med-X system developed in New Mexico[24] uses a set of antemortem symptoms to determine autopsy performance. The system's syndromic approach to postmortem diagnosis allows alerting of public health authorities to specific constellations of autopsy findings that could represent infectious agents before the specific agent is identified. Diseases caused by biologic terrorism agents are rare. To enhance surveillance for these conditions, a matrix of potential pathology-based syndromes (Table 12.1) has been developed to guide autopsy pathologists in recognizing potential cases.[24]
- Electronic information and data systems should be designed to allow rapid recognition of excess mortality—incorporating the ability to

assess possible commonalities among cases—and rapid communication/notification of such information to public health authorities who can use the information for effective response.

- Close working relationships should be developed between ME/Cs and local or state health departments to facilitate two-way communication that includes alerts to ME/Cs of possible outbreaks or clusters of nonfatal infectious diseases, which might have unrecognized fatal cases, and appropriate reporting by ME/Cs to public health authorities of notifiable disease conditions. Additionally, public health authorities should notify ME/Cs of the epidemiology of biologic terrorism-associated and other emerging infectious diseases in their community.

ME/C's Role in Data Collection, Analysis, and Dissemination

For public health surveillance, criminal justice, and administrative purposes, ME/Cs should promptly, accurately, and thoroughly collect, document, electronically store, and have available for analysis and reporting, case-specific death-investigation information. Initially, depending upon local resources and legal restrictions, all aspects of data management and use might not need to occur in-house. Recognizing that numerous entities use medicolegal death-investigation data, ME/Cs should establish collaborations with public health and law enforcement professionals to achieve the goal of complete, accurate, and timely case-specific death-investigation data. Advance planning and policy development should also clarify to whom such data may be released and under which circumstances. To facilitate this process, the following steps should be taken:

- Death-investigation information should be documented on standard forms that are consistent in content, at a minimum, with the Investigator's Death Investigation Report Form (IDIRF) and Certifier's Death Investigation Report Form (CDIRF).[95]
- Death-investigation data should be stored in an electronic database consistent with, at a minimum, the content outlined in the Medical Examiner/Coroner Death Investigation Data Set (MCDIDS).[96] These data elements should be updated periodically.

- Electronic death-investigation data sets should include the results of laboratory tests that are performed in the case in question.
- Entry of data into an electronic database should be prompt so that the database is current.
- Electronic databases should allow searching for and grouping of cases by disease or injury and circumstances of death.
- Electronic death-investigation data should be stored in open, non-proprietary formats so that it can be shared as needed.
- Death-investigation records should be stored in accordance with state or local regulations. Ideally, these records should be stored in perpetuity in a format that ensures future retrieval. The format or media of electronic records might require periodic updating.
- Mechanisms should be in place to ensure that electronic death investigation data can be shared with public health authorities, law enforcement agencies, and other death-investigation agencies while providing for appropriate confidentiality and control of the release of information to authorized personnel or organizations only.
- ME/Cs should have specific policies that outline the organizations and agencies that are authorized to receive death-investigation information and the conditions in which such information may be released.
- Policies and mechanisms should be in place to avoid releasing death-investigation information inappropriately and to avoid withholding information that should be available to the public.
- ME/C offices should consider establishing links with state or local public health agencies, academic institutions, or other health organizations to promote epidemiologic analysis and use of their medicolegal death-investigation data in an ongoing manner. Certain ME/C offices have determined that employing a staff epidemiologist is beneficial.

Jurisdictional, Evidentiary, and Operational Concerns

Federal role

On February 28, 2003, Homeland Security Presidential Directive 5 (HSPD-5) modified federal response policy.[97] Under the new directive, the Secretary of Homeland Security is the principal federal official for domestic incident management. Pursuant to the Homeland Security Act of

2002 (Public Law 107-296), the Secretary of the U.S. Department of Homeland Security (DHS) is responsible for coordinating federal operations within the United States to prepare for, respond to, and recover from terrorist attacks, major disasters, and other emergencies. The Secretary will coordinate the federal government's resources used in response to or recovery from terrorist attacks, major disasters, or other emergencies if and when any one of the following four conditions applies: (1) a federal department or agency acting under its own authority has requested the assistance of the secretary; (2) the resources of state and local authorities are overwhelmed and federal assistance has been requested by the appropriate state and local authorities; (3) more than one federal department or agency has become substantially involved in responding to the incident; or (4) the Ssecretary has been directed to assume responsibility for managing the domestic incident by the president.

HSPD-5 further stipulates that the U.S. Attorney General, through the FBI, has lead federal responsibility for criminal investigations of terrorist acts or terrorist threats by persons or groups inside the United States, or directed at U.S. citizens or institutions abroad, where such acts are within the federal criminal jurisdiction of the United States. The FBI, in cooperation with other federal departments and agencies engaged in activities to protect national security, will also coordinate the activities of the other members of the law enforcement community to detect, prevent, preempt, and disrupt terrorist attacks against the United States. In the event of a weapons of mass destruction (WMD) threat or incident, the local FBI field office special agent in charge (SAC) will be responsible for leading the federal criminal investigation and law enforcement actions, acting in concert with the principal federal officer (PFO) appointed by the U.S. Department of Homeland Security and state and local officials.

The FBI has a WMD coordinator in each of the agency's fifty-six field offices (Appendix 12.B). These persons are responsible for pre-event planning and preparedness, as well as responding to WMD threats or incidents. ME/Cs are encouraged to contact their local FBI WMD coordinator before an incident to clarify roles and responsibilities, and ME/Cs should contact the coordinator in any case where concerns or suspicions exist of a potential WMD-related death.

The FBI assertion of jurisdiction at the scene of a terrorist event would not necessarily usurp (or relieve) ME/Cs from their statutory authority and responsibility to identify decedents and determine cause and manner of death. Such an arrangement is consistent with the performance of medicolegal death investigation where other federal crimes are involved. ME/Cs who conduct terrorism-associated death investigations should be prepared to present their medicolegal death investigation findings in federal court.

Public health agency authority

State public health laws might establish the health department's specific authority to control certain aspects of operations, personnel, or corpses in a public health emergency. For example, the Center for Law and the Public's Health at Georgetown and Johns Hopkins Universities, at the request of CDC, has created a model state emergency health powers act for adoption by states.[98] Different states have either enacted versions of this act or are in the process of introducing similar legislative bills.[99] ME/Cs should know specifically how existing state laws might provide for the health department to take control and dictate the disposition of human remains (burial or cremation). A state's emergency health powers act might also provide for

- mandatory medical examinations for ME/C personnel;
- isolation and quarantine of the public or ME/C personnel;
- vaccination against and treatment for illnesses among ME/Cs; and
- control, use, and destruction of facilities.

ME/Cs and health departments should work together as part of the emergency planning process to determine which emergency health powers might be established by the health department and under what circumstances these might be invoked for each potential biologic terrorism agent. Determining how health departments and ME/C operations can best interact, including documenting concerns regarding the availability of death-investigation personnel and the control and disposition of human remains, should be emphasized. ME/Cs should take part in community exercises to clarify and practice their role in the emergency response process.

General operations

In the majority of terrorism-associated scenarios, ME/Cs are responsible for identifying remains and determining the cause and manner of death. To that end, ME/Cs might need to enlist additional local, state, or federal assistance while maintaining primary responsibility for death investigation. ME/Cs should request this assistance from the local or state emergency operations center (EOC), as appropriate. The probable source of federal assistance is the Disaster Mortuary Operational Response Team (DMORT). However, DMORT has not yet developed capacity to respond to events precipitated by the release of biologic agents (further details regarding DMORT and other federal agencies are discussed in following sections).

Where possible, postmortem examinations for identifying remains and determining cause and manner of death should occur within the local or state jurisdiction where victims have died. Local resources dictate whether the statutory ME/C system can accomplish this with existing personnel and within existing facilities, or whether additional local, state, or federal assistance is necessary. Moving substantial numbers of human remains, particularly those contaminated by a biologic agent (known or unknown) to locations considerably distant from the scenes of death is neither feasible nor safe. Two potential strategies can be used to augment the biosafety capacity of local agencies having limited resources. One strategy would be to develop a mobile Biosafety Level 3 autopsy laboratory. Another strategy would be to develop regional Biosafety Level 3 autopsy centers that can handle cases from surrounding jurisdictions or states. A combination of the two approaches will probably achieve the best coverage of national needs.

Postmortem examinations and evidence collection

A large-scale biologic event might create more fatalities than combined local, state, and federal agencies can store and examine.[15] Small or rural jurisdictions might be overwhelmed by a relatively limited number of fatalities, whereas larger state or city ME/C offices could conceivably process greater numbers of human remains. No formulas exist that can be used to determine in advance the autopsy rate and the extent of autopsy that might be needed. In the event of a biologic event, ME/Cs should perform complete autopsies on as many cases as feasible on the basis of case volume and biosafety risks. These autopsies should meet the standards that forensic pathologists usually meet for homicide cases. Conferring with the FBI and appropriate prosecutorial authorities early in the process will ensure that appropriate documentary and diagnostic maneuvers are employed that will support the criminal justice process. Similarly, interacting with public health authorities early in the death-investigation process should ensure that appropriate diagnostic evaluations are conducted to support the public health investigation and response.

After the etiologic agent has been determined, certain (or all) other potentially related fatalities can be selectively sampled to confirm the presence of the organism in question. ME/Cs should coordinate the decision to transition from complete autopsies to more limited examinations with law enforcement and public health professionals. Selective sampling could include skin swabs and needle aspiration of blood or other body fluids, tissues for culture, or biopsies of a particular tissue or organ for histologic diagnostic tests (e.g., immunohistochemical procedures and electron microscopy). The required specimens from a limited autopsy and the diagnostic procedures employed will be dictated by the nature of the biologic agent. Guidelines for targeted organs or tissues for culture or analysis were discussed previously. As with all homicides, chain-of-custody for specimens should be maintained at all times.

Whenever a complete autopsy is performed, the goals should be to (1) establish the disease process and the etiologic agent; (2) determine that the agent or disease is indeed the cause of death; and (3) reasonably rule out competing causes of death. When limited autopsies or external examinations are performed, ME/C personnel should

- identify the deceased;
- document the appearance of the body;
- establish that the presenting clinical symptoms and signs are consistent with the alleged etiologic agent;
- confirm the presence of the etiologic agent in the body;
- state with reasonable probability that the alleged agent was the underlying cause of death (e.g., inhalational anthrax infection); and
- state with reasonable probability the likely immediate cause of death (e.g., pneumonia, meningitis, or mediastinitis).

Forming a reasonably sound medical opinion regarding cause and manner of death can be accomplished with knowledge of the presenting syndrome and circumstantial events, external examination of the body, and testing of appropriate specimens to document the etiologic agent. For example, in a confirmed smallpox outbreak, identifying the deceased, externally examining the body and photographing the lesions, and obtaining samples from the lesions for culture or electron microscopy might be adequate.

Biologic evidence obtained at autopsy can be sent to local or state health department laboratories, and other physical evidence can be sent to the usual crime laboratory, unless otherwise instructed by the FBI. Laboratories within LRN, as described previously, are responsible for coordinating the transfer of evidence or results to the FBI, U.S. Attorney General, or local and state legal authorities, as appropriate. Consistent with routine practice, ME/Cs should document all evidence transfers adequately.

Cause and Manner of Death Statements

Death certificates are not withheld from the public record, even when the cause of death is terrorism-related. The cause of death section should be used to fully explain the sequence of the cause of death (e.g., "hemorrhagic mediastinitis due to inhalational anthrax"). If death resulted from a terrorism event, the manner of death should be classified as homicide. The "how injury occurred" section on the death certificate should be completed, and it should reflect how the infectious agent was delivered to the victim (e.g., "victim of terrorism; inhaled anthrax spores delivered in mail envelope"). The place of injury should be the statement of where (i.e., geographic location) the agent was received.

Reimbursement for Expenses and Potential Funding Sources

Additional funding for ME/Cs might be needed for either preparedness or use during an actual biologic terrorism event. ME/Cs should prepare financially for potential future terrorist events that might be similar to the anthrax attacks of October–November 2001. In crisis situations, funding is retroactive but no less a concern.

Preparedness funding can support multiple activities, including training of ME/Cs for large-scale terrorism events. Certain activities involving training of ME/Cs have occurred through DMORT, a program authorized by the DHHS Office of Emergency Preparedness to rapidly mobilize ME/Cs to respond to incidents of mass fatality. Preparedness funding can also support surveillance activities in ME/C offices. As part of the Bioterrorism Preparedness and Response cooperative agreements with state health departments, CDC has provided funding to New Mexico and other states that are pursuing ME/C surveillance systems as an enhancement to their traditional surveillance systems. The New Mexico Office of the Medical Investigator has been a recipient of this funding through the New Mexico Department of Health since the inception of the cooperative agreement program. This funding has supported development of specialized surveillance techniques for deaths caused by potential agents of biologic terrorism[24] and recognition of ME/Cs as a key resource for all phases—early detection, case characterization, incident response and recovery—of a public health emergency response. CDC encourages pursuit of this enhanced (ME/C) surveillance capacity through cooperative agreements with states, if the state has made adequate progress with other critical capacity goals.

ME/Cs might obtain preparedness funding by integrating their response activities into the existing EOCs that have been established at selected state and county levels (integration of ME/C offices into this framework is discussed in Communications and the Incident Command System). When ME/C offices are integrated into the emergency response system, ME/Cs have an opportunity to make emergency management officials aware of ME/C emergency responsibilities and resource needs.

The sources of funding for consequence management, including medicolegal death investigation, will depend on the scope of the terrorism event. In events with a limited number of deaths, funding for activities related to the detection and diagnosis might remain at the office level. Because terrorism deaths are homicides, these deaths will contribute to an office's jurisdictional workload, and future planning for preparedness funding should be considered. Certain ME/C offices are already a part of the local or state public health department or are already affiliated with an EOC. ME/C offices, health departments, and EOCs are strongly encouraged to forge links for effective preparedness and response and to participate in joint training exercises to maximize preparedness funding.

In events with multiple deaths, a federal emergency might be declared. As long as ME/Cs' offices are officially working through the state or local EOC, certain expenses associated with the response (e.g., cost of diagnostic testing) can be submitted to the Federal Emergency Management Agency (FEMA) for reimbursement. In the majority of localities, these requests for resources required for appropriate response during an event should be submitted through local emergency management agencies that are part of state and local EOCs. Costs will probably be covered by the agency that has jurisdiction over the disaster (e.g., FEMA). In cases where a presidential disaster declaration is made, testing costs, victim identification, mortuary services, and those services that are covered by the National Disaster Medical System (a mutual aid network that includes DHHS, the Department of Defense, and FEMA)[100] are reimbursable under Emergency Support Function 8 (Health and Medical) of the Federal Response Plan (FRP).

Under FRP, FEMA covers 75 percent of reimbursement costs; the remaining 25 percent are covered by the state through emergency funds or in-kind reimbursement. FEMA also supports state emergency funds through the DHHS electronic payments management system. In an emergency, all requests for reimbursement flow from their point of origin, in this case from an ME/C, through the state EOC/emergency management agency, to FEMA.§ Before an event, ME/Cs should clarify the procedures to follow to ensure that they will be reimbursed for expenses incurred as part of their emergency response.

DMORT

DMORT is a national program that includes volunteers, divided into ten regional teams responsible for supporting death investigation and mortuary services in federal emergency response situations involving natural disasters and mass fatalities associated with transportation accidents or terrorism. Team members are specialists from multiple forensic disciplines, funeral directors, law enforcement agents, and administrative support personnel. Each team represents a FEMA region. DMORT members are activated through DHS after mass fatalities or events involving multiple displaced human remains (e.g., a cemetery washout after a flood).

The primary functions of DMORT include the identification of human remains, evidence recovery from the bodies, recovery of human remains from the scene, and assisting with operation of a family assistance center. Whenever possible, identification of the bodies is made by using commonly accepted scientific methods (e.g., fingerprint, dental, radiograph, or DNA comparisons).

Upon activation, DMORT members are federal government employees. When DMORT is activated, representatives from DHS are also sent to manage the logistics of deployment. The FBI most commonly staffs the fingerprint section of the morgue. The Armed Forces DNA Identification Laboratory in Rockville, Maryland, has traditionally performed DNA analyses; the arrangements for this testing are negotiated separately with the local ME/C.

After a request for DMORT assistance has been made, one of two Disaster Portable Morgue Units (DPMUs) and DMORT staff are sent to the disaster site. DPMUs contain specialized equipment and supplies, prestaged for deployment within hours to a disaster site. DPMUs include all of the equipment required for a functional basic morgue with designated workstations and prepackaged equipment and supplies. DPMUs can operate at Biosafety Level 2, but do not have the ventilatory capacity necessary to protect prosectors and other nearby persons from airborne pathogens. DPMUs also contain equipment for site search and recovery, pathology, anthropology, radiology, photography, and information resources, as well as office equipment, wheeled examination tables, water heaters, plumbing equipment, electrical distribution equipment, personal protective gear, and temporary partitions and supports. DPMUs do not have the materials required to support microbiologic sampling. When a DPMU is deployed, members of the DPMU team (i.e., a subset of DMORT) are sent to the destination to unload the DPMU equipment and establish and maintain the temporary morgue. Additional equipment is required locally after DMORT activation. At a minimum, this equipment includes a facility in which to house the morgue equipment, a forklift to move the DPMU equipment into the temporary morgue facility, and refrigerated trucks to hold human remains.

ME/Cs can request DMORT response after a mass fatality or after an incident resulting in the displacement of a substantial number of human remains. ME/Cs should follow state protocols for DMORT requests.

Typically, ME/Cs contact the state governor's office, which then requests DMORT from DHS.¶ The request should include an estimate of how many deaths occurred (if known), the condition of the bodies (if known), and the location of the incident. When deployed, DMORT supports ME/Cs in the jurisdiction where the incident occurred. All medicolegal death investigation records created by DMORT are given to ME/Cs at the end of the deployment, and ME/Cs are ultimately responsible for all of the identifications made and the documents created pertaining to the incident.

DMORT-WMD Team

The DMORT-WMD team is composed of national rather than regional volunteers. The primary focus of DMORT-WMD is decontamination of bodies when death results from exposure to chemicals or radiation. DMORT-WMD is developing resources to respond to a mass disaster resulting from biologic agents. However, this team might have difficulty in responding to such an event if the deaths occur in multiple locations.

The major forensic disciplines (i.e., forensic dentistry, forensic anthropology, and forensic pathology) as well as funeral directors, law enforcement, criminalists, and administrative support persons are represented on the DMORT-WMD team. Members of DMORT-WMD undergo specialized training that focuses on chemical and radiologic decontamination of human remains. The DMORT-WMD unit has separate equipment, stored separately from the DPMU, including PPE (up to and including level A suits), decontamination tents, and equipment to gather contaminated water. DMORT-WMD teams are requested and deployed in the same manner as general DMORTs.

Communications and the incident command system

ME/Cs are key members of the biologic terrorism detection and management response team in any community and should be integrated into the comprehensive communication plan during any terrorism-associated event. Routine and consistent communication among ME/Cs and local and state laboratories, public health departments, EOCs, communication centers, DMORT, and other agencies, is critical to the success of efficient and effective biologic terrorism surveillance, fatality management, and public health and criminal investigations. Planning for different emergency scenarios and participation in disaster response exercises are necessary to ensure effective response to a terrorism event.

Each state and certain counties have some type of emergency operation center that has been organized to provide a coordinated response during a terrorism event. ME/Cs should verify their jurisdiction's EOC contact point and work with them periodically regarding concerns related to preparedness and response.

All EOCs follow the Incident Command System (ICS) (100), an internationally recognized emergency management system that provides a coordinated response across organizations and jurisdictions. The ICS structure allows for individual EOC decision making and different information flow in each state. ME/Cs should determine how the EOC functions in their jurisdiction.

Each ICS is composed of a managing authority that directs the response of health department, law enforcement, and emergency management officials during a planning exercise, emergency, or major disaster. In addition to assessing the incident and serving as the interagency contact, ICS also coordinates the response to information inquiries and the safety monitoring of assigned response personnel. The ICS organizational framework, includes planning, operations, logistics, and finance/administration sections.[101] ME/Cs are most likely to participate in the operations team, which makes tactical decisions regarding the incident response and implements those activities defined in action plans. This team might also include public health, emergency communications, fire, law enforcement, EMS, and state emergency management agency staff.

During a suspected terrorism event, ME/Cs should be responsible for the following actions to facilitate communication:

- Promptly inform laboratory, public health, and law enforcement personnel of findings of investigations of suspected biologic terrorism-related deaths as well as personnel needs and new developments. To expedite information exchange, ME/Cs should familiarize themselves with the appropriate contact persons and agencies for response in their jurisdictions.
- Answer the EOCs' requests to collect and report data in a timely manner.

- Coordinate communication of their activities with the state emergency management agency and EOCs for their jurisdiction to avoid release of confidential or speculative information directly to the public or media.[102]

Conclusion

ME/Cs are essential public health partners for terrorism preparedness and response. Despite state and local differences in medicolegal death-investigation systems, these investigators have the statutory authority to investigate deaths that are sudden, suspicious, violent, and unattended, and consequently play a vital role in terrorism surveillance and response. Public health officials should work with ME/Cs to ensure that these investigators can assist with surveillance for infectious disease deaths possibly caused by terrorism and provide confirmatory diagnoses and evidence in deaths linked to terrorism. This process should involve an assessment of local ME/C standards for accepting jurisdiction of potential infectious disease deaths and performing autopsies, laboratory capacity for making organism-specific diagnoses, and autopsy biosafety capacity. Ideally, ME/Cs should

- perform complete autopsies with histologic sampling of multiple organs in deaths potentially caused by biologic terrorism agents, given the constraints of case volume and biosafety concerns;
- have access to routine microbiologic testing for organism-specific diagnoses in potential infectious disease deaths;
- ensure protection from both airborne and bloodborne pathogens for all occupants of the autopsy facility (Biosafety Level 3);
- participate in a standardized ME/C surveillance model for infectious disease mortality (e.g., Med-X); and
- document death investigative information on standard forms that are stored in an searchable electronic format and that can be shared with public health authorities.

If biologic terrorism-related fatalities occur, ME/Cs are responsible for identifying remains and determining the cause and manner of death. Routine and consistent communication among ME/Cs and local and state laboratories, public health departments, EOCs, law enforcement, and other agencies is critical to the success of efficient and effective biologic terrorism surveillance, fatality management, and public health and criminal investigations. To prepare for this possibility, ME/Cs should

- contact their local FBI WMD coordinator to clarify roles and responsibilities;
- understand how local public health laws might impact ME/C function;
- become familiar with the capacity of local or state EOCs, ICS, and the process for submitting response-associated expenses for federal reimbursement;
- be aware of the process for submitting biologic and physical evidence in potential biologic terrorism-related fatalities;
- understand the procedure for writing cause and manner of death statements in terrorism-related fatalities; and
- identify appropriate health department officials for the reporting of notifiable or suspicious infectious diseases or potential biologic terrorism-related deaths.

The majority of ME/C facilities do not have the capacity to perform autopsies at Biosafety Level 3 as a consequence of facility design features that are expensive to fix. In addition, DMORT does not have the capacity to respond to events precipitated by the release of biologic agents. These limitations might affect local, state, and national surveillance for infectious disease deaths of public health importance, including those deaths potentially caused by terrorism. Two potential strategies might be used in the future to augment the biosafety capacity of local agencies having limited resources. One strategy would be to develop a mobile Biosafety Level 3 autopsy laboratory. Another strategy might be to develop regional Biosafety Level 3 autopsy centers that can handle cases from surrounding jurisdictions or states. A combination of the two approaches will probably achieve the best coverage of national needs.

Acknowledgments

This report was prepared with the assistance and support of the members of NAME, Michael A. Graham, M.D., President. The concept for this report originated with Lynda Biedrzycki, M.D. (member of NAME), of the

Waukesha County, Wisconsin, Medical Examiner's Office. The preparers of this report appreciate the early organizational efforts of John Teggatz, M.D., of the Milwaukee County, Wisconsin, Medical Examiner's Office, and the editorial comments of Victor Weedn, M.D., J.D., Carnegie Mellon University; Mary Ann Sens, M.D., Ph.D., University of North Dakota School of Medicine and Health Sciences; Samuel L. Groseclose, D.V.M., CDC. The preparers also thank Aldo Fusaro, M.D., of the Cook County, Illinois, Medical Examiner's Office for compiling Appendix 12.B.

† Additional information is available by contacting CDC by telephone (404-639-3133) or by fax (404-639-3043).

§ Robert T. Stafford Disaster Relief and Emergency Assistance Act, as amended by Public Law 106-390, October 30, 2000, United States Code, Title 42, The Public Health and Welfare, Chapter 68, Disaster Relief.

¶ State requests should be directed to the Department of Homeland Security, National Disaster Medical System Section, by telephone at 301-443-1167 (or 800-USA-NDMS) or by fax at 301-443-5146 (or 800-USA-KWIK)

The Authors

1. University of New Mexico School of Medicine, Albuquerque, New Mexico; 2. Division of Public Health Surveillance and Informatics, Epidemiology Program Office, CDC; 3. Fulton County Medical Examiner's Office, Atlanta, Georgia; 4. Epidemiology and Surveillance Division, National Immunization Program, CDC; 5. Immunization Services Division, National Immunization Program, CDC; 6. Georgia Bureau of Investigation, Trion, Georgia; 7. Hennepin County Medical Examiner's Office, Minneapolis, Minnesota; 8. Sparrow Hospital, Lansing, Michigan; and 9. Division of Viral and Rickettsial Diseases, National Center for Infectious Diseases, CDC. * Member of the National Association of Medical Examiners (NAME).

Appendix 12.A
Contact Information for State Public Health Laboratory Response Network (September 2002)

Contact information and laboratory specimen-collection systems are subject to change. Before sending specimens to a state laboratory, this information should be verified. Contact the Association of Public Health Laboratories by telephone at 202-822-5227 or by Internet at http://www.aphl.org/Public_Health_Labs/index.cfm.

Alabama
Bureau of Clinical Laboratories
State Department of Public Health
8140 University Drive
Montgomery, AL 36130-3017
Phone: 334-260-3400
Fax: 334-244-5083

Alaska
Alaska Department of Health and Social Services
Division of Public Health Laboratory
4500 Boniface Parkway
Anchorage, AK 99507
Phone: 907-334-2100
Fax: 907-334-2161

American Samoan
Department of Health Services
Government of American Samoa
LBJ Tropical Medical Center
Pago Pago, AS 96799
Phone: 684-633-4606
Fax: 684-633-5379

Arizona
Bureau of State Laboratory Services
Arizona Department of Health Services
1520 West Adams Street
Phoenix, AZ 85007
Phone: 602-542-0357
Fax: 602-542-0760

Arkansas
Arkansas Department of Health
4815 West Markham Street
Little Rock, AR 72205
Phone: 501-661-2191
Fax: 501-661-2310

California
California State Department of Health Service
2151 Berkeley Way, Room 703
Berkeley, CA 94704
Phone: 510-540-2408
Fax: 510-540-3075

Colorado
Colorado Department of Public Health and Environment
P.O. Box 17123
Denver, CO 80217
Phone: 303-692-3096
Fax: 303-692-3008

Connecticut
Division of Laboratories
Connecticut Department of Public Health
P.O. Box 1689

10 Clinton Street
Hartford, CT 06144
Phone: 860-509-8500
Fax: 860-509-8697

Delaware
Delaware Public Health Laboratory
P.O. Box 1047
Smyrna, DE 19977-1047
Phone: 302-653-2870
Fax: 302-653-2877

District of Columbia
Department of Health—Public Health Laboratory
300 Indiana Avenue, NW
Suite 6154
Washington, DC 20001
Phone: 202-727-8956
Fax: 202-724-1455

Florida
Department of Health
Bureau of Laboratories
P.O. Box 210
Jacksonville, FL 32331-0042
Phone: 904-791-1550
Fax: 904-791-1567

Georgia
Georgia Public Health Laboratory
Department of Human Resources
1749 Clifton Road
Decatur, GA 30033-4050
Phone: 404-327-7900
Fax: 404-327-7919

Guam
Inactive (as of 11/09/01)
Department of Public Health and Social Services
P.O. Box 2816
Agana, GU 96910
Phone: 671-735-7102
Fax: 671-734-5910

Hawaii
Laboratory Division
State of Hawaii Department of Health
2725 Wiamano Home Road, 3rd Floor
Pearl City, HI 96782
Phone: 808-453-6652
Fax: 808-453-6662

Idaho
Department of Health and Welfare
2220 Old Penitentiary Road
Boise, ID 83712
Phone: 208-334-2235
Fax: 208-334-2382

Illinois
Illinois Department of Public Health
825 North Rutledge Street
P.O. Box 19435
Springfield, IL 62794-9435
Phone: 217-782-6562
Fax: 217-524-7924

Indiana
Indiana State Department of Health
635 North Barnhill Drive
Indianapolis, IN 46202
Phone: 317-233-8006
Fax: 317-233-8003

Iowa
University Hygienic Laboratory
University of Iowa
H 101 Oakdale Hall
Iowa City, IA 52242
Phone: 319-335-4500
Fax: 319-335-4600

Kansas
Division of Health and Environmental Laboratories
Kansas Department of Health and Environment
Forbes Building, No. 740
Topeka, KS 66620
Phone: 785-296-1619
Fax: 785-296-1641

Kentucky
Department for Public Health
100 Sower Boulevard
Frankfort, KY 40601
Phone: 502-564-4446
Fax: 502-564-7019

Louisiana
State Office Building, Central Laboratory
325 Loyola Avenue, 7th Floor
New Orleans, LA 70112
Phone: 504-568-5375
Fax: 504-568-5393

Maine
Department of Human Services
221 State Street, Station 12
Augusta, ME 04333
Phone: 207-287-2727
Fax: 207-287-6832

Maryland
State Department of Health and Mental Hygiene
P.O. Box 2355
Baltimore, MD 21203
Phone: 410-767-6100
Fax: 410-333-5403

Massachusetts
State Laboratory Institute
305 South Street
Boston, MA 02130
Phone: 617-983-6201
Fax: 617-983-6927

Michigan
Michigan Department of Community Health
2250 North MLK Boulevard, Building 44
Lansing, MI 48909
Phone: 517-335-8063
Fax: 517-335-9631

Minnesota
Minnesota Department of Health
717 Delaware Street, SE
Minneapolis, MN 55440
Phone: 612-676-5331
Fax: 612-676-5514

Mississippi
State Public Health Laboratory
Mississippi Department of Health
570 East Woodrow Wilson Drive
Jackson, MS 39215-1700
Phone: 601-576-7582
Fax: 601-576-7720

Missouri
State Public Health Laboratory
Missouri Department of Health
P.O. Box 570
Jefferson City, MO 65102
Phone: 573-751-3334
Fax: 573-751-7219

Montana
Public Health Laboratory
P.O. Box 6489
Helena, MT 59601
Phone: 406-444-3444
Fax: 406-444-1802

Nebraska
Public Health Laboratory
University of Nebraska Medical Center
600 42nd Street
Omaha, NE 68198
Phone: 402-559-4116
Fax: 402-559-4077

Nevada
Nevada State Laboratory
University of Nevada School of Medicine
1660 North Virginia Street
Reno, NV 89503-1738
Phone: 775-688-1335
Fax: 775-688-1460

New Hampshire
Office of Community and Public Health
6 Hazen Drive
Concord, NH 03301
Phone: 603-271-4657
Fax: 603-271-4783

New Jersey
Public Health Laboratories
John Fitch Plaza, 4th Floor, P.O. Box 361
Trenton, NJ 08625-0361
Phone: 609-292-7783
Fax: 609-292-9285

New Mexico
New Mexico Department of Health
Scientific Laboratory Division
P.O. Box 4700
Albuquerque, NM 87196-4700
Phone: 505-841-2500
Fax: 505-841-2543
New York
Wadsworth Center
New York State Department of Health
P.O. Box 509
Albany, NY 12201
Phone: 518-474-7592
Fax: 518-474-3439

North Carolina
State Laboratory of Public Health
P.O. Box 28047
Raleigh, NC 27611-8047
Phone: 919-715-5874
Fax: 919-733-8695

North Dakota
Division of Microbiology
North Dakota Department of Health
P.O. Box 5520
Bismarck, ND 58506
Phone: 701-328-5262
Fax: 701-328-5270

Northern Mariana Islands
Inactive (as of 11/09/01)
Department of Public Health
Commonwealth Health Center
P.O. Box 409 CL
Saipan, MP 96950
Phone: 670-234-8950
Fax: 670-234-8930

Ohio
State Department of Health
P.O. Box 2568
Columbus, OH 43216
Phone: 614-644-4590
Fax: 614-752-9863

Oklahoma
Public Health Laboratory Services
State Department of Health
P.O. Box 24106
Oklahoma City, OK 73214

Phone: 405-271-5070
Fax: 405-271-4850

Oregon
Oregon Health Division
Center for Public Health Laboratories
P.O. Box 275
Portland, OR 97207
Phone: 503-229-5296
Fax: 503-229-5682

Pennsylvania
Bureau of Laboratories
Pennsylvania Department of Health
P.O. Box 500
Exton, PA 19341-0500
Phone: 610-280-3464
Fax: 610-594-9972

Puerto Rico
Institute of Health Laboratory
Department of Health
Commonwealth of Puerto Rico
Building A—Call Box 70184
San Juan, PR 00936-8184
Phone: 787-274-7817

Rhode Island
Rhode Island Department of Health
50 Orms Street
Providence, RI 02904-2283
Phone: 401-222-5554
Fax: 401-222-3332

South Carolina
Harold Dowda, PhD
Director, Bureau of Laboratories
Department of Health & Environmental Control
P.O. Box 2202
Columbia, SC 29202
Phone: 803-896-0800
Fax: 803-896-0983

South Dakota
Michael Smith
Laboratory Director
615 East Fourth Street
Pierre, SD 57501
Phone: 605-773-4757
Fax: 605-773-6129

Tennessee
Tennessee Department of Health
630 Hart Lane
Nashville, TN 37247
Phone: 615-262-6300
Fax: 615-262-6393

Texas
Texas Department of Health
110 West 49th Street
Austin, TX 78756
Phone: 512-458-7318, ext. 2418
Fax: 512-458-7221

Utah
Division of Epidemiology and Laboratory Services
46 North Medical Drive
Salt Lake City, UT 84113-1105
Phone: 801-584-8450
Fax: 801-584-8486

Vermont
Vermont Department of Health
108 Cherry Street
P.O. Box 70
Burlington, VT 05420-0070
Phone: 802-863-7246
Fax: 802-865-7701

Virgin Islands
Inactive (as of 11/09/01)
Roy L. Schneider Hospital
P.O. Box 7309
Charlotte Amalie, VI 00801

Phone: 340-776-8311
Fax: 340-714-6314

Virginia
Division of Consolidation Laboratory Services
Commonwealth of Virginia
One North 14th Street, Room 231
Richmond, VA 23219
Phone: 804-786-7905
Fax: 804-371-7973

Washington
Washington State Department of Health
Public Health Laboratories
1610 NE 150th Street
P.O. Box 550501
Shoreline, WA 98155-9701
Phone: 206-361-2885
Fax: 206-361-2904

West Virginia
Office of Laboratory Services
State of West Virginia
Department of Health & Human Resources
167 11th Avenue
South Charleston, WV 25303-1137
Phone: 304-558-3530
Fax: 304-558-2006

Wisconsin
State Laboratory of Hygiene
William D. Stovall Building
465 Henry Mall
Madison, WI 53706
Phone: 608-262-3911
Fax: 608-262-3257

Wyoming
Wyoming Public Health Laboratory
517 Hathaway Building
Cheyenne, WY 82002
Phone: 307-777-6066
Fax: 307-777-6422

Appendix 12.B
Federal Bureau of Investigation
Field Office Telephone Numbers

Alabama
Birmingham
205-326-6166

Mobile
334-438-3674

Alaska
Anchorage
907-258-5322

Arizona
Phoenix
602-279-5511

Arkansas
Little Rock
501-221-9100

California
Los Angeles
310-477-6565

Sacramento
916-481-9110

San Francisco
415-553-7400

Colorado
Denver
303-629-7171

Connecticut
New Haven
203-777-6311

Delaware
Baltimore, MD
410-265-8080

Florida
Jacksonville
904-721-1211

Miami
305-944-9101

Tampa
813-273-4566

Georgia
Atlanta
404-679-9000

Hawaii
Honolulu
808-521-1411

Idaho
Salt Lake City, UT
801-579-1400

Illinois
Chicago
312-431-1333

Springfield
217-522-9675

Indiana
Indianapolis
317-639-3301

Iowa
Omaha, NE
402-493-8688

Kansas
Kansas City, MO
816-221-6100

Kentucky
Louisville
502-583-3941

Louisiana
New Orleans
504-816-3000

Maine
Boston, MA
617-742-5533

Maryland
Baltimore
410-265-8080

Massachusetts
Boston
617-742-5533

Michigan
Detroit
313-965-2323

Minnesota
Minneapolis
612-376-3200

Mississippi
Jackson
601-948-5000

Missouri
Kansas City
816-221-6100

St. Louis
314-231-4324

Montana
Salt Lake City, UT
801-579-1400

Nebraska
Omaha
402-493-8688

Nevada
Las Vegas
702-385-1281

New Hampshire
Boston, MA
617-742-5533

New Jersey
Newark
973-792-3000

Philadelphia, PA
215-418-4000

New Mexico
Albuquerque
505-224-2000

New York
Albany
518-465-7551

Buffalo
716-856-7800

New York City
212-384-1000

North Carolina
Charlotte
704-377-9200

North Dakota
Minneapolis, MN
612-376-3200

Ohio
Cincinnati
513-421-4310

Cleveland
216-522-1400

Oklahoma
Oklahoma City
405-290-7770

Oregon
Portland
503-224-4181

Pennsylvania
Philadelphia
215-418-4000

South Carolina
Columbia
803-551-4200

South Dakota
Minneapolis, MN
612-376-3200

Tennessee
Knoxville
423-544-0751

Memphis
901-747-4300

Texas
Dallas
214-720-2200

El Paso
915-832-5000

Houston
713-693-5000

San Antonio
210-225-6741

Utah
Salt Lake City
801-579-1400

Vermont
Albany, NY
518-465-7551

Virginia
Norfolk
757-455-0100

Richmond
804-261-1044

Falls Church
703-762-3000

Washington
Seattle
206-622-0460

West Virginia
Pittsburgh, PA
412-471-2000

Wisconsin
Milwaukee
414-276-4684

Wyoming
Denver, CO
303-629-7171

Appendix 12.C
Terms and Abbreviations Used in This Report

APHL	Association of Public Health Laboratories
CDIRF	Certifier's Death Investigation Report Form
DFA	direct fluorescent assays
DHHS	U.S. Department of Health and Human Services
DHS	U.S. Department of Homeland Security
DMORT	Disaster Mortuary Operational Response Team
DPMU	Disaster Portable Morgue Unit
EPA	Environmental Protection Agency
EOC	emergency operations center
FBI	Federal Bureau of Investigation
FDA	Food and Drug Administration
FEMA	Federal Emergency Management Agency
FRP	Federal Response Plan
H&E	hematoxylin and eosin
HAZMAT	Hazardous materials
HEPA	high-efficiency particulate air
HSPD 5	Homeland Security Presidential Directive 5
ICS	Incident Command System
IDIRF	Investigator's Death Investigation Report Form
IHC	immunohistochemical
LRN	Laboratory Response Network
MCDIDS	Medical Examiner/Coroner Death Investigation Data Set
ME/Cs	medical examiners and coroners
NAME	National Association of Medical Examiners
NDMS	National Disaster Medical System
PAPRs	powered air-purifying respirators
PCR	polymerase chain reaction
PFO	principal federal officer
PPE	personal protective equipment
SAC	special agent in charge
USAMRIID	United States Army Medical Research Institute of Infectious Diseases
WMD	weapons of mass destruction

Appendix 12.D
Medical Examiners, Coroners, and Biologic Terrorism Committee Members

Andrew M. Baker, M.D., NAME and Hennepin County Medical Examiner's Office, Minneapolis, Minnesota; Michael Bell, M.D., CDC, Atlanta, Georgia; Ed Bond, International Association of Coroners and Medical Examiners; Scott Bowen, M.P.H., CDC, Atlanta, Georgia; Wayne Brathwaite, CDC, Atlanta, Georgia; David Bressler, M.S., CDC, Atlanta, Georgia; Joyce L. DeJong, D.O., NAME and Sparrow Hospital, Lansing, Michigan; Richard Ehrenberg, M.D., CDC, Atlanta, Georgia; Aldo Fusaro, D.O., NAME and Cook County Medical Examiner Office, Chicago, Illinois; Bill Greim, M.P.H., CDC, Atlanta, Georgia; Sam Groseclose, D.V.M., CDC, Atlanta, Georgia; Jeannette Guarner, M.D., CDC, Atlanta, Georgia; Randy L. Hanzlick, M.D., NAME, Fulton County Medical Examiner's Office, and CDC, Atlanta, Georgia; Harvey Holmes, Ph.D., CDC, Atlanta, Georgia; Bruce Lin, M.P.H., CDC, Atlanta, Georgia; Dennis E. McGowan, NAME and Fulton County Medical Examiner's Office, Atlanta, Georgia; Denise McNally, NAME Executive Director, Atlanta, Georgia; Kurt B. Nolte, M.D., NAME, CDC, and University of New Mexico School of Medicine, Albuquerque, New Mexico; William R. Oliver, M.D., NAME and Georgia Bureau of Investigation, Trion, Georgia; Allen Paris, M.D., University of London School of Hygiene and Tropical Medicine, London, United Kingdom; Lisa Rotz, M.D., CDC, Atlanta, Georgia; Wun-Ju Shieh, M.D., Ph.D., CDC, Atlanta, Georgia; John Teggetz, M.D., NAME and Milwaukee County Medical Examiner's Office, Wisconsin; John Watson, Federal Bureau of Investigation/Joint Terrorism Task Force, Atlanta, Georgia; Angela Weber, M.S., CDC, Atlanta, Georgia; David Williamson, Ph.D., CDC, Atlanta, Georgia; and Sherif R. Zaki, M.D., Ph.D., CDC, Atlanta, Georgia.

References

1. CDC. Biological and chemical terrorism: strategic plan for preparedness and response; recommendations of the CDC Strategic Planning Workgroup. *MMWR* 2000;49(No. RR-4):1–14.

2. Hanzlick R, Combs DL. Medical examiner and coroner systems: history and trends. *JAMA* 1998;279:870–4.

3. Brachman PS. Bioterrorism: An update with a focus on anthrax. *Am. J. Epidemiol.* 2002;155:981–7.

4. Török TJ et al. A large community outbreak of salmonellosis caused by intentional contamination of restaurant salad bars. *JAMA* 1997;278:389–95.

5. Jernigan JA et al. Bioterrorism-related inhalational anthrax: the first 10 cases reported in the United States. *Emerg. Infect. Dis.* 2001;7:933–44.

6. Borio L et al. Death due to bioterrorism-related inhalational anthrax. *JAMA* 2001;286:2554–9.

7. Bush LM et al. Index case of fatal inhalational anthrax due to bioterrorism in the United States. *N. Engl. J. Med.* 2001;345:1607–10.

8. CDC. Update: Investigation of bioterrorism-related inhalational anthrax: Connecticut, 2001. *MMWR* 2001;50:1049–51.

9. Combs DL, Parrish RG, Ing R. *Death Investigation in the United States and Canada, 1995*. Atlanta, GA: U.S. Department of Health and Human Services, CDC, 1995.

10. Nolte KB, Yoon SS, Pertowski C. Medical examiners, coroners, and bioterrorism. *Emerg. Infect. Dis.* 2000;6:559–60.

11. Nolte KB. Medical examiners and bioterrorism. *Am. J. Forensic Med. Pathol.* 2000;21:419–20.

12. Nolte KB. Evaluation of inhalational anthrax. *JAMA* 2002;287: 984–5.

13. Luke JL, Halpern M. Sudden unexpected death from natural causes in young adults. *Arch. Pathol.* 1968;85:10–7.

14. Nolte KB, Simpson GL, Parrish RG. Emerging infectious agents and the forensic pathologist: The New Mexico model. *Arch. Pathol. Lab. Med.* 1996;120:125–8.

15. O'Toole T, Mair M, Inglesby TV. Shining light on "Dark Winter." *Clin. Infect. Dis.* 2002;34:972–83.

16. Inglesby T, Grossman R, O'Toole T. A plague on your city: Observations from TOPOFF. *Clin. Infect. Dis.* 2001:32:436–45.

17. Schwartz DA, Bryan RT, Hughes JM. Pathology and emerging infections–quo vadimus? *Am. J. Pathol.* 1995;147:1525–33.

18. Walker DH, Yampolska O, Grinberg LM. Death at Sverdlovsk: What have we learned? *Am. J. Pathol.* 1994;144:1135–41.

19. Dworetzky M. Smallpox, October 1945. *New Engl. J. Med.* 2002;346:1329.

20. CDC. Update: investigation of anthrax associated with intentional exposure and interim public health guidelines, October 2001. *MMWR* 2001;50:889–93.

21. CDC. Update: Investigation of bioterrorism-related anthrax and interim guidelines for exposure management and antimicrobial therapy, October 2001. *MMWR* 2001;50:909–19.

22. CDC. Update: Investigation of bioterrorism-related anthrax and interim guidelines for clinical evaluation of persons with possible anthrax. *MMWR* 2001;50:941–8.

23. CDC. Update: Investigation of bioterrorism-related anthrax and adverse events from antimicrobial prophylaxis. *MMWR* 2001;50: 973–6.

24. Nolte KB et al. Medical examiner surveillance for bioterrorism mortality [Abstract]. Presented at the National Association of Medical Examiners Annual Meeting, October 2001, Richmond, Virginia; 39–40.

25. Grinberg LM et al. Quantitative pathology of inhalational anthrax, I: Quantitative microscopic findings. *Mod. Pathol.* 2001;14:482–95.

26. Abramova FA et al. Pathology of inhalational anthrax in 42 cases from the Sverdlovsk outbreak of 1979. *Proc. Natl. Acad Sci. U.S.A.* 1993;90:2291–4.

27. Albrink WS et al. Human inhalation anthrax: A report of three fatal cases. *Am. J. Pathol.* 1960;36:457–71.

28. Jaax NK, Fritz DL. Anthrax [Chapter 41]. In: Conner DH et al., eds. *Pathology of Infectious Diseases*, Vol 1. Hong Kong: Appleton and Lange Co., 1997;397–406.

29. Perl DP, Dooley JR. Anthrax [Section 5, Chapter 1]. In: Binford CH, Conner DH, eds. *Pathology of Tropical and Extraordinary Diseases*, Vol. 1 Washington, DC: Armed Forces Institute of Pathology, 1976;118–23.

30. Guarner J et al. Immunohistochemical detection of Yersinia pestis in formalin-fixed, paraffin-embedded tissue. *Am. J. Clin. Pathol.* 2002;117:205–9.

31. Jones AM, Mann J, Braziel R. Human plague cases in New Mexico: Report of three autopsied cases. *J. Forensic. Sci.* 1979;24:26–38.

32. Finegold MJ. Pneumonic plague in monkeys: An electron microscopic study. *Am. J. Pathol.* 1969;54:167–85.

33. Finegold MJ et al. Studies on the pathogenesis of plague: Blood coagulation and tissue responses of Macaca mulatta following exposure to aerosols of Pasteurella pestis. *Am. J. Pathol.* 1968;53:99–114.

34. Smith JH, Reisner BS. Plague [Chapter 79]. In: Conner DH. et al., eds. *Pathology of Infectious Diseases*, Vol 1. Hong Kong: Appleton and Lange Co., 1997;729–38.

35. Smith JH. Plague [Section 5, Chapter 3]. In: Binford CH, Conner DH, eds. *Pathology of Tropical and Extraordinary Diseases*, Vol 1. Washington, DC: Armed Forces Institute of Pathology, 1976:130–4.

36. Guarner J et al. Immunohistochemical detection of Francisella tularensis in formalin-fixed paraffin-embedded tissue. *App. Immunohistol. Molec. Morphol.* 1999;7:122–6.

37. Evans MA et al. Tularemia: A 30-year experience with 88 cases. *Medicine* 1985;64:251–69.

38. Schmid GP et al. Clinically mild tularemia associated with tick-borne Francisella tularensis. *J. Infect. Dis.* 1983;148:63–7.

39. Gallivan MV et al. Fatal-cat transmitted tularemia: Demonstration of the organism in tissue. *South. Med. J.* 1980;73:240–42.

40. Geyer SJ, Burkey A, Chandler FW. Tularemia [Chapter 92]. In: Conner DH et al., eds. *Pathology of Infectious Diseases*, Vol 1. Hong Kong: Appleton and Lange Co., 1997;869–73.

41. Schwartz DA, Geyer SJ. Clostridial infections [Chapter 54]. In: Conner DH et al., eds. *Pathology of Infectious Diseases*, Vol 1. Hong Kong: Appleton and Lange Co., 1997;517–32.

42. Henderson DA. Smallpox and monkeypox [Chapter 103]. In: Guerrant RL, Walker DH, Weller PF, eds. *Tropical Infectious Diseases: Principles, Pathogens, and Practice*. Philadelphia, PA: Churchill Livingstone, 1999;1095–108.

43. Cruickshank JG, Bedson HS, Watson DH. Electron microscopy in the rapid diagnosis of smallpox. *Lancet* 1966;2:527–30.

44. Murray HGS. Diagnosis of smallpox by immunofluorescence. *Lancet* 1963;1:847–8.

45. Bras G. Morbid anatomy of smallpox. *Doc. Med. Geog. Trop.* 1952;4:303–51.

46. Councilman WT, Magrath GB, Brinckerhoff WR. Pathological anatomy and histology of variola. *J. Med. Research* 1904;11:12–134.

47. Cockerell CJ. Poxvirus infections [Chapter 29]. In: Conner DH et al., eds. *Pathology of Infectious Diseases*, Vol 1. Hong Kong: Appleton and Lange Co., 1997;273–9.

48. Strano AJ. Smallpox [Section 1, Chapter 14]. In: Binford CH, Conner DH, eds. *Pathology of Tropical and Extraordinary Diseases*, Vol 1. Washington DC: Armed Forces Institute of Pathology, 1976;65–7.

49. Zaki SR, Shieh WJ, Greer PW et al. Novel immunohistochemical assay for the detection of Ebola virus in skin: implications for diagnosis, spread, and surveillance of Ebola hemorrhagic fever. *J. Infect. Dis.* 1999;179(Suppl 1):S36–47.

50. Zaki SR, Kilmarx PH. Ebola virus hemorrhagic fever [Chapter 17]. In: Horsburgh CR, Nelson AM, eds. *Pathology of Emerging Infections*. Washington, DC: American Society for Microbiology, 1997;299–312.

51. Zaki SR, Goldsmith CS. Pathologic features of filovirus infections in humans. In: Klenk HD, ed. *Marburg and Ebola Viruses*. Berlin, Germany: Springer-Verlag, 1998;97–116.

52. Gubler DJ, Zaki SR. Dengue and other viral hemorrhagic fevers [Chapter 3]. In: Nelson AM, Horsburgh CR, eds. *Pathology of Emerging Infections* 2. Washington, DC: American Society for Microbiology, 1998;43–72.

53. Zaki SR, Peters CJ. Viral hemorrhagic fevers [Chapter 37]. In: Conner DH et al., eds. *Pathology of Infectious Diseases*, Vol 1. Hong Kong: Appleton and Lange Co., 1997;347–64.

54. Child PL. Viral hemorrhagic fevers [Chapter 2]. In: Binford CH, Conner DH, eds. *Pathology of Tropical and Extraordinary Diseases*, Vol. 1. Washington DC: Armed Forces Institute of Pathology, 1976;5–11.

55. CDC. *Summary on the Laboratory Response Network.* Atlanta, GA: US Department of Health and Human Services, CDC, 2002. Available at http://www.cdc.gov/cic/functions-specs/function4Docs/nLRNvision-summary.doc.

56. CDC. *Laboratory Response to Biological Terrorism.* Atlanta, GA: US Department of Health and Human Services, CDC, 2002. Available at http://www.cdc.gov/programs/bio.htm.

57. Robinson-Dunn B. Microbiology laboratory's role in response to bioterrorism. *Arch. Pathol. Lab. Med.* 2002;126:291–4.

58. Weilbaecher Jr JO, Moss ES. Tularemia following injury while performing post-mortem examination on human case. *J. Lab. Clin. Med.* 1938;24:34–8.

59. Alibek K, Handelman S. *Biohazard: The Chilling True Story of the Largest Covert Biological Weapons Program in the World—Told from the Inside by the Man Who Ran It.* NY: Random House, Inc., 1999.

60. White HA. Lassa fever: A study of 23 hospital cases. *Trans. R. Soc. Trop. Med. Hyg.* 1972;66:390–401.

61. Heymann DL et al. Ebola hemorrhagic fever: Tandala, Zaire, 1977–1978. *J. Infect. Dis.* 1980;142:372–6.

62. Culley AR. Smallpox outbreak in South Wales in 1962. *Proc. R. Soc. Med.* 1963;56:339–43.

63. Benn EC. Smallpox in Bradford 1962: A clinical review. *Proc. R. Soc. Med.* 1963;56:345.

64. Pospisil L. Contribution to the history of glanders in the Czech Republic. *Veterinarni Medicina* 2000;45:273–6.

65. Pike RM. Laboratory-associated infections: Incidence, fatalities, causes, and prevention. *Annu. Rev. Microbiol.* 1979;33:41–66.

66. MacCallum FO, Marmion BP, Stoker MGP. Q fever in Great Britain: Isolation of Rickettsia burneti from an indigenous case. *Lancet* 1949;2:1026–7.

67. Harman JB. Q fever in Great Britain: Clinical account of eight cases. *Lancet* 1949;2:1028–30.

68. Robbins FC, Rustigian R. Q fever in the Mediterranean area: Report of its occurrence in allied troops. IV. A laboratory outbreak. *Am. J. Hyg.* 1946;44:64–71.

69. Commission on Acute Respiratory Diseases. Laboratory outbreak of Q fever caused by the Balkan grippe strain of *Rickettsia burneti. Am. J. Hyg.* 1946;44:123–57.

70. Beck MD et al. Q fever studies in southern California, II: An epidemiological study of 300 cases. *Public Health Rep.* 1949;64:41–56.

71. Nolte KB, Taylor DG, Richmond JY. Biosafety considerations for autopsy. *Am. J. Forensic. Med. Pathol.* 2002;23:107–22.

72. Holzer VE. Botulismus durch inhalation [German]. *Med. Klin.* 1962; 41:1735–40.

73. CDC, Association for Professionals in Infection Control. Bioterrorism readiness plan: A template for healthcare facilities. Atlanta, GA: U.S. Department of Health and Human Services, CDC, 1999. Available at http://www.cdc.gov/ncidod/hip/Bio/13apr99APIC-CDCBioterrorism.PDF.

74. Sewell DL et al. Protection of laboratory workers from occupationally acquired infections; approved guideline, 2d ed., Vol 1, No. 23. Wayne, PA: National Committee for Clinical Laboratory Standards (NCCLS), 2001. Publication no. M29-A2.

75. Garner JS. Guideline for isolation precautions in hospitals. Hospital Infection Control Practices Advisory Committee. *Infect. Control Hosp. Epidemiol.* 1996;17:53–80.

76. CDC, National Institutes of Health. *Biosafety in Microbiological and BioMedical Laboratories*, 4th ed. Washington, DC: U.S. Department of Health and Human Services, U.S. Government Printing Office, 1999. Available at http://www.cdc.gov/od/ohs/biosfty/bmbl4/bmbl4toc.htm.

77. Garner JS. Guideline for isolation precautions in hospitals, Part I: Evolution of isolation practices. Hospital Infection Control Practices Advisory Committee. *Am. J. Infect. Control* 1996;24:24–31.

78. Jewett DL et al. Blood-containing aerosols generated by surgical technique: A possible infectious hazard. *American Industrial Hygiene Association Journal* 1992;53: 228–31.

79. Green FHY, Yoshida K. Characteristics of aerosols generated during autopsy procedures and their potential role as carriers of infectious agents. *Appl. Occup. Environ. Hyg.* 1990;5:853–8.

80. Kembach-Wighton G, Kuhlencord A, Saternus KS. Knochenstaube bei der autopsie: Entstehung, ausbreitung, kontamination (Sawdust in autopsies: Production, spreading, and contamination) [Article in German]. *Der Pathologe* 1998;19:355–60.

81. Johnson GK, Robinson WS. Human immunodeficiency virus-1 (HIV-1) in the vapors of surgical power instruments. *J. Med. Virol.* 1991;33:47–50.

82. Pippin DJ, Verderame RA, Weber KK. Efficacy of face masks in preventing inhalation of airborne contaminants. *J. Oral Maxillofac. Surg.* 1987;45:319–23.

83. National Institute of Occupational Health and Safety. Final rule: Respiratory protective devices. 42 CFR Part 84. *Federal Register* 1995;60:3035–98.

84. CDC. Guidelines for preventing the transmission of Mycobacterium tuberculosis in healthcare facilities, 1994. *MMWR* 1994;43(No. RR-13):1–132.

85. Shieh W-J et al. High risk autopsy of fatal Lassa fever cases in Sierra Leone [Abstract 857]. *Lab. Invest.* 78,147A. 1998.

86. Nolte KB, Foucar K, Richmond JY. Hantavirus biosafety issues in the autopsy room and laboratory: Concerns and recommendations. *Hum. Pathol.* 1996;27:1253–4.

87. Inglesby TV et al. Plague as a biological weapon: Medical and public health management. *JAMA* 2000;283:2281–90.

88. Peters HJ. Morgue and autopsy room design [Chapter 9]. In: Hutchins GM, ed. *Autopsy Performance and Reporting*. Skokie, IL: College of American Pathologists, 1990; 51–4.

89. American Institute of Architects. *Guidelines for Design and Construction of Hospital and Healthcare Facilities*. Washington, DC: American Institute of Architects Press, 2001.

90. CDC, National Institutes of Health. *Primary Containment for Biohazards: Selection, Installation and Use of Biological Safety Cabinets*, 2nd ed. Washington, DC: U.S. Government Printing Office, 2000.

91. CDC. Recommendations for using smallpox vaccine in a pre-event vaccination program: supplemental recommendations of the Advisory Committee on Immunization Practices (ACIP) and the Healthcare Infection Control Practices Advisory Committee (HICPAC). *MMWR* 2003;52(No. RR-7):6.

92. CDC. Prevention of plague: Recommendations of the Advisory Committee on Immunization Practices (ACIP). *MMWR* 1996;45(No. RR-14):1–15.

93. Mallak CT, Ritchie EC. Investigation, identification, and repatriation of contaminated fatalities [Abstract G46]. Presented at the American Academy of Forensic Sciences annual meeting, February 16–21, 2004, Dallas, Texas.

94. Nolte KB. Emerging infectious agents and the forensic pathologist: making organism specific diagnoses. *N.A.M.E. News* 1997;5(6):4.

95. Hanzlick R, Parrish RG. Death investigation report forms (DIRFs): generic forms for investigators (IDIRFs) and certifiers (CDIRFs). J Forensic Sci 1994;39:629–36.

96. CDC. Medical Examiner/Coroner Death Investigation Data Set (MCDIDS), January 1995. Atlanta, GA: US Department of Health and Human Services, CDC, 1995. Available at http://www.cdc.gov/epo/dphsi/mecisp/forms/MCDIDS95A.doc.

97. Bush GW. Homeland security Presidential directive/HSPD-5: Management of domestic incidents. Washington, DC: the White House, 2003. Available at http://www.fas.org/irp/offdocs/nspd/hspd-5.html.

98. Center for Law and the Public's Health at Georgetown and Johns Hopkins Universities. Model State Emergency Health Powers Act, as of December 21, 2001. Washington, DC: Center for Law and the Public's Health, 2002. Available at http://www.publichealthlaw.net/MSEHPA/MSEHPA2.pdf.

99. Gostin LO et al. Model State Emergency Health Powers Act: Planning for and response to bioterrorism and naturally occurring infectious diseases. *JAMA* 2002;288:622–8.

100. Federal Emergency Management Agency. Basic Incident Command System (ICS). Emmitsburg, MD: Federal Emergency Management Agency, 2003. Available at http://training.fema.gov.

101. Dekalb County Board of Health Center for Public Health Preparedness. Dekalb and Fulton counties bioterrorism response plan. Atlanta, GA: Dekalb County Board of Health, 2001. Available at http://www.dekalbhealth.net.

102. CDC. *Smallpox Response Plan and Guidelines* (version 3.0). Atlanta, GA: US Department of Health and Human Services, CDC, 2002. Available at http://www.bt.cdc.gov/agent/smallpox/response-plan/index.asp.

Chapter 13

Scene Investigation: The Role of Law Enforcement and Forensic Scientists

Henry C. Lee, Ph.D., Major Timothy M. Palmbach, M.S., J.D., and Major John J. Buturla

Synopsis

13.1 Introduction

America is at war. A war we are engaged in simply because of the increase in domestic and international terrorist attacks. These attacks have threatened our fundamental American way of living in a free and democratic society with open borders.

This war has necessitated that the front line on American soil is our police, fire departments, emergency medical services, forensic professionals, public health departments, national guard, emergency management and, of course, our citizens. Although the response to an incident will often involve all emergency personnel, the responsibility for preventing and investigating terrorist acts rests primarily with law enforcement personnel.

There is no mistaking that there is a shift in the paradigm for law enforcement in the twenty-first century. Preventing and solving crime had followed traditional roles and methods. Resources remained constant and were easily identified and procured, and were personnel trained. The shift is now away from tradition. To rely on the abilities and experiences of the past would mean a failure in the responsibility of law enforcement and crime scene investigators, today and in the future, to respond to acts of domestic and international terrorism.

This shift in the paradigm is not only warranted, it is overdue. In the twenty-year period between 1981 and 2001, there was an annual average of 369 terrorism related incidents worldwide.[1] Although improvised explosive devices are commonplace weapons, law enforcement has faced increasing use of nontraditional chemical and biological weapons. Formerly a concern only for the military, law enforcement must now recognize their vulnerability and the viciousness of these attacks. The use of chemical, biological, or other weapons of mass destruction, and the individual groups or organizations using them have a singular purpose: to cause mass casualties and destroy a peaceful society.

Domestic and international terrorism have become daily events in the modern world. Hundreds and thousands of deaths occur as the result of terrorist actions. Commonly the identity of the suspects is found by determining the type of weapons used in the attack. Therefore, maintaining scene integrity and searching for physical evidence are extremely important for the first responder and investigator. Certainly there are differences in the scene techniques required at rape, robbery, or homicide cases in contrast to a scene involving a terrorist attack. Yet the basic guidelines and procedures are the same.

This chapter addresses some of the most important aspects of scene investigation of terrorist incidents. The first, and most urgent of steps, is establishing a working protocol from the point of initial notification of the

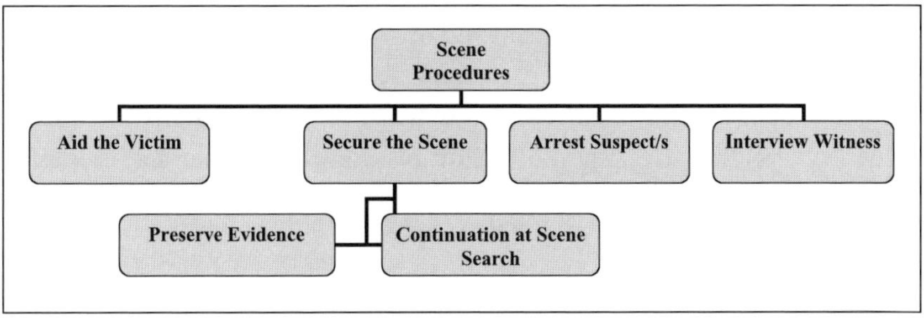

Figure 13.1 *General scene procedures*

incident through the collection and preservation of evidence. All law enforcement, fire, and emergency service personnel should be trained and knowledgeable of these protocols. Second, any successful terrorism investigation needs the cooperation of federal, state, and local agencies. A team and systematic approach of crime scene investigation is essential for all of the participants. See Figure 13.1.

A. Initial notification

Reports of an incident of chemical or biological weapon usage may come from several sources. The notification for chemical weapon dispersal will likely be an overt act. This overt act will inundate 911 dispatch centers with reports of noxious odors, and incapacitated or dead people and animals. All operators must have a protocol to follow to insure they are obtaining as much information as possible and disseminating it to all emergency responders as quick as possible. Failure to do so will result in the "blue canary" syndrome. The first responding law enforcement officers will enter the hazardous situation blindly and succumb to the weapon. Responding fire and EMS units will note the "blue canary" and equip themselves accordingly for proper response.

Biological weapons will likely have a covert dispersal and notification of their use will be made through different methods. Emergency dispatchers will be replaced by emergency room physicians and public health disease surveillance systems. The communication between law enforcement and public health officials must be present to insure timely reporting. Biological weapons, with their incubation periods, will require a different response by government officials.

Whether overt or covert, a threat or a hoax, those charged with the protection of our citizenry and investigation of the crime must respond.

This response must be coordinated and be by trained and equipped law enforcement, EMS and forensic personnel. All available resources must be used. The scene or potential scene requires thorough examination, documentation, preservation and collection by trained forensic and evidence technicians.

B. Response

The initial report will no doubt yield a significant multidisciplinary response. These responders must work collectively, in a unified command structure, to effectively and efficiently mitigate and manage an event. Although fire departments have long had training, experience and the appropriate equipment to respond to hazardous material calls, law enforcement and emergency medical services must now be on par. All have a role and responsibility and must understand their own and each others functions.

The initial response will quickly establish whether local resources are overwhelmed and county, state and federal assistance may be required. With the implementation of Homeland Security, Presidential Directive 5 (HSPD-5) all responders will understand the importance of a seamless function in the emergency. HSPD-5 establishes the National Response Plan (NRP) and National Incident Management System (NIMS) for adoption and integration by emergency response personnel. It further establishes that any deliberate terrorist act requires an investigation by law enforcement personnel. Although large-scale acts will rest with federal law enforcement, state, county and local law enforcement have jurisdictional authority with the adoption of state terrorism laws. Most states passed legislation after 9/11 to give law enforcement the ability to actively pursue actual, suspected or hoax chemical or biological weapons incidents, in the absence of a federal investigation or with the consent of the United States Attorney.

The response to these incidents must be made in the safest and most effective manner possible.

1. Establish a clear protective zone

These zones, designated as "hot" "warm" and "cold" will be established to determine the required functions within the zones and level of protection required. See Figure 13.2.

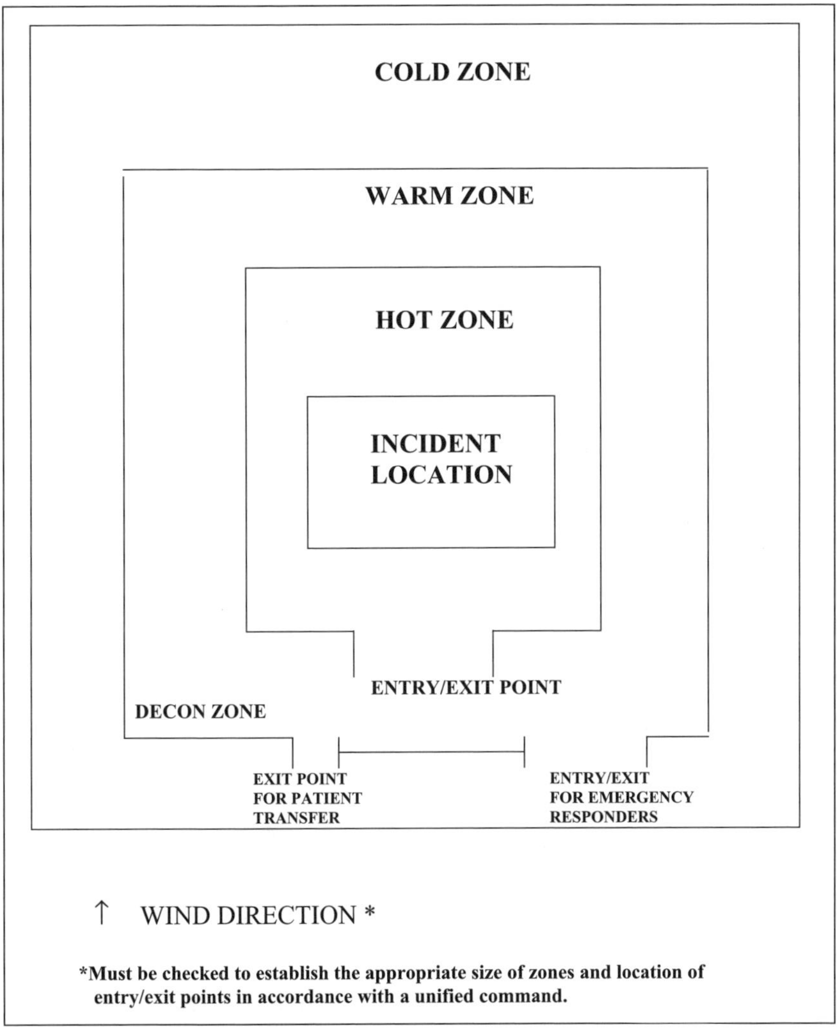

Figure 13.2 *Protective zones*

The cold zone will function as an area in which protective equipment is available or may be required. The purpose of personnel in this tier of scene management is to provide support to those entering the "warm" or "hot" zones and to insure scene security. The duties will also include triage assistance to the fire and EMS personnel.

The "warm" zone will function as a decontamination area. This area will essentially function as a screening point for law enforcement. As a function of decontamination, exposed victims will be required to remove personal effects that may contain evidence of the chemical or biological weapons or material. Law enforcement personnel, working with fire and EMS personnel, will be required to separate, catalogue, identify, and package potentially hazardous material.

2. Develop protective zones

Protocols identifying these procedures should be established and exercised long before an incident. They must demonstrate a unified approach to patient care, without compromising potential evidence. Trained crime scene personnel should be part of the warm zone team to alleviate the burden of decontamination personnel and insure integrity of belongings.

3. Develop special protocols related to the following issues

- Allowing citizens to collect their small items of personal belongings, such as wallets, purses, cell phones, and keys
- Segregating and appropriately labeling clothing and personal effects
- Keeping all items in the warm zone until examined or decontaminated
- Removing sensitive law enforcement equipment before entering the warm zone and securing it with supervisory personnel
- Having personnel and clean items sufficient for the duration of the mission
- Securing items that may contain secondary devises or delivery systems
- Rotating crime scene personnel in the area to reduce fatigue associated with wearing personal protective equipment
- Consulting with federal or state prosecutorial authorities regarding search and seizure warrant requirements

C. The crime scene

As discussed, the crime scene may encompass a variety of areas, individuals, items and locations. There are many challenges associated with chemical or biological weapon scenes that must be managed to effectively prosecute responsible parties. One of these challenges is the "hot" zone and the intricacies associated in this area.

The hot zone encompasses the actual incident site. It may be a bus, plane, train, home, mail facility, office building or individual. It is only limited by one's imagination. Therefore, adequate training and exercising is essential for all emergency responders in a variety of conditions in order to improve their safety and that of the public.

The entry will be performed only by trained hazmat or EOD teams. These teams should be trained in scenarios that familiarize them with rules and responsibilities, including that of crime scene and forensic personnel. Crucial steps are taken in the evidentiary process by these teams that greatly influence the criminal investigation. The hazmat or EOD team will be required to obtain initial samples only as part of preliminary screening of the suspected materials. National Guard Civil Support Teams or FBI, ATF, and other specially trained response teams can also be used for this function. Subsequent scene examination must be by trained law enforcement crime scene, forensic laboratory or public health laboratory personnel.

Careful consideration must be given to insure established crime scene procedures are adhered to. These procedures include the following.

- Using appropriate personal protective equipment
- Instructing hazmat teams to only collect quantities required for initial screening
- Using GPS devices to mark locations of evidence for diagram purposes
- Using photographic equipment capable of being decontaminated, such as commercially available underwater equipment, or disposable cameras
- Following chain-of-custody procedures for all samples and evidentiary items
- Securing unknown materials in packaging that is capable of being decontaminated prior to site removal to the laboratory

Following are procedures for general processing of crime scene related to biological and chemical weapon incidents.

13.2. Processing a Crime Scene Containing Biological or Chemical Weapons

Despite other significant health concerns for the general public and investigative personnel a policy and procedure must be in effect that recognizes the critical need to treat incidents that involve hazardous agents as crime scenes. Therefore, fundamental crime scene procedures involving recognition, documentation, collection and preservation of evidence must be followed. Of course modification to routine procedures will be necessary to protect personnel and equipment.

First, the scene must be secured and contained by properly trained and equipped personnel. Many uses or threatened uses of biological or chemical weapons depend on a hazardous deployment device. Thus, personnel trained in handling explosive or hazardous devices are essential. Once that threat is mitigated the suspected agent must be contained and secured. Preliminary field presumptive tests may be conducted to give scene personnel and investigators an idea as to what they are dealing with and how best to proceed. While recent advances in these field tests have occurred it must be emphasized that these are presumptive tests only, susceptible to false negatives and positives. A positive and negative control should be run with each test. Any samples must be handled with all precautions until which time laboratory analysis confirms the preliminary negative test results.

If biological or chemical agents are suspected, the following general sequence should be followed.

A. Containment of affected areas

Containment of potentially infected areas can be best accomplished by multiple levels of access or control zones, as previously described. The scope and configuration of these zones will be determined by the nature of the actual or perceived threat as well as the general structural or topography considerations. Moreover the design and structure of the physical barrier or zone boundary will vary. It may be as simple as blocking access to a roadway with police personnel or as complex as constructing an encompassing physical barrier.

Any citizens in the affected areas should be evacuated to a safe area as soon as practical. However, individuals should not be transplanted from the area until it is determined that they are not potential transport agents. If necessary these individuals will have to undergo a personal decontamination process. The extent of the evacuation plan is dependent on the nature and degree of the chemical or biological agent. Moreover, the manner in which the agent was deployed, and prevailing environmental factors such as wind, will also dictate the evacuation plan. In addition to controlling individual access, the protected area must also be restricted to vehicular and air traffic.

B. Decontamination facility

To protect both people and equipment exposed or potentially exposed to these biological or chemical agents a decontamination area or facility need to be established. The decontamination area must be sufficiently close to the affected areas to prevent further spread or contamination, but removed enough that true decontamination can occur. These facilities are essentially portable and constructed on the selected sites.

The specific design will depend on the magnitude of the event, how many individuals and what equipment will need to be decontaminated. These facilities need to be designed and managed by specifically trained personnel.

C. Scene management

Crime scenes must be properly managed to ensure proper procedures are followed and that the integrity of the scene is preserved (see Figure 13.3). Management needs to be directed through a unified command post. This command center should be located near to the event site or scene, but far enough removed not to interfere with scene functions and integrity, and far enough away so it does not endanger personnel at the command post. It must always be outside of the protective zones. The command post may be established in an available facility or room, or may be a mobile command center brought to the location. Mobile command centers are beneficial in that they are a known entity, stocked in advance with necessary supplies and communications equipment. If it will take significant time to get the long-term command post to the scene, a temporary staging area or command center should be established as soon as possible. This may be as simple as a patrol vehicle with communications capabilities. All information should be processed through the command post. In addition, person-

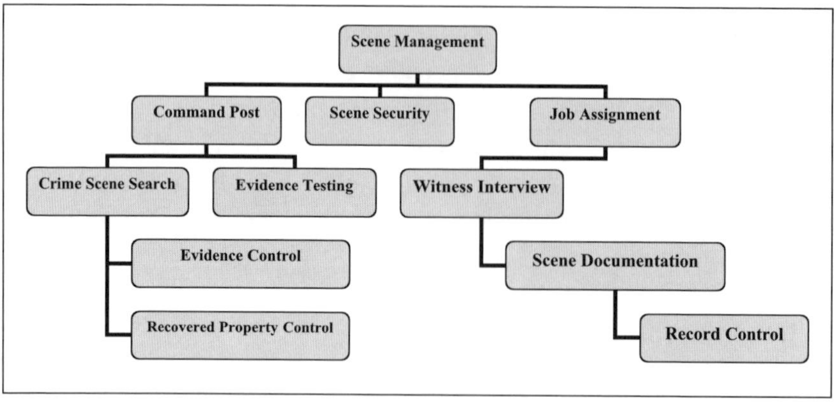

Figure 13.3 *General scene management*

nel availability and assignments should be coordinated through the command center.

After the emergency aspects of the scene have been adequately addressed and contamination and decontamination issues resolved, the command center can begin directing the scene activities relevant to processing the crime scene. First, experienced crime scene and forensic personnel should conduct a preliminary scene survey. Essentially this will require a personal inspection or walk-through. With scenes involving the use or potential use of chemical or biological agents, personnel entering the scene must wear adequate protection and undergo decontamination afterward. During this survey, the process of evidence recognition will begin. All forms of evidence should be noted. Types of evidence likely to be encountered include examples of the following five general categories of evidence.

Conditional evidence. This is evidence that is the result of an action or event such as the size or color of the flame, the degree of destruction, and the condition of victims.

Transient evidence. This type of evidence is temporary in nature and may be easily lost or destroyed, such as an odor, color, smoke and fire.

Pattern evidence. Examples of pattern evidence include fire burn pattern, explosive damage pattern, victim injury pattern, building destruction pattern and glass fracture pattern.

Transfer or trace evidence. This type of evidence occurs when objects come in contact with one another and there is a mutual exchange of material between the items such as explosives, gun powder, biological agents, deployment devices, cigarettes, glass, blood, hairs, fingerprints, footprints and tire marks.

Associative evidence. This type of evidence helps establish links among the scene, vehicle, device, victim, suspect, and physical evidence associated with the case.

Systematic documentation must occur as soon as the scene process commences and continue throughout the entire process (see Figure 13.4). Documentation can be accomplished in many forms, and often requires the use of these varied formats as each form has its own attributes and weaknesses. These formats include photography, video taping, sketching and diagramming, and general note-taking—written or audio. With contaminated scenes these procedures have many additional challenges. It may be difficult to operate some of this documentation equipment with the protective suits and respiratory equipment. In addition, the equipment used must be capable of operating in the environment and being decontaminated. Generally, that would require the equipment to be in watertight capsules or the use of disposable equipment. Otherwise, the equipment will need to be properly discarded or quarantined until it can be determined that there are no residual biological or chemical agents on it.

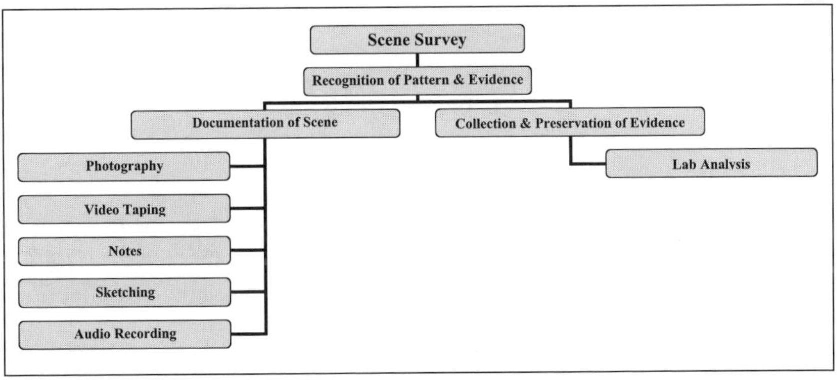

Figure 13.4 *A proper scene survey leads to the recognition, documentation, collection, preservation, and analysis of evidence.*

After the scene has been thoroughly documented, the collection process can begin. While general collection and packaging procedures establish a basic framework, there will need to be modifications made, because of contamination issues. As with documentation equipment, collection tools will need to be in protective shields capable of decontamination processes, or disposable. Packaging and handling procedures may also have to be modified to prevent contamination. Essentially, packaging containers must be secure and airtight. This type of packaging may conflict with other evidentiary concerns. For example, standard protocol dictates that items containing biological materials should not be placed in airtight containers since that may result in bacterial growth and sample degradation. Despite these additional concerns, special biohazard or chemical explosive labeling and documentation must be done to establish a chain of custody, protecting the integrity of the collected evidence.

Generally, scene investigators should expect to find evidence in one or more of the following general classifications of evidence:

- Bodies or body parts
- Other forms of biological material
- Chemical matter
- Biological, chemical or nuclear-based weapons of mass destruction
- Explosive materials or hazardous devices
- Trace evidence: hair, fibers, tissue, debris and so forth
- Imprint or impression evidence
- Various forms of pattern evidence
- Vehicles or vehicle parts
- Clothing, valuables and personal belongings

Each piece of evidence should be marked on a diagram and photographed. These steps are extremely important for further reconstruction. Based on the nature of the evidence, condition of the evidence, contamination of the evidence, and questions to be resolved the precise collection, preservation, and analysis schemes may vary somewhat.

13.3 The Role of the Forensic Scientist

Successfully preparing for and working through a biological or chemical weapon attack requires collaboration of a diversified team. A key component of that team is the forensic scientist. Forensic science is a broad based discipline and likely will require the assistance of several forensic specialists representing various key subdisciplines. Generally, these scientists will focus on several aspects of the incident involving the use of weapons of mass destruction. Roles include recognition of a biological or chemical attack, victim identification, determination of symptoms and exposure or manner and cause of death, scene analysis and reconstruction, examination of physical evidence, classification and identification of biological or chemical agents or weapons, tracing the chemical or biological fingerprint, and linking suspects to the case.

A. Recognition of a biological or chemical attack

Many times the use or threatened use of a biological or chemical agent will be telegraphed or easily identified. Terrorists who employ these types of weapons thrive on the fear and chaos that accompanies their use, so they clearly mark or identify these agents. Most often the essential task is to confirm the stated threat and scientifically confirm the structure of the agent. However, forensic scientists, emergency personnel, and healthcare workers need to be prepared to rapidly and correctly identify the symptoms and characteristics of these agents in the event that they are used without warning or public knowledge. The diversity of these agents makes this a very daunting mission.

Recognition starts at the scene of a suspicious a substance or package that may be used to contain or disseminate these agents. Next, immediate precautions must be taken to contain the contaminated areas and begin isolation and decontamination of potentially infected individuals and objects. Reliable and sensitive field testing kits or portable testing equipment should be used to screen for the common chemical or biological agents. Finally, the materials must be properly collected, preserved, and transported to a qualified laboratory for additional testing.

B. Identification of victims

Identification of a victim's remains can be challenging under normal settings; potential contamination with biological or chemical agents further complicates the process. Positive identification of the remains is a necessary legal and investigative requirement, and this may be accomplished by a variety of means. Generally, two methods of identification should be used. How identification will be accomplished often depends on the conditions of the remains, and the available resources or alternatives. Use of witnesses who can visually identify the victim is relatively rapid and reliable. However, the state of remains, or difficulty in presenting contaminated remains, may pose a significant hurdle. With contamination issues, use of quality photographic or video images is recommended.

If identification of the actual remains is not possible or practical, it may be possible for an individual closely associated with the victim to effect identification by examination and verification of the victim's personal belongings. These must be sufficiently unique to allow for a reliable identification—such as identification documents, photographs, clothing, jewelry, keys, badges, and other miscellaneous accessories.

External markers also provide a means of identification. Facial characteristics, and anthropological measurements and findings may be obtained by a forensic anthropologist. Computer programs can reconstruct facial features based on anthropological measurements and characteristics obtained from the skull. Careful examination of the remains may also detect birthmarks, birth defects and deformations, or surgical markings. If the friction ridge skin on the fingers and palms is intact it may provide the means of identification. If known inked impressions are not available for the person's fingerprints, they can be entered into a national automatic fingerprint identification system (AFIS) in hope that the individual was fingerprinted in some capacity in his lifetime. Individuals are fingerprinted for a variety of reasons, such as arrests, military or government employment, applications for classified jobs, pistol permits, special licenses or permits and so on. Also, tattoos can be a means of identification through either a friend or family member, or the artist who created it.

As examination of the remains continues internal markings can be studied and documented. Comparison of dentition to dental records is a common means of identification. However, this method depends on the recovery of dental materials and the ability to obtain current quality dental records and x-rays. Other medical records and radiographs can also be used to identify bodies or remains. Surgical records or artificial organs can also provide valuable information.

With advances in DNA typing, the use of genetic markers has become a method for positive identification. The sensitive and discriminating characteristics of STR-based (short tandem repeat) methods can provide a definitive identification even with a very small amount of remains. When only minute body parts are available, or the body is significantly decomposed or degraded, alternate methods such as mitochondrial DNA analysis may be required to provide a genetic profile. However, mitochondrial DNA typing is not as discriminating as STR typing and is only effective for establishing maternity links. DNA samples should be collected from family members and personal belongings of the victim; these samples can be used to create a data bank. Each piece of recovered body part or biological sample should be preserved and typed.

C. Determination of symptoms and exposure: Manner and cause of death

A health professional's first obligation is to the welfare of the patient. However, a timely and proper diagnosis provides investigators and scientists with information that they will use to identify the actual agents used, likely methods of dissemination, and links in the effort to trace the origin of the biological or chemical materials.

For both medical and legal reasons, the manner and cause of death for each victim must be correctly established. Therefore, it is essential to develop early communications with medical examiner's or coroner's offices. Teams of experienced forensic pathologists should be formed to conduct the autopsies. Communication is essential within the medical community so that illness or deaths associated with biological or chemical agents are not inadvertently attributed to normal causations (e.g., pneumonia or influenza).

D. Examination of physical evidence and classification and identification of agents

Examination of physical evidence suspected of being a biological or chemical weapon, or other evidence contaminated with these materials, poses many challenges to a forensic science laboratory. There are two major issues with this type of evidence. First, the material must be identified. While this type of testing can be done with existing laboratory protocols, it must be conducted in a facility that can safely handle these hazardous materials; only qualified laboratories should conduct this type of analysis. Laboratories are classified by levels that delineate what types of materials they may safely handle. The following is the Centers for Disease Control and Prevention's guidelines for laboratory capacity with chemical agents.

Level-one laboratories. These facilities can collect and ship human blood and urine specimens in response to a chemical terrorism incident.

Level-two laboratories. These facilities can analyze human samples for level-two industrial chemicals, selected chemical threat agents (such as heavy metals, lewisite, and cyanide), or their metabolites.

Level-three laboratories. Theses facilities can analyze human samples for chemical threat agents that require a higher level of analytical expertise. Level-three chemical agents include nerve agents, mustards, mycotoxins, and selected toxic industrial chemicals.

Until laboratory testing has deemed the specimen as a nonbiological or chemical threat, stringent laboratory precautions must be followed. Once the material is deemed as a safe or routine material, the sample may be handled with normal precautions. This may facilitate the use of additional instruments or methods, or transferring the sample to another, more analytically sophisticated laboratory that was not capable of conducting examinations for biological or chemical agents.

In addition to identifying the compound there is often the need to conduct a variety of other forensic examinations on the submitted physical evidence. Examples of this analysis would include processing objects for latent fingerprints, examination of machine or tool marks on devices, and visualizing any labels or writings. Collection and analysis of a wide variety of trace evidence on the objects can also provide investigators with leads. Trace components may be biological or chemical in nature, and may include materials suitable for DNA analysis, hair, fibers, or a variety of trace chemical components. This type of laboratory analysis can provide important investigative leads, identify suspects, prove or disprove alibis, or establish links between the victim, suspect, crime scene, and evidence. A real concern is to ensure that the evidence is properly collected and preserved throughout the entire process to prevent its alteration or destruction. This will require a coordinated plan with the scene personnel who will be handling the contaminated materials, as well as with the laboratory that will first examine the evidence.

E. Tracing the chemical or biological fingerprint

Once the material is identified, analytical schemes should be considered that may yield information about the origin of the material. For example, with some biological agents, such as anthrax, a DNA analysis can be conducted to determine the specific genetic fingerprint of that particular strain of bacteria. Thus, that anthrax may be linked with other anthrax samples of known or unknown origins. Even if the origin is unknown, the association of samples from several different cases is invaluable to investigators. This same type of analytical tracing can be conducted on certain chemical agents as well. Manufacturing impurities or additives that can be identified and quantified may help scientists link several samples. Unfortunately, currently there are no worldwide databases that contain this type of information. Therefore, tracing biological or chemical agents will require significant inquiries outside the realm of modern artificial intelligence resources. A global database should be established to trace all traditional chemical and biological weapons.

F. Linking a suspect to the case

Linking a suspect to a specific sample containing a chemical or biological agent can occur by various means. Classification and identification of the storage container or dissemination device should be a priority. The components used, or the manner in which they were assembled, may provide a signature of the individual or group who manufactured the weapon. In a general sense, the overall *modus operandi* (method of operation), if systematically determined, may help associate different events, and provide potential investigative links. In addition, these related objects should be processed for latent prints and trace evidence. It may be possible to obtain trace residues with sufficient material to develop a suspect's DNA profile. This may have occurred as the suspect handled certain components of the device. If envelopes were used, genetic material may have been transferred if the suspect licked the adhesive flap. Hair and trace evidence often will render class characteristics that may assist in including or excluding a certain suspect or provide some genetic trait of the suspect. Moreover, mt-DNA typing can be used on hair samples. If the hair includes a follicle, then traditional STR analysis can be conducted. If there is no follicle then the only option is mitochondrial DNA analysis. If documents were seized during the investigation, then document and handwriting analysis can provide leads to potential suspects.

Document examination may focus on the paper or envelopes, including type of material, watermarks, or other physical characteristics, such as the manner in which the paper was folded. Analysis of the ink or toner used to create the document may also provide leads. In addition the content or language may be evaluated to help determine likely educational, cultural, or other characteristics of the author. As with any type of forensic examination nondestructive methods should be employed first and subsequent destructive methods used only if necessary. Nondestructive methods for document examination include macro and microscopic examination, use of various forensic lighting sources, and ESDA (electrostatic document analysis).

13.4 Scene Analysis and Reconstruction

Despite the concerns and particular issues associated with scenes involving the use or threatened use of these weapons it must be emphasized that these are nothing more than another form of crime scenes. Therefore, all standard precautions and procedures must be considered. Too often there is an emphasis on and panic related to the biological or chemical weapon materials. As a result, traditional evidence is overlooked. This evidence includes transient evidence, conditional evidence, pattern evidence, transfer evidence, and associative evidence. In the final analysis the case will likely be solved and successfully prosecuted only if the basic investigation and crime scene procedures are followed.

Proper crime scene analysis requires the recognition, documentation, collection, and preservation of all types of evidence. Failure to conduct these foundational tasks will greatly restrict, if not totally prohibit, a subsequent crime scene reconstruction.

Reconstruction is the process of establishing or eliminating certain events and actions that occurred at the scene through analysis of scene patterns, the location and position of physical evidence, laboratory examination of physical evidence, and analysis of relevant information. This process is conducted following the basic scientific method (see Figure 13.5) and logical reasoning. The scientific method is comprised of five sequential steps: data collection, conjecture, hypothesis formulation, testing and, finally, theory formation.

The information that is incorporated into the process comes from a variety of sources. These sources include crime scene documentation in all forms, such as notes, photographs, sketches, and video tapes. Relevant investigative reports and documents should also be considered. If appropriate, medical or autopsy reports and photographs should also be evaluated. Reconstruction can be conducted through various levels or means. These levels include direct scene examination, review of records and documents, examination of physical evidence, and a review of documentary materials such as photographs, sketches, and videos. Finally, the ultimate product will depend on the amount of information available as well as the extent of inquiry or unresolved issues. Thus, reconstructions can be partial, limited, or full-scale.

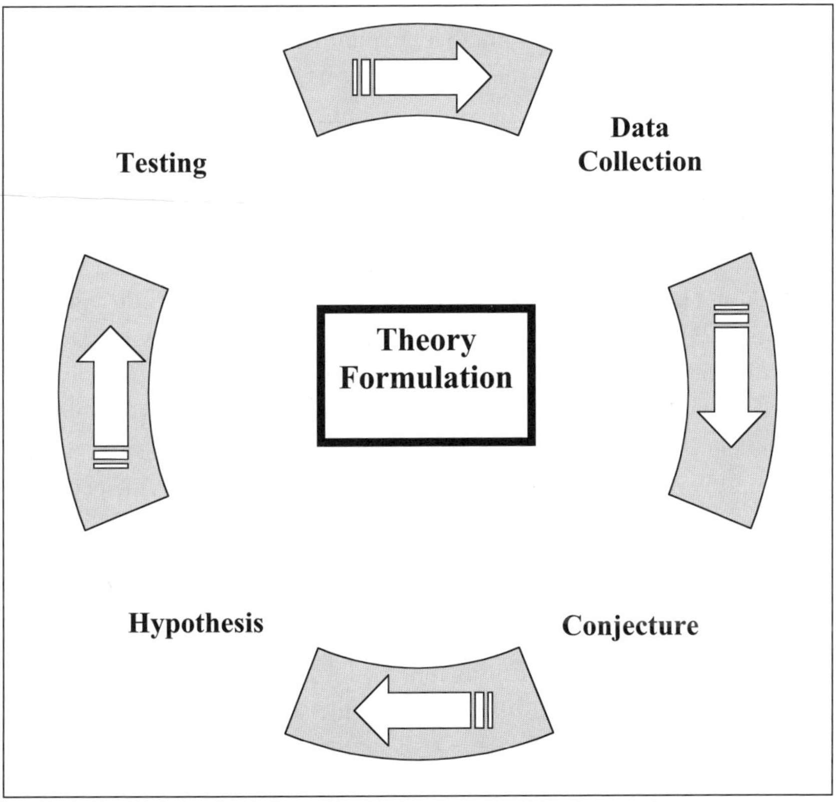

Figure 13.5 *The scientific method*

13.5 Case Example: Oxford Connecticut, Anthrax Incident

Within months of the tragic 9-11 events, the United States was confronted with the need to respond to the threat and actual use of anthrax as a weapon of potential mass destruction. In a short period of time five individuals succumbed to the deadly effects of anthrax inhalation. These individuals consisted of a sixty-three-year-old photo editor from Florida, two Washington D.C. postal workers (forty-seven and fifty-five years old), a sixty-one-year-old postal worker from New York, and a ninety-four-year-old retiree from a small community in Connecticut.

A. Information management and notification procedures

Ottilie Lundgren, a ninety-four-year-old female, retiree, living in Oxford, Connecticut, appeared to be a very unlikely target. On November 14, 2001, she became sick with flu-like symptoms. By November 16th her sickness progressed to the point that hospitalization was required, and she was admitted with pneumonia. The following day, blood tests indicated the possibility of anthrax in her system. Connecticut's Department of Public Health was notified through an existing disease surveillance system. An additional test for anthrax was administered on November 18th, but was inconclusive. However, by November 20th the governor of Connecticut responded with a public announcement regarding Ms. Lundgren's diagnosis, and he ordered her Oxford home quarantined. The following day, November 21, 2001, Ottilie Lundgren died, and the Centers for Disease Control confirmed that she had died as a result of exposure to anthrax. The CDC began its investigation into the matter, and offered Cipro to relatives or associates of Ottilie, as well as to postal workers at the Seymour post office and Wallingford postal facility where the anthrax was suspected of having originated.

An extensive search was initiated to locate the source of anthrax. A background into Ottilie's daily contacts revealed that she led a fairly isolated life and there were only a few potential sources of exposure outside of her residence. After confirming that her local church, hair salon, bakery and grocery store were not likely sources, the search focused on her residence. Moreover, trace amounts of anthrax were identified at the Wallingford postal facility, where Ottilie's mail was routed.

B. Searching the suspected scene

Officials from the CDC and the Connecticut Department of Public Health conducted an extensive search of Ottilie Lundgren's house for trace amounts of anthrax. Samples were taken from both inside and outside the house; these included samples from filters in air ducts located within the residence. Finally, handheld devices were used to obtain air samples. Large fans were brought into the residence to assist in getting any particles airborne during some of the air testing procedures. All the testing failed to detect any anthrax spores.

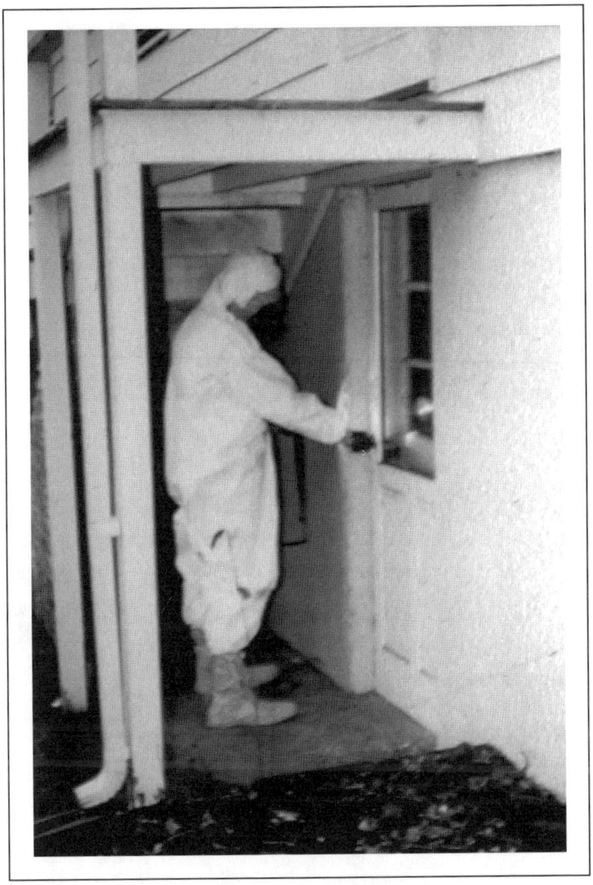

Figure 13.6 *Crime scene personnel conduct an exterior examination of the Lundgren residence. Note that this location is within the hot zone, thus protective equipment is required.*

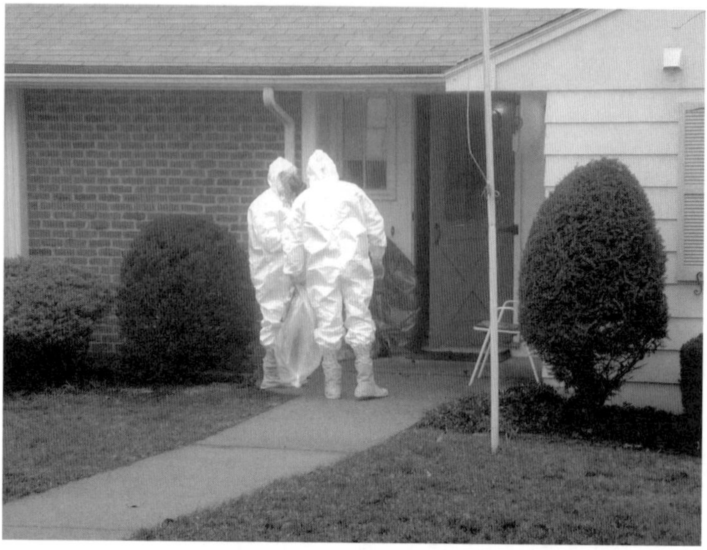

Figure 13.7 *Scientists prepare to enter the residence to begin the scene survey process. All items brought into the hot zone must be decontaminated. A clipboard and pencil are in the large, clear plastic bag.*

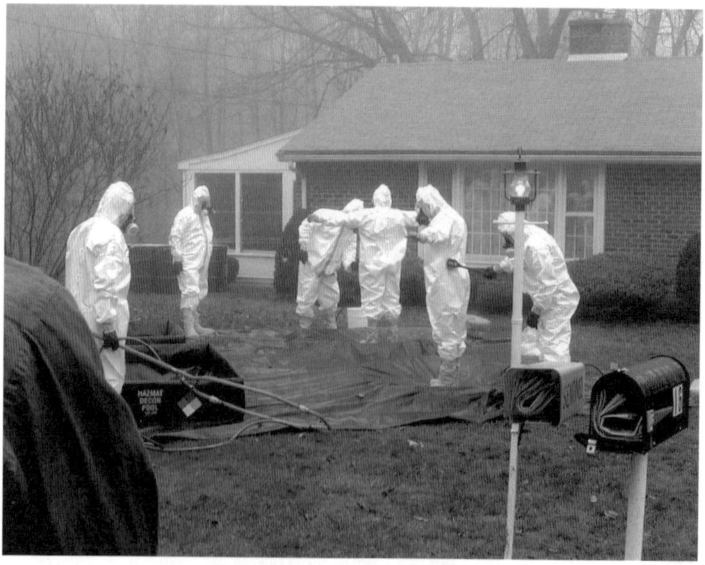

Figure 13.8 *Crime scene personnel and laboratory scientists undergoing decontamination after exiting the residence.*

There came a point in the investigation when it was determined that a traditional crime search of the Lundgren house might provide investigative leads. Thus, trained crime scene personnel were dispatched to the home to conduct a systematic crime scene search and documentation. However, the home was still a potential biological incident location and had to be treated as a hot zone. Personnel conducting the scene search had to wear protective suits and subject themselves and their equipment to decontamination (Figures 13.6–13.8).

C. Investigative efforts

Follow-up investigation into the trace amounts of anthrax detected at the post office indicated that the mail system was the likely source of the anthrax that had resulted in Ottilie Lundgren's demise. Very small amounts of anthrax were associated with mail that was delivered in areas adjacent to the Lundgren residence. A trail of the mail through the sorting facility was determined by postal inspectors.

While it was never conclusively demonstrated where Ottilie Lundgren had been exposed to anthrax, it was determined that most likely she was exposed to a small number of spores on mail that had been tainted at the nearby postal facility and delivered to her residence. Medical experts hypothesized that, because of her age and related health status, she was more vulnerable and so contracted anthrax from the inhalation of a very few spores—too few to detect in the subsequent examination of her residence. These findings, in conjunction with further examination results by FBI and state police forensic laboratories, indicated that this case was an isolated incident. Ms. Lundgren was likely not targeted by an anthrax letter, but was exposed through a secondary contact. Additional DNA testing on the anthrax may provide a genetic profile that can be used to establish associations with other anthrax investigations or known sources of anthrax. This can be accomplished by using DNA testing to identify a particular strain of DNA by its unique DNA profile.

Bibliography

Bioterrorism: A Guide for First Responders (Springfield, IL: Imaginatics, 2003).

Butler, Jay C. et al. "Collaboration between public health and law enforcement: New paradigms and partnerships for bioterrorism planning and response," *Emerging Infectious Diseases* 8(10), 2002.

Chemical/Nuclear Terrorism: A Guide for First Responders (Springfield, IL: Imaginatics, 2003).

Counterterrorism Office, U.S. Department of State. *Patterns of Global Terrorism 2001* (Washington, DC: U.S. Department of State, 2002).

Lee, Henry C., Timothy Palmbach and Marilyn T. Miller. *Henry Lee's Crime Scene Handbook* (San Diego: Academic Press, 2001).

Sidell, Frederik R., William C. Patrick III and Thomas R. Dashiell. *Jane's Chem-Bio Handbook* (Alexandria, VA: Jane's, 1998).

U.S. Army Soldier and Biological Chemical Command (SBCCOM), *Law Enforcement Officers Guide for Responding to Chemical Terrorist Incidents*, (U.S. Army Soldier and Biological Chemical Command, 2003).

Chapter 14

Psychopathy, Media and the Psychology at the Root of Terrorism

Michael Welner, M.D.

Synopsis

14.1 Introduction and Definitions

What is terrorism? Is it defined differently today? Should it be? Engaging the psychology of terrorism requires a clear acceptance and understanding of what terrorism actually is.

The challenge of understanding terror confronts decision makers and thought-leaders who sometimes enjoy the comfort of remoteness from terror acts. The news media's abandonment of focus on fact for the sympathies of its reporters[1] has nurtured ambiguity into contemporary understanding of the definition of terrorism. The by-product of this whitewashing has included attaching moral equivalence between terror and the actions of terrorists' targets;[2] or, validating such terror as an acceptable stimulus to change.[3]

The visceral impact of terror ensures that targets of terrorism will never need to be educated as to the meaning of the word "terrorism." Furthermore, as the very goals of terror include chaos and confusion, it behooves all of us to revisit what terror is, and its aims, in order not to be indeed victimized by terror's less vivid objectives.

This chapter is written with the objective of maintaining purity in use of the word "terrorism," for it is the flip exploitation of "terrorism" that cleverly handicaps efforts to expose terror. To appreciate the meaning of terror is to recognize the urgency to eliminate it as one of the lowest, most disgusting forms of human expression. But emotion must be dispensed with in the belly of the beast—for it is emotion of the victim that terror seeks to manipulate as well. Discipline and resolve is needed for the study of anything incendiary, lest we mishandle something explosive and cause untimely and unwanted damage.

Terrorism, as defined for the application of this chapter, is a strategy of action through which, in target, timing, significance, or substance, aims at a broader unknown civilian society by design in such a way as to inspire fear and anxiety, and to intentionally affect a population to cause them to avoid conventional actions of their daily life. The intended targets of violence are not only the physical targets; rather, the broader society.

A common distinction, however erroneous, is that terrorism does not occur as part of a military action or war.[4] That distinction, however, ignores the goals of war and those organizations that employ terrorism as a strategy. War is designed to a strategic end, of capturing land, strategic targets, and resources, or defending the same. The endpoint of war is not a primary targeting of civilians in order to inspire a traumatic, terrorized effect on them. Terrorism may be part of war—it is a strategy of war declared by terrorists.

Small organizations with no sovereignty haven't the luxury of formally declaring war. Without clarification, virtually anything violent that such non-sovereign organizations do might then be considered terror. And likewise, if some special allowance is made for the context of war, governments in wartime would therefore have moral allowance to exploit the conditions of war to carry out genuine terrorism. However, the human condition transcends issues of statehood with standing armies as opposed to ragtag guerillas. Terrorism is as terrorism does.

For these reasons, parsing out the setting of "war" from consideration of terror serves only the convenience of avoiding suggesting allegiances that inspire charges of bias of one's view of a particular conflict. But what good is academic consideration of terrorism if it cowers to fear of unjustified criticism, and ignores the trauma of so many affected by what should genuinely be considered terrorism? This chapter aims to preserve a consistency in defining terror so that it may be held accountable long after the covers of this book are closed.

The term "terror" is occasionally used interchangeably with "revolutionary." This, too, is inexact—for revolution is radical change, and can be brought about by a variety of means, nonviolent or violent. Even violent means need not necessarily inspire fear and disruption in the lives of uninvolved civilians. "Revolution" is, in actuality, a term of respectability, as change has been the engine of progress for many societies. Terrorism euphemizes itself by ascribing its motives as revolutionary; there is nothing reformatory about terror for the sake of destruction or personal aggrandizement. And terror has proven to fall far short of revolution. History reflects that revolution has followed the will of the masses, not the savaging of those masses through terrorist acts.

The forensic psychiatric perspective on terror borrows from evaluations of criminal responsibility. Defendants who present for psychiatric assessment in the American justice system have acknowledged involvement in a crime, and seek to mitigate responsibility in presenting themselves and their rationale to psychiatrists. As such, articulate rationale and poignant explanations are native to virtually all criminal defendants, regardless of education. All criminals—whether sane or insane—are people who can, when pressed, provide some digestible explanation for their actions if not driven from frank intoxication. The importance of psychology to terrorism, in leadership, ideology, recruitment, training, targeting, and methods of action, demands investigative verification of motives and behaviors as integral components of what distinguishes terrorism from other controversial policies or crimes.

Science lends itself to the study of terrorism by diving underneath canned advocacy to untangle the forces driving an organization, its adherents, its helpers, its targets, its timing, its actions, and its outcomes. Evidence and collateral information-gathering is a necessary part of this exercise, just as it is in every credible investigation. What falls short of this diligence perpetuates terror by misidentifying it and negating the impact that defines it.

Terrorism pursues the goal of power: real, perceived, and financial. Its modus operandi for achieving these ends has features common across cultures and conflicts. The success of that terror, however, depends very much on the leadership of a specific terror organization, its financing, how the terror group goes about achieving its impact, and the complex relationship terrorists have with the media that observes and frames that impact for the public that terrorists wish to reach.

14.2 Media as a *Modus Operandi*

Terror creates fear and confusion in the community of the target, making routine activity difficult or avoided. This tumult causes a broader society to focus on the terrorism and to consider the legitimacy of the terrorists' agenda. To maximize the likelihood of such an end, terror must be exceptionally media-sensitive, targeting symbols, dates, images, and influencing perceptions directly and subtly.

Like the most cynically devised political campaigns, terror specifically focuses on attention-seeking, bringing the terrorists notoriety, perceived omnipotence, and through that, validity to the terrorist group. Terror creates an exaggerated perception of a gang's influence in broader society and then, generates momentum among sympathetic observers to more actively enlist in that gang.

Terrorism is sometimes chosen to achieve sociopolitical end by militant groups who haven't the resources, diplomatic credentials, or might to confront an enemy militarily. Attention-seeking acts of seemingly spectacular or symbolic scope therefore counterbalance the realities that a given terror group may have only a small number of hard-core adherents.

Mass media is therefore the oxygen and an essential ingredient of terror. Free press, and the antiestablishment spirit that drives acknowledgment in news organizations today, is readily manipulated by terror organizations that cloak themselves in rhetoric that claims to speak for the dispossessed masses.

Why, in fact, has there been so little terrorism germinating in Communist China, and North Korea, two of the most repressive societies on earth? Because the press in those countries is so repudiating to disorder and nonconformity that any successfully destructive terrorist initiative would gain no traction, glamorization, or consideration from the press beyond the act itself.

For this reason, terror goes where the press is, goes where the press goes. Charles Manson targeted Hollywood, and his Manson family became legend for it. Colombia's FARC and the Phillipines' Abu Sayyaf kidnapped and executed Americans on several occasions. President

Akhmad Kadyrov of Chechnya was blown up during an official 2004 state celebration that was being covered by world media.

Before the media age, and in particular before communications linked the world with such immediacy, the potential for spectacular destruction to inspire anxiety in a surviving community was far more limited. Thus, small organizations with little substance or sincerity could not gain a foothold in any society without a clear ideology behind them, and a more deliberate method of attracting followers. That was an age of poets and writers, of orators and intellectuals who inspired through ideas. Now, fireballs and blood-soaked images are used to recruit[5] and inspire consideration of ideas, whose power carries an endorsement of the capacity to end life, or the security of a way of life.

Terrorism, for this reason, has become far more widespread with the increasing appreciation of mass media and public information as the real instruments of power. American political campaigns raise money and orchestrate appearances to maximize exposure to the voting public and citizenry. A media magnate is the Prime Minister of Italy. Public relations companies that engage news organizations are essential arms of foreign policy.[6]

It should therefore not be surprising that terrorists measure their achievement by their ability to gain widespread attention for themselves. Terrorists would live in a cave for months to years to hide from police, but can always be found by the Associated Press for an interview. Al-Manar, the official television station of Hizbullah, reaches 10 million homes and is one of the five most-watched television stations in the entire Arab World.[7]

Terrorism is "spin" in its most destructive form. You will not see, for example, exclamations of pain from Spanish victims of the 2004 Madrid train bombings in the mosques of Morocco, where the terror was planned. However, impact of Spain's national fear of Islamic power is celebrated as a victory.

Terror has a psychological underpinning—but there is no sensitivity to those suffering terror. The notion that terrorists seek to have their enemies experience their helplessness, inferiority, humiliation, and terror is spurious; for the planned actions depersonalize victims and do not embrace their feelings. Rather, terror focuses on the media and mass response to the event. Bombing is a sensational crime: Explosions, along with dramatic assassinations, have been used to dramatic effectiveness by the IRA in Northern Ireland and Great Britain, the Liberation Tigers of Tamil Eelam (LTTE) in Sri Lanka, and elsewhere.

Moslem terrorists, Arab Moslem terrorists in particular, have made suicide bombing unique to their contemporary honored culture. The inspiration for suicide bombing, however, and the impact of its terror spectacle, cannot ignore the impact of the LTTE (also known as the Tamil Tigers) and the perversity of their modus operandi.

The Tamil Tigers had a penchant for recording, through videos and photography, their political assassinations. The Tamil's filming of the 1991 assassination of India's Prime Minister Rajiv Gandhi enabled the solving of that case, as the photographer perished in the suicide bomb attack but his film somehow survived.[8]

Terror targets communities in such a way as to maximize horror, shock, dismay, and grief. Numbers tell part of the story; attacks may be selected to defile religious holidays and worship, target charity or rescue workers, or students and children.[9] The impact extends and amplifies anxiety in the surviving community, and may also communicate a message within the terror organization or the community of its supporters.[10]

Impact enables the terror organization to extend far beyond its sheer numbers. For example, Peru's Senderoso Luminoso (Shining Path) never claimed more than several thousand adherents in its heyday. Yet, in the 1980s, rebels of the Shining Path took over larger sections of the Peruvian countryside by killing villagers en masse, often hacking them with machetes. The most formidable terror movement of its time, Shining Path inspired fears of shaking the very foundation of the government of Peru, and was responsible for an estimated 30,000 deaths.[11]

There is no need to identify with terrorism and the stated missions of its leaders in order to understand them. For much of the rationalization and philosophy attached to terrorism originates from sympathetic writers and thinkers who seek to make sense of the unthinkable after it happens. Goetzel termed these individuals "radical theorists."[12] Some of these radical theorists are even showcased in respectable texts as experts in terrorist theory, and use such platforms to heap historical revisionism into near-delusional reconsideration of whom terrorists actually are. By instilling confusion in the otherwise well-armed potential targets of terrorism, these radical theorists and their benefactors in academia[13] and the media[14] are facilitators, providing air cover to future terror cells who exploit passivity in interdiction efforts. Resolve weakens, and the cooperative relationship between law enforcement and the community that is so needed to ferret out criminals in hiding becomes sorely undermined.

The terror-leaders themselves are more concerned with attention-seeking, and reaping the rewards of a successful terror operation. As such, the academic discourse of terrorism has in certain circles done much to encourage and foster terror, by creating an intellectual foundation for seemingly antiestablishment causes that those thinkers may identify with. With no theory or ideology well-articulated, terror is more readily appreciated for its true essence—violent crime.

Sometimes, the leaders of such terror movements have hardly advanced their own theories beyond street philosophy. The press and academia then add the agenda for them. Prabhakaran even recruited a journalist to write an ideological manifesto, long after establishing his Tamil Tigers.[15] This backward development of ideology illustrates the fundamental dishonesty of the purported link between terrorism and problem resolution that radical theorists advance to negate appreciation of terrorism as unacceptably subhuman.

One example where terror advocacy has gathered little traction because it has not inspired support among the antiestablishment press is the American white supremacist movement. Author William Pierce published novels which have been gobbled, manifesto-like, by adherents.[16] Rather than looking for "root causes" of his agenda, the leftist press has appropriately dismissed Pierce, whatever his education and ability to compose a coherent tome, as an annihilationist who simply exploited the disaffected contemporary white male to promote overt race and religious war. Far more oxygen of rationalization and justification is given, by comparison, to rationalizations for the nihilism of Palestinian nationalism.

14.3 Terrorist Leaders

The most successful leaders of terrorism organizations are often examples of psychopathy. The psychopath, on a personal scale, has the exquisite sensitivity to tap into the soft spots of the person and soul he wishes to seduce. On a smaller scale, the psychopath's target is money, sex, or drugs—essentially, the ingredients of hedonism. More sophisticated tastes drive some psychopaths to seek power as an aphrodisiac.

The essence of psychopathy is disruptive. Cold, remorseless, exploitative, impulsive, and grandiose in scope, often violent, lawless, diversely criminal, and relating to others as objects rather than people, the psychopath is a fundamentally destructive, callous temperament. The West German terrorist, Michael Baumann, recalled reacting to Charles Manson as "quite funny."[17] Given the tool for a functional or constructive path, the terror leader-psychopath cannot help but to create chaos, and to be functionally disruptive. A psychopath leader's core dysfunction is often the reason why terror movements do not endure.

Some have invoked malignant narcissism as a model for terrorist leaders, particularly when their brutality is also accompanied by signs of competent leadership.[18] When the grandiosity of psychopathy and malignant narcissism attaches (1) purpose to (2) sizeable scope of destruction, and (3) gains control of others, terror movements are born. In such circumstances, terror leaders effortlessly exploit sensitive religious and political issues to enlist devotees.

Nihilism is at the core of malignant narcissism. For the grandiosity and exploitation organizes around a hatred and an exaggerated paranoia for a target enemy. Malignant narcissists are more functionally capable of leading than psychopaths, even if their agenda so involves terror. Many leaders from even recent history, with legacies of inspiring terror among their own peoples and others, were malignant narcissists who could successfully negotiate a number of aspects of leadership. The apparent gains of Germany, for example, were testament to Adolf Hitler's capabilities long before the dominant influence of his nihilism became universally appreciated.

Malignant narcissism grows from a youth of subjugation, repression, and powerlessness. Ascribing the origins of psychopathic terror-leaders to their own experience of trauma and oppression is, however, disingenuous. Vellupilai Prabhakaran, founder of the Tamil Tigers of Sri Lanka, was educated, doted on, and experienced his parents as loving, if strict. Osama bin Laden emerged from a privileged family to cofound al-Qa'eda with Mahmoud Salim, an engineer; Ayman al-Zawahiri, a pediatrician, led the virulent strain of Egyptian Jihad Islami that later folded into bin Laden's network. Likewise, the disingenuousness of the "disenfranchised" characterization extends to non-Moslem terror as well. Abimael Guzman, son of a prosperous businessman and top student in a Catholic school, grew up to found Shining Path in Peru.

Prabhakaran, whatever his healthy example, cultivated a fascination with death which initially limited itself to killing animals. But he became king of the hill when he hunted human game, murdered a moderate mayor, and drew others who fell under the spell of his shocking violent brazenness into the Tamil Tigers liberation movement.

As a matter of political predation, Prabhakaran had no peer; he was responsible for killing many political figures, including India's Prime Minister Rajiv Gandhi (1991), Sri Lankan President Ranasinghe Premadasa (1993), and numerous elected members of the Sri Lankan Parliament. Prabhakaran readily acknowledged in his earlier days, however, that he had no ideological underpinning, and was more motivated by action and excitement.[19] Asked at one time to name his heroes, he cited Clint Eastwood's personification. No one has doubted Prabhakaran's operational savvy; yet victims of the Tamil Tigers included Tamils who were inclined to more peaceful means of achieving Tamil autonomy in Sri Lanka.

How is a nihilistic terror leader able to advance such a malignant agenda beyond being isolated as a homicidal crackpot? Because no matter how unusual that terror leader is, he is distinguished by his ability to hold others under his sway, with the charisma of his personal appeal, the power of his communication, and his exquisite capacity to manipulate. Prabhakaran has, for example, inspired highly dedicated and disciplined cadres of followers, austere and conserving of resources.

How, then, are psychopath terrorist leaders different from successful politicians, or even malignant narcissists? After all, successful political movements routinely exploit populist sentiments in order to ascend. Politicians guided by the aim of public service, however, do serve the needs of public when given the opportunity. The psychopath terrorist leader, even when improbably given authority and autonomy, will not successfully transition into a servant of his community, but rather a more elaborated terrorist leader, or simply a person who profits and exploits what he has been given for material aggrandizement.

Psychopaths satisfy a penchant for destruction as antisocial personalities by proxy. Antisocial personality by proxy refers to the capacity of one person to satisfy criminally destructive aims by inspiring others to cultivate destructiveness within themselves.[20]

Yasser Arafat is a stunningly vivid study in psychopathy, and the life cycle of the psychopath as terrorist leader. An Egyptian bourgeois turned into a devoted Marxist by KGB foreign intelligence, he committed his first murder at age twenty. The KGB had trained him at its Balashikha special-ops school east of Moscow and in the mid-1960s decided to groom him as the future PLO leader.[21]

Ion Pacepa, former head of Romanian Intelligence, and the highest ranking former Soviet bloc intelligence officer to ever defect to the West, chillingly wrote of the creation of Arafat,

> In 1972, the Kremlin put Arafat and his terror networks high on all Soviet bloc intelligence services' priority list, including mine. Bucharest's role was to ingratiate him with the White House. We were the bloc experts at this . . . KGB chairman Yuri Andropov in February 1972 laughed to me about the Yankee gullibility for celebrities. We'd outgrown Stalinist cults of personality, but those crazy Americans were still naïve enough to revere national leaders. We would make Arafat into just such a figurehead and gradually move the PLO closer to power and statehood. Andropov thought that Vietnam-weary Americans would snatch at the smallest sign of conciliation to promote Arafat from terrorist to statesman in their hopes for peace.[22]

The KGB attached Arafat to the grievances of Arabs displaced by lost wars attempting to destroy the nascent state of Israel. Since pan-Arab pride successfully suffused with vehement anti-Zionism passions, Arafat emerged in 1968 as a solitary alternative to Arab armies that had been repeatedly proven impotent to achieve the mission of an oil-wealthy region.

Financed by the deep pockets of the Soviet bloc and Arab governments, and successful at employing the necessary brutality to eliminate political alternatives, Arafat eventually assumed leadership of a people, who came to be known as Palestinians, to ascribe to his methods for achieving their political self-determination.

After being expelled from Syria in 1968, he based himself in Jordan, where he and his Fatah faction soon began terrorizing the local people, running extortion rackets against businesses, and undermining the Jordanian regime. Black September followed in 1970: Jordan's King Hussein launched a huge and bloody war against the Palestinians, killing thousands and leading to the expulsion of Arafat and his army in 1971. In Lebanon a decade later, with Palestinian thugs looting banks and destroying the local government,[23] Arafat was later expelled to Tunisia.[24]

Ultimately, Arafat masterminded the biggest hijacking (four aircraft at once), the largest number of hostages (3,000 at one time), the largest ransom extorted ($5 million from Lufthansa) and the greatest number and variety of terrorist targets (forty civilian aircraft, five passenger ships, thirty embassies or diplomatic missions and schools).[25]

Recalled Pacepa,

> We Romanians were directed to help Arafat improve his extraordinary talent for deceiving. The KGB chief of foreign intelligence, General Aleksandr Sakharovsky, ordered us to provide cover for Arafat's terror operations, while at the same time building up his international image. 'Arafat is a brilliant stage manager,' his letter concluded, 'and we should put him to good use.' In March 1978 I secretly brought Arafat to Bucharest for final instructions on how to behave in Washington. You simply have to keep on pretending that you'll break with terrorism and that you'll recognize Israel—over, and over, and over.[26]

Facing elimination by Israel in Beirut, Arafat succeeded in gaining American protection for his transfer to Tunisia—only months before 243 Marines were killed in a suicide bomb attack by Hizbullah. And in 1993, Arafat was bestowed political leadership of the Palestinian Authority under an Oslo peace treaty that eventually won him a Nobel Peace Prize.

His consolidation of legitimized power, from 1993, enabled Arafat to leverage and to successfully embezzle those monies showered upon his people by Israel, the United States and the international community, perpetuate the poverty of many of his people,[27] while manipulating additionally extending and deepening the enmity of the Palestinians toward Israel. By maintaining poverty and creating an identity of disempowerment of internal repression, invoking religious symbols and objectives such as the spurious deification of Jerusalem, and finally, the attachment of empowerment to "martyrdom," Arafat exploited his control to trick the Arabs under his control to buy into terror and nihilism on an unprecedented scale. He constructed, within his media and education systems, a foundation of fundamental demonization of Israel, from which Arafat could create symbols of Palestinian empowerment through self-destruction—notwithstanding that his ascent to legitimacy through the 1993 Oslo Accords, was predicated upon his fostering a sense of peaceful coexistence among his people.

Arafat transformed the identity of "Palestinians" into a cause that transcended any semblance of reality or proportion, and thus Arafat brilliantly seduced the international community into showering him with unprecedented largesse and protection. Specifically, from the Oslo Accords until the end of 2001, more than $5.5 billion was given to the PA in aid. This translates to $1,330 a Palestinian. In comparison, the Marshall Plan to rebuild Europe after World War II provided each European with $272 in today's dollars.[28] All this while terror continued unabated.

However, like any psychopath, Arafat had no constitutional wherewithal for leadership of a country. He was not programmed, after all, as a leader of men, but rather an exploiter of men.

In the twenty years before the Oslo Accords, gave Yasser Arafat sovereign authority, the number of Israelis killed by Palestinian terrorists was approximately 400. In the ten years that followed, that number was approximately 1,600, nearly 1,000 of which came during the war initiated by Arafat in 2000 and dubbed the "intifada."[29] Arafat's preparation, financing, coordination, and launching[30] of the offensive in 2000 has, as of this writing, accounted for almost 4,000 deaths (approximately 75 percent of which are Palestinian),[31] including the deaths of Palestinians who blew themselves up in 113 separate incidents.[32] Nothing compares in scale. In so doing, despite being a beneficiary of financial support of the billions of the Arab world, Arafat successfully cultivated—even among Israelis—the perception that the people in his control, the nominal Palestinians, were a "David" fighting an asymmetrical war against a Goliath, Israel.

According to *Forbes* magazine, Yasser Arafat is today the sixth wealthiest among the world's "kings, queens and despots," with more than $300 million stashed in Swiss bank accounts.[33] Others actually estimate that figure to be much higher.[34] Yet unlike despots who also appeared on that list, such as Saddam Hussein, Arafat had no oil reserves to exploit; rather, the only asset he has is a media-created cause from which he draws hundreds of millions from Europe,[35] Asia, the Arab world,[36] the U.S.,[37] Israel, and the U.N.[38] The IMF disclosed that its own audit uncovered the fact that Arafat, between 1995 and 2000, diverted fully $591 million from the PA budget into a special bank account under his personal control.[39]

As such, Yasser Arafat represents, at this writing, the most successful psychopath terrorist leader in history. Any aspiring terrorist leader would do well to study his life as a how-to guide for achieving any and all aims of terrorism, including astonishing longevity. Remembering that Arafat was shaped by intelligence agencies, students of terrorism must recognize that intelligence agencies may create weapons of mass destruction that actually have a heartbeat.

Terrorist leaders may successfully gain sanctuary from posing as symbolic martyrs. Such psychopaths successfully manipulate with baseless rhetoric that they should not be killed, lest they inspire others in multiple.[40] Yet these terror leaders—simply because they lead terrorism but nothing more, contribute so little materially to the lives of those they ostensibly advocate for that they are rendered irrelevant by the placid history that follows their passing.

Extortionists that promise protection of organized crime, for example, are not replaced by crime waves. Charles Manson was not replaced by multiples of his antiestablishment cause. Neither was Sheikh Ahmed Yassin, obliterated former founder of Hamas. Once Yassin's successor, Ahmed-Abdel Rantisi, was blown up by the Israeli military three weeks later, there followed no great rush to assume the throne of Hamas. Although Shining Path's Abimael Guzman was replaced by Oscar Ramirez Durand, the latter could never inspire more than a few hundred followers in an underground movement, before eventually being captured.[41]

Old as terrorism is, there is no prevailing legacy of a terrorist whose "martyred" legacy has inspired future generations to terror. Rather, terror leaders do their inspiring while they have the living identity and the validation of attention to inspire those to whom they are exposed.

Now dead, the psychopath terrorist leader can no longer employ the techniques of manipulation that emotionally and materially enslave his followers. Free from such haze, and finding tranquility in the aftermath of their leader's demise, followers discover that there is nothing inspiring about the nihilistic life of yesteryear.

Cinque, of the Symbionese Liberation Army, was such an example. Years after he captured national attention with the kidnapping of newspaper heiress Patty Hearst, and was later killed, Cinque inspired no one.

William Harris, one of his devotees who survived the crime spree that inspired intervention by law enforcement and ended in a Waco-style conflagration, later observed, "I wish everyone would forget us."[42]

14.4 Terrorist Followers and Soldiers

Terrorist soldiers are obviously not born terrorists, nor made terrorists by their eventual targets. Their hatred and depersonalization of their victims, and their sacrifice for an agenda is shaped by the terror leaders they answer to.

Some terror followers may originate from poverty, and from powerlessness. Their anger and disenfranchisement is sharpened into an experience of feeling attacked. Then, the terror follower is focused by manipulative terror-leaders into viewing violence as the only remaining solution.[43]

Other terror-followers are spiritually driven souls who are cause-driven and eschew the material world that is nevertheless available to them. John Walker Lindh may have ended up in an Afghan rat hole, but he certainly did not grow up in one. These pathways are best dissected on an individual-by-individual basis.

It is easier to recruit terror followers from angry, alienated or marginalized populations, for these folks exist in identities that offer them little. Civil disobedience in disenfranchised workers proved to be a fertile soil for the later seeds of leftist terror organizations from Kurdistan to Colombia. Likewise, for this reason, Muslim terror recruitment from American prisons is so successful.[44]

It is not necessarily because they are broken that the disaffected opt for terror. Rather, the acceptance of their lot, within a radicalized if "righteous" life path, fosters their identification with the terror leader, their openness to his ultimate agenda, and channels their well-credentialed anger. The seduction is never the terror itself; rather, a legal, often pious purpose becomes the foundation for acquainting with the terror follower. But the terror leaders cannot help but view people with a violent past as ripe and especially desirable recruiting targets.

Do terror followers really differ, substantially, from other violent criminals? After all, prisons are littered with disaffected, violent, powerless, alienated men and women. A Northern Ireland study that compared politically-driven murderers compared to other murderers found that the former were of average intelligence and educational background, more psychologically stable, with less likelihood of substance abuse.[45] Of course, these conclusions reflect that as a group, terrorists are noticeably less damaged than common criminals, and therefore warrant even less sympathy than common murderers. Such data also distinguishes the more pronounced overall wretchedness of the common murderers' earlier life experiences.

Nevertheless, individuals who are not yet violent or criminal may be sensation-seeking, yearning to be part of something befitting their education and privileged upbringing, gnawing at the opportunity to buck convention, or to confront authority. The terror leader need only manipulate the raw ingredients, once he realizes they are there. The deeper that the terror group member sinks into activities of the group, the more alienated from the enemy—be it the government, organized society, even his or her former self—that the terror group member becomes. At that point, identification with the terror leader becomes that much more cemented, even as the repressiveness or brutality of the terror leader manifests itself.

The extant literature has provided little understanding on the significance of life events on inspiring terrorists to violence. The poignant stories we imagine of powerless folk who are terribly abused, who rise up to engage in terrorism to avenge, do exist. However, those stories are far more associated with members of terror groups who join in order to engage in paramilitary activities, such as Northern Ireland residents might join the IRA to fight British troops or loyalists.

Those terror followers who attack civilian targets, however, killing strangers in spectacular numbers or ghoulishly desecrating them, such as Shining Path was known to do, were never tormented by those innocent villagers they terrorized and slaughtered. What, then, inspired them to such carnage?

The same dynamic, in fact, that inspires members of the IRA or Chechens or Basques, who have not experienced death or direct aggression at the hands of their victims. When terror leaders exploit symbolism, demonize and dehumanize the enemy, value destruction in accordance with its magnitude, manipulate a sense of urgency, and isolate terror members from the outside world, including their peripheral sympathizers, even families, focus enables the mission to divest itself of conscience. Suicide bombers are even able to relinquish the fundamental human instinct of survival, having bought into the fraud of receiving seventy-two virgins and heaven as a reward for blowing one's self up.

Successful con artistry is why terror movements cannot be inspired without psychopaths; for terror followers are much more than mere property-destroying political advocates, more violent than assaultive paramilitaries. They are terrorists carrying out terror, carrying out unconscionable acts of depravity that they were never born to do, nor were reared by parents and spouses who loved them, to do. What Tamil woman is reared to hack a baby to death with a machete? Only a sinister guiding infrastructure can groom the terrorist and shape and train him or her for the mission.

Thus, there is no terror follower without terror leaders; for no matter what the follower has witnessed, no matter how banal killing has come, no matter the abuse, the billions of people who live these daily realities do not submit themselves as soldiers in the War on Terror. Namibia is not a hub of suicide bombing, nor is Cambodia. Raped women the world over have not mobilized to armed attack on facilities housing sex offenders. Israelis who have watched their children blown to bits do not themselves hijack Saudi Air planes and fly them into a Mecca Hilton during the Hajj. But if each of these peoples' traumas and grievances were exploited, and they inspired by messianic, charismatic psychopathic leaders, they would embrace a terror agenda. (Charisma, however, has its limits; even Prabhakaran of Sri Lanka has swelled his ranks by the forced recruitment of scores of children as young as ten years old.[46])

Such exploitation of the zealotry of followers is on full display in the Palestinian Authority, where terror leaders rarely, if ever, submit themselves or their children to suicide bomb. In a letter to the editor of the London Arabic-language daily *Al-Hayat*, Abu Saber M.G., the father of a young Palestinian who carried out a suicide bombing in an Israeli city, wrote:

> Four months ago, I lost my eldest son when his friends tempted him, praising the path of death. They persuaded him to blow himself up in one of Israel's cities. When the pure body of my son was scattered all over, my last signs of life also dispersed, along with hope and my will to exist. Since that day, I am like [an] apparition walking the earth, not to mention that I, my wife, and my other sons and daughters have become

> displaced since the razing of the home in which we lived. But the last straw was when I was informed that the friends of my eldest son the martyr were starting to wrap themselves like snakes around my other son, not yet seventeen, to direct him to the same path towards which they had guided his brother, so that he would blow himself up too to avenge his brother, claiming "he had nothing to lose."
>
> Do the children's lives have a price? Has death become the only way to restore the rights and liberate the land? And if this be the case, why doesn't a single one of all the sheikhs who compete amongst themselves in issuing fiery religious rulings, send his son? Why doesn't a single one of the leaders who cannot restrain himself in expressing his joy and ecstasy on the satellite channels every time a young Palestinian man or woman sets out to blow himself or herself up send his son?[47]

This lament is the essence of the aforementioned antisocial personality by proxy, the mechanism by which a terror leader is able to manipulate followers to do his or her destructive bidding.[48] Similar dynamics occur in criminal enterprises, when a predatory instigator may inspire an explosive follower to effect the destruction he could not do, or do alone. Or, the leader inspires the actor so that he or she may evade direct responsibility for the crime.

Both qualities manifest themselves in terrorism. Psychopathic leaders like Charles Manson whipped up violent inspiration his followers, enabling carnage far more dramatic than anything the diminutive Manson could have ever accomplished on his own. Moreover, by remaining physically removed from a number of the crime scenes of the terrorism he inspired, Manson was able to assert that he was not involved and could not be held responsible.

Studies of terrorist followers show them, like their leaders, to be preoccupied with power, absolute in their thinking, and to externalize the causes of their personal problems, as well as potential solutions for those difficulties.[49] Terror enables them to transfer from a meaningless sense of identity to an omnipotent one.[50]

Terror followers gain strength from believing that what they are doing is right; the illegality of their actions may be known to them, but they reach a point in their indoctrination that they no longer care. In the case of the Tamil Tigers, their intensity may be such that they are prepared to die for the sake of the group. Each regular member of the LTTE carries a cyanide pill and is pledged to committing suicide rather than being captured by the enemy.[51]

Adherence is cultivated by a variety of means. A leader who establishes a brutal control over adherents mutes internal discourse and potential derailment of objectives.[52] The PKK's Abdullah Ocalan was quoted as saying, "I establish a thousand relationships every day and destroy a thousand political, organizational, emotional and ideological relationships. No one is indispensable for me. Especially if there is anyone who eyes the chairmanship of the PKK. I will not hesitate to eradicate them. I will not hesitate in doing away with people."[53]

The terror leader answers to no one, in order to maintain control. It is a delicate dance for the terror leader to maintain an identity of piety and righteousness among his following in the face of what might be obviously destructive actions.

That terror recruits are more educated, from more cultivated backgrounds, is understandable. After all, in order to carry out terror intimate to the enemy and at times, in an international setting, a recruit has to have the constitution and skills to blend into a strange environment.[54]

Why are followers young men? Men because males are more given to destruction as an expression of masculine identity. Young because idealism in the more naive outpaces the capacity for skepticism of life experience. Young because the older and more personally entangled haven't the freedom to cast aside other responsibilities unless the cause has sufficient real urgency, and terror movements do not. Not surprisingly, when asked of his earlier experiences in the Weathermen, former activist Bill Ayers observed, "We were young with an edge of certainty and arrogance that I would be hard-pressed to recreate or even fully understand again."[55]

The Sri Lankan experience, however, uniquely demonstrates how women have been incorporated into terror. The practical needs of assembling enough able bodies to overcome an organizational mandate that LTTE members kill themselves upon capture overcomes gender bias. In so doing, the LTTE demonstrates that women may not be naturally given to banal killing, but indoctrination overcomes all.[56] Not surprisingly, LTTE propaganda rails at the oppression of women in Sri Lankan society, hailing female recruitment to terror as an alternative to caste oppression.[57]

Unfortunately, radical theorists and those intellectuals who parrot them are not so willing to dismiss such destructiveness as the product of foolhardy youth or exploited certitude until many years and many wasted lives later. And the attention these academics give, in its platitudes and substance, becomes a sustaining nutrient for the otherwise nonviable integrity of terror.

14.5 Ideology

Terror followers show a willingness to submit to the governing ideology. Faith-based and capable of strong conviction, they have the qualities that make for successful soldiers being dispatched to battle. It is the service of the greater ideology that allows for their willingness to break the laws of the state or to even risk their lives. Terrorist leaders create the perception of urgency. Perception of urgency will capture the idealistic; urgency will capture all. For this reason, themes of existential threats are frequently manipulated by terror leaders.

Ideologies underlying terror have traditionally been political. While religious themes are readily invoked by the Islamofascist global terror initiative, their objective of a global theocracy is clearly political. The use of violence to terrorize, therefore, is best understood by discerning the power goals of those who plot and instigate it.

Italian terrorism in the 1970s was dominated from the right by the (*Ordine Nuovo*) New Order, which sought to mobilize an authoritarian identity in Italy modeled on German Nazism. To do so required creating chaos, and a yearning among the people to restore order, by any means necessary. New Order and (*Avanguardia Nazionale*) National Vanguard, rather than seek attention for their crimes, blamed far-left groups in order to foment tension.[58]

This modus operandi actually reflects the blueprint actually developed by Carlos Marighella for organizing, funding, and carrying out terror operations to the end of leftist revolution.[59] Marighella proposed that terror attacks would inspire a repressive response from forces in power, brutal to the point of aligning the population with the leftists seeking to overthrow the government.

Sometimes ideology attaches closely to the attention-seeking agenda. The leftist Red Brigades, operating in Italy in the 1970s and 1980s, kidnapped and murdered rightist and centrist political figures it deemed symbolic to worsening the plight of the working class. While the Red Brigades avoided bombings and other mass casualty attacks so frequently employed by terrorists, the group's high profile killings—the most stunning of which was former Italian Prime Minister Aldo Moro in 1978—attempted to instigate wider political impact. The media's repudiation for the spectacle of their criminality, however, thwarted any hopes that sensationalism would inspire a following, and the Red Brigades dwindled to irrelevance.

Contemporary attention to terror focuses on Islamofascism because its tentacles have extended across oceans and continents. Islamofascist terror, most notoriously embodied by al-Qa'eda, is the most internationalized, most well-financed, most-ambitious (in political objectives and in weapons acquisition) such effort in history. Consequently, Islamofascist terror has inspired unprecedented international cooperation in law enforcement and transaction monitoring.

Islamofascism, sponsored financially by legitimate[60] and illegitimate businesses[61,62] and through direct financial or logistical support from countries such as Iran, Syria,[63] and Saudi Arabia,[64] characteristically aims at a Muslim fundamentalist dominance to the host government. That agenda is reflected in attacks directed at the state—or targeting Western or non-Moslem (particularly Jewish) influences.

Suicide terror has been optimized by Islamofascism (Dar es-Salaam, Iraq, Istanbul, Beirut, Buenos Aires, Casablanca, Nairobi, Russia, Chechnya, Bali) through truck and vehicle bombs. In 2002 in Bali, nightclubs were bombed.[65] In Tanzania and Kenya in 1998, it was U.S. embassies that were attacked,[66] in Istanbul and Tunisia, synagogues,[67] in Nairobi, an Israeli-owned hotel,[68] and in Casablanca, a Jewish club.[69]

Even in Moslem countries, Islamofascists have used terror to overthrow influences that were more moderate in their orientation. Anwar el-Sadat of Egypt was killed by the Muslim Brotherhood.[70] Even though that crime was vigorously prosecuted, and Egypt remains essentially a non-fundamentalist dictatorship, Islamofascist terror organizations have persisted in Egypt over the past two decades, just as they has in other prominent Arab countries such as Saudi Arabia.

In Northern Iraq, Ansar al-Islam, seeded by al-Qa'eda and comprised of Moslems from around the Arab world, has fomented jihad in autonomous Iraqi Kurdistan since just before the 9/11 attacks.[71] More recently, Ansar al-Islam has been implicated in attacks against those countries in Iraq who support the U.S. presence there.

In Pakistan, General Pervez Musharraf has survived several assassination attempts by Islamofascist terrorists from Harkat ul-Mujaheddin al-Almi. Also in Pakistan, over seventy Shiite physicians have been killed by terrorists in recent years,[72] and numerous attacks have targeted Christians, including charity workers.[73]

In Indonesia, Islamists terrorist initiatives to impose Islamic Law, or Sharia, have contributed to over 19,000 deaths since 1999. Christians have been targeted for forced circumcision and conversion, and otherwise isolated and intimidated. A similar agenda in Bangladesh has also targeted Buddhists and Hindus, subjecting them to amputations, rapes in front of family, and religious institutions torched and destroyed.[74]

Abu Sayyaf, operating in the south of the Phillipines, seeks an independent Islamic state in the Mindanao province. That group has garnered international notoriety for kidnapping foreigners, including American nationals, despite a membership of no more than a thousand fighters. Abu Sayyaf operates independently from the much more numerous Moro National Liberation Front (MNLF), though their common advocacy for Moslem autonomy, and financial support from al-Qa'eda, solidify the Abu Sayyaf presence in spite of vigorous Phillipine government efforts to stamp them out.[75]

While Chechnya attracts little attention relative to other terror stages, Chechen Islamofascists have been responsible for some of the most deadly terror attacks of recent years. Only this year, Chechens carried out a suicide bombing on a Moscow subway,[76] and more recently, assassinated the country's President Kadyrov, a Moslem who rejected the fundamentalist direction of the terror movements.[77] Acting in concert with Arab Islamofascists, the Chechens have a long track record for spectacular terror, including a hostage takeover of a Moscow theater in 2002 that ended in the deaths of nearly 100 hostages at the hands of Russian police.

The very fatal resolution to that hostage takeover, which involved the use of a ventilated gas, was endorsed by Russian President Vladimir Putin, who warned of Islamofascist efforts to create a "worldwide caliphate."[78] Said Putin to a reporter from *Le Monde*, "If you want to become an Islamic radical and have yourself circumcised, I invite you to come to Moscow. I would recommend that he who does the surgery does it so you'll have nothing growing back afterward."[79] In that regard, President Putin reflected the exasperated, perhaps desperate reaction of a society already subjected to its share of terrorist attacks. That is the very point of terror—to create anxiety and unease through spectacular civilian destruction.

Terror failed to generate supportive traction for leftist organizations like Germany's Baader-Meinhoff gang and Italy's Red Brigades, and nationalist groups like the ETA. Yet terror has been quite successful for many of the Islamofascist movements, certainly for the Palestinian nationalist terrorists. The difference appears to be that the Islamofascists have intimidated the media into silence, rather than a response of repudiation as the press demonstrated in Europe and South America, and the United States in earlier years. Palestinian terrorists have succeeded in actually cultivating support in the media by a remarkably successful creation of false history and fabrications[80] on which to cast themselves as victims, and to generate external support.

It is easy to understand why the tools of inspiration for terror are often religious, especially given research findings that terror followers are generally more intelligent, more educated, and less psychiatrically impaired than other violent criminals. Scripture is hard to find dispute with, and traditionally more viscerally affecting than nationalism.

Some political terror employs philosophical reference, enough that the leader creates a perception of his brilliance for the mastery of such inscrutable writings. Likewise, it is difficult to argue—at least successfully—with a zealous and charismatic leader who displays an unusual command of subject matter, which others normally equate with great intellect and wisdom. The terror leaders, insights overidealized, pull the strings of the vulnerabilities of their followers, be they a background of poverty, social alienation, romantic rejection, or class disenfranchisement.

It may be more difficult, however, to fathom why the educated would work themselves up to the end of self-destruction simply because a government is not religious enough, or a Western presence competes against the local religious influence. For this, leaders pulling the intellectual strings of Islamofascist terror have borrowed from the writings of such well-credentialed professors as Edward Said, late of Columbia University. Said, in his well-read book *Orientalism*, blamed the very progress of the West for the shortcomings and developmental retardation of the Arab world.[81] As such, the book provided vigorous intellectual argumentation for the now widely adopted idea of Arabs being a victimized people. In Arabic academia, scores of externalizing scholars provide readily available theological and philosophical sophistry to fuel the nihilistic barbarism that has metastasized around the world. As such, one can understand why the very existence of the West is reason enough for the nuclear-minded Islamofascists to eliminate the advanced world as we know it.

Blaming the successful, empowered establishment is a familiar canard of terrorists, be their agenda religious or political. The inspiration for IRA terror was the exclusion of Catholics from opportunity and representation in Protestant-run Northern Ireland, as well as ongoing violent confrontation with Protestant militants. The Marxist Shining Path gained adherents among the indigenous peoples of Peru who felt the ruling government perpetuated their poverty.

Timothy McVeigh, for example, can readily be accepted at his representation—or, by the assertions of those who share his ideology: a person driven to his Oklahoma City destruction by the U.S. government's handling of the Waco incident. Yet, McVeigh was neither personally affected by the Waco inferno, nor an adherent of David Koresh's Branch Davidian church.[82] McVeigh was a disenfranchised military veteran whom closer scrutiny exposes as simply a person who found the notion of spectacular destruction enticing. Attached to an expedient grievance, he transitioned from a dead-end military vet into a trained killer who, rejected for the Green Berets, did find expression of his skills in a sufficiently empowering manner. But does that say he was powerless? And rendered powerless by the U.S. government? Or only that McVeigh perceived himself to be powerless unless he could act out his homicidal fantasies?

It is easier to dismiss the sincerity of McVeigh's rejoinder than it is the Islamofascists' assertions only because the latter have the luxury of many miles of distance from the accountability of honest scrutiny. Still, closer consideration exposes the fact that the insatiable Western appetite for oil empowers a society that has contributed little technology, humanities, or science to the rest of the world, nor itself. Just as Western medicine and agriculture provides improved quality of life, and indeed, life, to the Arab and Moslem world.

Suicide bombing utilized by groups like Hamas, Islamic Jihad, and Arafat's Al-Aksa Brigades and Fatah in the conflict between Israelis and Palestinians, reflects dynamics unique to its participants. Citizens of the

Palestinian Authority are indoctrinated to the degree that killing themselves in the furtherance of the elimination of Israel is the highest honor one can achieve;[83] there are those who seek death for is spiritual and material rewards (from heaven to seventy-two virgins to monies for their families).

Those allowed proximity to the process of brainwashing suicide bombers observed just how important it is for the best and brightest to be brainwashed into self-destruction. In a London *Times* article, Hala Jaber wrote of what he learned of the selection of bombers during his visit to the Gaza hideout of an al-Aksa Brigades cell.

> Those who excel militarily and show steely composure in stressful situations are most likely to be chosen. The young men must be reasonably religious, convinced of the meaning of "martyrdom and jihad (holy war)" . . . The commander observes candidates over several days as they go about their routine business in public and at home. If the assessment is positive, he informs them of their selection.
>
> An intense twenty-day period of religious study and discussion ensues between the commander and each candidate. Verses from the Koran about a martyr's attainment of paradise are recited constantly.
>
> The candidate is reminded of the good fortune that awaits him in the presence of prophets and saints, of the unimaginable beauty of the houri, or beautiful young woman, who will welcome him and of the chance he will have to intercede on behalf of seventy loved ones on doomsday. Not least, he is told of the service he will perform for his fellow countrymen with his sacrifice.
>
> "Of course I am deeply saddened when I have to use a suicide attacker. I am very emotional and at times I cry when I say good-bye to them," the commander said softly. "These men were not found on the streets. These are educated men who under normal circumstances would have the potential of being constructive members of society. If they did not have to carry out such a mission, they could have become a doctor, a lawyer or a teacher."
>
> Once the bomber's preparations are complete, he is collected by another member of the unit who accompanies him on the final journey to his target. It is only just before the assault that he is told the details of his operation, whether he will be a bomber or will attack with grenades and guns until he is shot dead. Ten to fifteen minutes before being dropped at the target, the bomber straps on a hand-tailored vest filled with about ten

> kilos of explosive and five kilos of nails and metal. He is then given his final instructions about the precise point at which he should detonate himself.
>
> The later he knows the better for the martyr, since he will not have much time to think of the target nor to experience doubts," the commander said.[84]

Other terror followers adopt the notion that death is inevitable, so best to die in a manner that is most advantageous, and most damaging to the Israeli enemy. Not surprisingly, Palestinian terror masters have also recruited those with terminal illnesses[85] and others with emotional crises.[86] Exploitation by psychopathy, of course, means that the end justifies the means. Exhorting[87] and deploying children[88] to kill themselves as they do, therefore, without regard to their capacity to consent to such a mission, reflects such *modus operandi.*

It is a fairly popular short-sightedness for some to engage terrorism by suggesting that it can be eliminated by addressing "root causes" of terror. That exercise serves the end of the psychopath terror leader, for placing the onus on the victim drives attention to an agenda, hereby legitimizing the terror leader in the eyes of previously skeptical; furthermore, it diverts attention from the enormity of a terrorist group's decision to victimize innocents who had no connection to their grievance; distracts the target of terrorism from the resolve to eradicate it; and completes the mission of the psychopath leader to provide him justification for the exercise of his fundamentally apocalyptic personality.

Indeed, disaffection has legitimate roots for some. For those who experience ongoing fear and direct oppression, it is easier to develop a sense that violence, even homicidal violence, is a necessary survival skill.[89] They are the ones who require less manipulation, less indoctrination with political theory. But any study of those who opt for political violence has never controlled for an underlying rageful personality that may have been driven by internal family dynamics, alcoholism, or an assortment of factors. Violence as an expression that the actor believes in still reflects a reservoir of anger, unique to that individual, that a "cause" provides a justifiable outlet for. Not surprisingly, research does show a higher incidence of nonpolitical criminality among paramilitary prisoners in Northern Ireland.[90]

Yet of those orphaned, nearly killed, or injured in American military actions that did not surgically avoid civilian casualties, none were among the nineteen air hijackers who perpetrated 9/11. Was it indeed the grievance, and only that? Would there have been a 9/11 if there were no madrassas and Afghanistan training camps to indoctrinate followers with an absolute approach to the world?

If grievances make terror, where are the Japanese terrorists who originated from Hiroshima-destroyed families? Perhaps if the Japanese media had the vehement externalization and manipulative nihilism seen in the Arab media, America would have seen far more dumped on its shores than cheap steel. Disaffection may have merit, but the disaffected may seek alienation as an end, as an identity. Terror-leaders, psychopathically attuned to such vulnerability, all too easily tap into such dead-end spirit to channel it into the history-altering destruction of their agenda of personal grandiosity.

Basque separatist terror gained initiative under the Spanish dictatorship of Generalissimo Francisco Franco. Basques had long struggled to resolve a wish for autonomy versus outright independence from Spain and France, with roots in preserving a Basque language and culture that Basques felt was threatened by immigrants' dilution and diminution. Franco traditionally responded violently to dissent, and violent response to Spain was thus more acceptable among Basques. This contributed to the popularity, in the 1960s, of the ETA (Euzkadi Ta Azkatasuna—Basque Nation and Liberty).

In the years following Franco's death, however, a far less repressive Spain and various aspects of autonomy and cultural preservation diminished the urgency for many to support violent terror against Spain. Yet even in recent years, in spite of a more conciliatory Spanish government affording Basques a number of areas of autonomy, incidents of terror continue as ETA has carried out a number of high profile political assassinations. The media has been clearly unsympathetic to the ETA in the wake of the assassinations, and their repudiation has interfered with the group's ability to translate high visibility and impact death into successful recruitment of new adherents.[91] The ETA example demonstrates that even as one addresses sensitive root causes, terror leaders with a destructive and nihilistic bent would prefer to retain the prerogative to remain apocalyptic.

The Tamil situation in Sri Lanka has some similarities to the Basque separatist movement. But so fierce and authoritarian was the LTTE that India harbored great concern about acceding to what may have been otherwise legitimate nationalistic aspirations of a disenfranchised people. Sometimes terror is so effective, therefore, that others are afraid to address its grievance for fear of further empowering what shows to be an unquenchable thirst for death.

Is poverty inspiring Islamofascist terror? Facts demonstrate otherwise. Economic downturns in Indonesia and Malaysia, for example, were not accompanied by upsurges in terror, and militant Islam is powered by the prosperous and educated of the more prosperous and educated Moslem nations.[92] On the other hand, economic downturn in Nigeria[93] has witnessed a turn to Islamic fundamentalism—albeit through changes in state laws, rather than enlistment in terror organizations.

A study of Hizbullah terrorists in Lebanon and Palestinian terrorists in Israel and the Palestinian Authority noted that no correlation was found between participation in violence and economic depression; violence increased when local economic conditions and optimism were getting better, and after a period during which education levels among young Palestinians had risen remarkably.[94]

Manipulating symbolism is a key component of successful development of a terror agenda. One example of the distortion of symbolism is seen in the exploitation of the concept of "humiliation" by those who explain contemporary Islamofascist terror. The United States is particularly flagellated for victimizing those soldiers of terror, for "humiliating" them. Yet, is there any more humiliated person in the Arab world than the Arab woman? Or the non-Moslem prevented from practicing his faith? Why, then, did we not see Buddhist terrorists driven by the humiliation of the destruction of the Bamiyan Buddhas by the Taliban Islamofascists?[95]

Because the realities of "humiliation" are exaggerated—the terror leaders exploit this word, however, to smartly manipulate people who are under their absolute or media control. "Eyewitness accounts" maximize the emotions of powerlessness and humiliation in viewers of such pan-Arab media as *al-Jazeera*, for example.[96]

Yet, historically oppressed peoples like American Indians, displaced, exterminated, disenfranchised, have not embraced terror as a vehicle for resolving their grievances. Why? Because there has not yet been a psychopath to emerge and exploit American Indian grievances to foment terror in White America.

Kuwait was liberated by the United States only recently, in 1991, from an occupying Iraq that pillaged the country. Yet only one decade later, Kuwaiti endorsement for the September 11th terror attacks on America as morally justifiable was by far more frequent than six other countries in the Arab world, and almost three times as frequent as among Iranians.[97] These astonishing figures were supplemented with Kuwaiti's greatest expressed resentment as U.S. policy toward the Palestinians. And yet, it was the Kuwaitis themselves who summarily evicted 300,000 Palestinians from their country at the end of Gulf War I. There had not been any Palestinian suicide bombings in Kuwait City; the Palestinians were thrown out simply because of their allegiance with Saddam Hussein.

Closer examination of the "root causes" then reveals the simpler truth that Kuwaiti power increasingly rests in the hands of fundamentalists who ideologically support the ambitions of the Islamofascists, yet are too disingenuous to explain their siding with terrorism any other way than to dream up a way to bring tiny Israel into their domestic affairs, from thousands of miles away. Such is the fraud of those who prefer simple homilies to more textured understandings of what drives alliances on a country-by-country, relationship-by-relationship basis.

Not all ideologies are such to outshine the attention created by the criminal activities of a given terror group. The Marxist Fuerzas Armadas Revolucionarios de Colombia (FARC) is known for its drug trafficking, kidnapping and extortion, operating in Colombia, Ecuador, Venezuela, and Panama. Its success as a profit-engineering rural-based crime operation eclipses its political substance. Terror as a modus operandi works for organized crime; visible attacks that send messages to the rest of the community are readily adaptable to terrorists who have an ostensible political agenda as well.

Terrorism exploits grievances of its adherents—or their inherent tendencies toward sensation-seeking behavior—in order to legitimize violence, to achieve more sinister or selfish motives. Those grievances may escalate to hatred for those responsible for the perceived injustice. When organized terrorism is at work, the grievance is manipulated to inspire an emotion of hatred. Why, then, do the adherents of some terrorist organizations hate the United States, for example? Because their leaders cleverly attach emotional pitch to grievances that may be legitimate, or features of the target that excite the solders-in-training.

Clearly, those from repressed, backward societies such as the Arab world generally have far more basis for growing up alienated and identifying with causes espousing chaos. But personal experiences of those growing up in developed nations, such as Europe, rendered the future followers of the Red Brigades, Manson Family, and Baader Meinhof every bit as vulnerable to the ministrations of a psychopath terror leader—whatever their political interest.

Manipulated hatred of terror becomes a rationalized expression that, viewed impassively, is entirely purposeless. For all his brilliance as the accomplished college professor, for example, what did Abimael Guzman's Shining Path accomplish by targeting the Peace Corps, social workers, priests, and leftist activists for public displays of grotesque brutality?

The value of exploring the stated "root causes" rests only, therefore, in confronting terror soldiers over time with the reality that their concerns are being co-opted and manipulated for a psychopathic leaders' aims, and that their needs are better met through nonterrorist means. Dr. William Pierce of the National Alliance suggested that whites in America face racial extinction because of forced ethnic diversification and imposed multiculturalism. What, then, does attention to solving the root cause of white supremacist terror do? Elimination of the Columbia School of Journalism for its ethnically diverse composition? Obviously not. But those same journalists have the power, viewing truth under stark light, to pour a bucket of cold water over the heads of the manipulated, whether they mistakenly envision the end of white America or the end of Islamic-dominated Saudi Arabia.

The psychopath terror leader thus exposed loses adherents, attention, and financial backing, and proceeds to self-destruction (as in the case of the Symbionese Liberation Army), prison (as in the case of the Manson family), or relative irrelevance (Shining Path).

It is for this reason that the resolute, even emphatic rejection of terror is a necessity. For such repudiation robs terror of the counterfeit romanticism its psychopathic leaders shroud it with. Such interdiction is not retaliation; rather it is crime prevention. In Israel, for example, eighty-three Israelis were killed by Palestinian suicide bombers between 1996 and

1997.[98] After Israel Prime Minister Benjamin Netanyahu let it be known to Palestinian Authority chairman Yasser Arafat that Israel was prepared to respond to terror with military might, only one Israeli died from a suicide bombing in the three years that followed—notwithstanding that Arafat's Palestinian Authority continued its policy of indoctrinating its own people to kill as many Israeli Jews as they could.[99]

Crime prevention can be carried out without sadism, just as law enforcement routinely respectfully apprehends even the most vicious killers and notorious killers. Psychopaths may operate with completely insensitive viciousness, but when confronted with firm limits, they respond with restraint borne of instinctual survivalism. Thus, terror ends when it becomes clear to the psychopath leader that his own survival, or his own symbolic notoriety, is no longer in his control and at the whim of those his terror organization victimizes.

As long as there will be religion, and the devotion to higher spiritual callings; as long as there will be haves and have-nots of any variety, there will always be an agenda that a terror leader can exploit, in order to foment the gaudy destruction of his fantasy. Eliminating the psychopaths who exploit agendas and ideologies, or isolating terror masters so that they no longer can draw attention—oxygen, eliminates terror. For psychopathy is the root of terrorism, not ideology.

Furthermore, terror's success advances with the paralysis of society. Therefore, it is necessary for a resolute response demonstrating that terrorist actions have not at all inspired fear and avoidance in the target society or community. Terror's end will result from the community that rejects the illusion of its paralysis that terrorists strive to orchestrate.

Endnotes

1. K. Lopez. "The media elite: Behind the ego." *New York Post*, November 2, 2003.

2. V. Hanson. "Why the Muslims misjudged us." *City Journal* 12(1) (2002).

3. V. Hanson. "The abuse of history." *National Review Online,* May 24, 2002.

4. W. Reid. "Controlling political terrorism: Practicality, not psychology." In *The Psychology of Terrorism: A Public Understanding,* C. Stout, ed. (Westport, CT: Praeger, 2002) p. 2.

5. "Terror, lies and videotape." CBSNews.com, May 15, 2002.

6. E. Kintisch. "Top D.C. lobbyists facing heat over Saudi ads." *Forward*, May 31, 2002.

7. A. Jorisch. "Al Manar: Hizbullah TV, 24/7." *Middle East Quarterly*, winter 2004.

8. "How LTTE murderers killed Rajiv Gandhi." *India Today*, July 7, 1996.

9. L. Beres. "The unique cowardice of Palestinian terrorism." Dept. Political Science, Purdue University, March 6, 2003.

10. R. Dowling. "Terrorism and the media: A rhetorical genre." *J. of Communication* 36(1):12–24 (1986).

11. *Patterns of Global Terrorism 2001*. U.S. Department of State, April 2002.

12. T. Goetzel. "Terrorist beliefs and terrorist lives." In *The Psychology of Terrorism: A Public Understanding,* C. Stout, ed. (Praeger Westport, CT: Praeger, 2002), p. 100.

13. T. Dalrymple. "A terrorist returns." *City Journal*, May 31, 2002.

14. M. Shaviv. "When terrorism is the story." *Jerusalem Post*, June 27, 2002.

15. A.S. Balasingham. *Liberation Tigers and the Tamil Eelam Freedom Struggle* (Madras, India: Liberation Tigers of Tamil Eelam, 1983).

16. Law Enforcement Agency Resource Network, ©2004 Anti-Defamation League.

17. M. Baumann. *Terror or Love? Bommi Baumann's Own Story of His Life as a West German Urban Guerilla* (NY: Grove Press, 1979).

18. R. Robins and J. Post. *Political Paranoia: The Psychopolitics of Hatred* (New Haven: Yale Press, 1997).

19. N. Swamy. *Tigers of Lanka, from Boys to Guerillas* (1994 Delhi: Konark, 1994).

20. T. Stawar. "Antisocial personality by proxy." *Journal of Psychology* 131(1) (1997).

21. I. Pacepa. "The KGB's man." *Wall Street Journal*, September 22, 2003.

22. Ibid.

23. D. Brooks. "A brief history of Yasir Arafat." *Atlantic Monthly*, July-August 2002.

24. D. Bossie. "Yasser Arafat: Nazi trained." *Washington Times*, August 9, 2002.

25. S. Lunev. "Just who are Arafat and the Palestinians?" Newsmax.com, June 27, 2002.

26. I. Pacepa. "The KGB's man." *Wall Street Journal*, September 22, 2003.

27. M. Charen. "The suffering Palestinians." Townhall.com, May 20, 2003.

28. R. Ehrenfeld. "Arafat's wrong turn." *New York Sun*, March 5, 2003.

29. E. Karsch. "Arafat's War." Address to Middle East Forum, Philadephia, PA December 2, 2003.

30. D. Warren. "Arafat's Cover is Now Truly Blown." *Ottawa Citizen* April 2, 2002.

31. Palestine Red Crescent Society, May 29, 2004.

32. Israel Foreign Ministry, May 29, 2004.

33. N. Vardi. "Auditing Arafat." *Forbes*, March 17, 2003.

34. Ibid.

35. "Swallow the Money." *Wall Street Journal Europe*, July 16, 2002.

36. R. Ehrenfeld. "U.S. vs. Arafat." *National Review Online*, September 19, 2003.

37. R. Ehrenfeld. "Arafat's purse." *National Review*, September 13, 2002.

38. D. Fischer. "What exactly is the U.N. doing in its refugee camps (with our money)?" *Weekly Standard*, May 13, 2002.

39. "Arafat's investments." *New York Post*, October 2, 2003.

40. A. Tamimi. "Advice for the U.S.: Don't make al-Qaeda's leader a martyr." *Time*, March 10, 2003.

41. "Shining Path leader taken without a shot." CNN.com, July 14, 1999.

42. Sterngold, J. "Four former radicals are charged in 1975 killing in bank robbery." *New York Times* Jan 17, 2002. pp. 1, 26.

43. Bell, S. "The unseen hand behind suicide bombers," *National Post*, May 20, 2002.

44. Thomas, C. "Radical recruiting in America's prisons," Tribune Media Services, June 20, 2002.

45. Lyons, H. and Harbison, H. "A comparison of political and non-political murderers in Northern Ireland 1974–1984." *Journal of Medicine, Science, and the Law* 26:193–197 (1986).

46. Gunaratna, R. "LTTE child combatants." *Jane's*, July, 1998.

47. Abu Saber, M.G. "Let Hamas and Jihad leaders send their own son," *Al-Hayat*, October 1, 2002.

48. Stawar, T. "Antisocial personality by proxy," *Journal of Psychology* 131(1) (1997).

49. Post, J. "Terrorist organization and motivation." Testimony before the Senate Armed Services Committee, November 2001.

50. Kfir, N. "Understanding suicidal terror through humanistic and existential psychology." In *The Psychology of Terrorism: A Public Understanding,* C. Stout, ed. (Praeger Westport, CT: Praeger, 2002).

51. Dixit, J.N. *Assignment Colombo* (Delhi, India: Konarak, 1998).

52. Volkan, V. *Bloodlines: From Ethnic Pride to Ethnic Terrorism* (NY: Farrar, Straus, and Giroux, 1997).

53. Witschi, B. "Who is Abdullah Ocalan?" CNN Interactive.

54. Kreuger, A. and Maleckova, J. "The Economics and the education of suicide bombers." *New Republic*, June 24, 2002.

55. Ayers, B. *Fugitive Days: A Memoir* (Boston: Beacon, 2001).

56. Harrison, F. "Up close with the Tamil Tigers." BBC January 29, 2002.

57. A. Ann. "Freedom birds of Tamil Eelam." http://www.eelamweb.com/women/.

58. M. von Tangen Page. *Prisons, Peace, and Terrorism: Penal Policy in the Reduction of Political Violence in Northern Ireland, Italy and the Spanish Basque Country, 1968–97* (London: MacMilllan, 1998) 90–118.

59. C. Marighella. *Minimanual of the Urban Guerilla* (Abraham Guillen Press, 1969).

60. D. McGrory. "Al-Qaeda bought $20M diamonds to hide finances." (London) *Times*, December 30, 2002.

61. "Islamic insurgency groups financed by drugs." *Middle East News Line*, March 14, 2002.

62. G. Wright. "Hizbullah suspects plead guilty: Six of ten accept U.S. Attorney deal on money laundering." *Charlotte Observer*, March 12, 2002.

63. "Syria number two terror sponsor, Gilmore Commission finds." World Tribune.com, January 8, 2003.

64. R. Ehrenfeld. "Trail of funds." *National Review Online*, September 16, 2003.

65. R. Peters. "The Bali attack is a sign of the terrorists' desperation." *Wall Street Journal*, October 15, 2002.

66. "Bombings in Nairobi, Kenya and Dar es-Salaam, Tanzania." August 7, 1998 www.state.gov, updated January 20, 2001.

67. "Tunisia synagogue blast kills 5." CNN.com, April 12, 2002.

68. "Al-Qaeda blamed for Kenya attacks." CNN.com, November 28, 2002.

69. "Car bombs explode in Casablanca." MSNBC.com, May 17, 2003.

70. "The swastika and the crescent." *Southern Poverty Law Center Intelligence Report*, http://www.splcenter.org/intel/intelreport/article.jsp?pid=242.

71. J. Schanzer. "Ansar al-Islam: Back in Iraq." *Middle East Quarterly*, winter 2004.

72. S. Inskeep. "Killing of doctors in Karachi, Pakistan." National Public Radio, March 19, 2002.

73. K. Khan. "7 Christians executed at charity in Pakistan." *Washington Post*, September 25, 2002.

74. D. Pipes and J. Schanzer. "Militant Islam's new strongholds." *New York Post*, October 22, 2002.

75. S. Rogers. "Beyond the Abu Sayyaf." *Foreign Affairs*, February, 2004.

76. J. Dougherty. "Moscow Metro blast kills 39." CNN.com, February 6, 2004.

77. "Chechen president killed by bomb." BBC News, May 9, 2004.

78. A. Evans-Pritchard and J. Strauss. "West in mortal danger from Islam, says Putin." *Daily Telegraph*, November 12, 2002.

79. "C'mon Vlad: Tell us how you really feel." *Wall Street Journal*, November 13, 2002.

80. J. Farah. "The Jews took no one's land." World Net Daily, November 19, 2002.

81. E. Said. *Orientalism* (NY: Vintage, 1979).

82. L. Michel and D. Herbeck. *American Terrorist: Timothy McVeigh and the Oklahoma City Bombing* (NY: Regan Books, 2001).

83. J. Kay. "The terrorist and Palestinian society feed off one another." *National Post*, September 11, 2003.

84. H. Jaber. "Inside the world of the Palestinian suicide bomber." (London) *Times,* March 24, 2002.

85. D. Rudge. "Report: Bomber was AIDS carrier." *Jerusalem Post*, June 18, 2002.

86. A. Fischman. "How Hamas turned adulteress into suicide bomber." *Yediot Ahronot*, January 18, 2004.

87. A. Lerner. "Arafat tells kids to die on Int'l Children's Day." *Jerusalem Post*, June 1, 2003.

88. T. Harnden. "I did it because people don't like me." *Daily Telegraph*, March 26 2004.

89. von Tangen Page, note 58, pp. 12–16.

90. Ibid.

91. "Violence marks 5th day of protests in Spain." CNN.com, July 15, 1997.

92. D. Pipes. "God and Mammon: Does poverty cause militant Islam?" *National Interest*, winter 2001–2002.

93. P. Lyman. "The U.S. can't allow 50 million Muslims to descend into extremism." *Wall Street Journal*, November 27, 2002.

94. D. Walker. "Education may be key to extremist actions." *Guardian*, July 29, 2002.

95. J. Mapes. "Explosions tear at Afghan statues." *National Geographic,* March 9, 2001.

96. R. Alt. "The al-Jazeera effect." *Weekly Standard*, April 21, 2004.

97. Gallup Organization. "Poll of the Islamic World." Washington D.C., March, 2002.

98. Israeli Ministry of Foreign Affairs.

99. C. Krauthammer. "How Arafat raised an entire generation to murder." *Washington Post*, March 29, 2002.

Chapter 15

The Biological and Chemical Threat to Aviation and Transportation Security

Kathleen M. Sweet, M.A., J.D., Lt. Col. (Ret.) USAF

Synopsis

15.1 Introduction

It is clear that airports, railroad stations, ports and mass transit services are all means of public transportation which terrorist covet as potential targets. Thousands of people may jam a terminal on any given day. Larger transportation facilities resemble small cities and definitely present a particularly enticing target for terrorists for several logistical reasons. First of all, they typically are crowded with people everyday. Secondly, modes of transportation move on a schedule in predictable geographic locations. Most important, they are public facilities providing a public service and are extremely difficult to harden as targets. They also provide ready made dispersal systems. Consequently, public transportation remains an attractive target in terms of difficulty in providing adequate physical, personnel and operational security.

Of primary importance to policy makers will be the ability to keep air clean, develop technology to quickly detect contaminates and lastly, to have the capability to shut down an entire transportation system at the first indication of a problem. The September 11 tragedy evidenced that the Federal Aviation Administration could rapidly stop air travel and that the New York transit system could be stopped from a central control room. The magnitude of the job, however, is daunting and currently would tax the aptitude of transportation facility operators, health officials and law enforcement. In November 2003, the Department of Homeland Security, initiated project "Biowatch" which is a $60 million sensor network to detect bioterrorism in thirty-one cities.

15.2 Biological and Chemical Threats

As the potential threat of chemical, biological and other unconventional weapons grows on the local, state and federal levels, preparation for such an event is rapidly becoming a significant issue to the private sector. Private security managers, medical practitioners, health administrators and law enforcement officials at all levels now need to address the age old question of "what if" as it pertains to a biological or chemical attack on a transportation facility; especially airports and mass transit. After the horrendous attacks of 9/11, Secretary of Defense Donald Rumsfeld announced that the United States was taking seriously the possibility that terrorists might engage the use of such unconventional weapons. Fatalities at even a midsize airport, railway station or port would be monumental, ranging from hundreds, to thousands, to tens of thousands depending on the agent, its dissemination rate and the adequacy and availability of effective medical response.

It is the stated purpose of this chapter to educate private practitioners to the fact that biologic, as well as chemical and nuclear threats are not just the concern of international policy makers and national level law enforcement. They are the concern of the private practitioner as well as local and state governments. More specifically, the silent partner of the weapons of mass destruction (WMD) triumvirate, "biologicals" could become the most insidious danger of the three. In March of 1996, the president of the International Association of Fire Chiefs informed the U.S. Senate that it would be the responsibility of local firefighting, police and emergency personnel to cope with any attack by biological weapons and that unfortunately they were not up to the task. Admittedly, since September 2001, emergency response agencies have been more focused in this area, but the extraordinary costs involved have delayed any valid effective countermeasures or the acquisition of appropriate response equipment and training programs. Additionally, advances in scientific discovery and technology have supplied the terrorist with a diversified array of very lethal and purely indiscriminate weapons requiring authorities and practitioners to recognize the diversity of response actually needed.

During the Cold War, both the U.S. and the former Soviet Union developed an extensive and comprehensive biological and chemical weapons program designed for use against each other. Regardless of the disintegration of the former Soviet Union, thousands of technical specialists and an extensive array of chemical and biological weapons are still proliferating. In fact, it is arguable that many governments continue extensive research in this sensitive area. The Russians are likely pursuing such efforts deep within the Ural Mountains at highly classified locations and rogue nations are also likely involved in such research. Furthermore, there is very little being done to collect intelligence on "biologicals" issues and even less being done to share the information between agencies. If any truly effective management of a biological or chemical incident is to be successful, renewed interagency cooperation and communication will be a crucial necessity relating both to prevention efforts and after action operations. In conjunction, private sector security managers, local health officials and medical practitioners must first recognize the threat as a credible one.

Currently, the Biological and Toxin Weapons Convention of 1972 prohibits the development, production and stockpiling of such substances. Nevertheless, the treaty recognizes the desire for governments to research and produce effective counter agents to any biologic threat. Consequently, there is only a threadbare difference between a lab producing a toxic agent and one producing the agent to counteract it. For the private practitioner, the existence of such substances and their availability to virtually anyone with the determination to use them constitutes a viable threat and must be taken into consideration as part of any prevention planning process.

Not only must the practitioner contemplate the inherent threat from a rogue state or individual but the even more threatening feasibility of the intentional or accidental release of an airborne biological from a legitimate lab. One infected individual can circumvent the entire globe is quite a short period of time considering today's global transportation network. Several years ago, for example, biologists at the Australian National University in Canberra sought to isolate a contraceptive vaccine for mice to reduce the pest population. They inadvertently transformed a virus into a highly lethal pathogen that was later even made more lethal by more research. Therefore, concern should not be restricted to efforts related directly to germ warfare but must also be expanded to include innocuous research that can be potentially misused.[1] The scientist themselves can constitute a threat without any malice whatsoever. Awareness and openness to any potentiality is key to a successful counter bioterrorism program.

The U.S. government has been collecting data on the dissemination of agents since 1949. In fact, more than 200 secret tests were conducted in populated areas to calculate the effects of such attacks within urban areas. For example, in the 1950s a U.S. Navy vessel sprayed bacteria off a two-mile stretch of coastline near San Francisco. The bacteria covered the city with a little help from the weather. Had the bacteria actually been lethal, untold numbers of people would have died. Additionally, military scientists actually tossed light bulbs filled with bacteria onto the underground tracks of the New York City subway just to test the dissemination rate of the agent in the 1960s. Airflows from the trains actually pushed the test bacteria through the subway cars and the underground tunnels. The publication[2] that such tests took place provoked outrage but also evidenced that the science of unconventional warfare has been underway for decades.

Since the development of nuclear weapons physicist have been "policed" in the name of national security. More recently, fears of bioterrorism may require a similar approach for biologists. In October 2003, the National Research Council issued recommendations for overseeing unclassified experiments that might assist a terrorist. The regulatory approach would be multilayered and envelop all sorts of experimentation including those designed to disable vaccines, confer resistance to antibiotics, enhance the virulence of a strain, or turn cells or proteins into weapons. However, to be effective any such controls would require an international approach.

Many scientists consequently support the establishment of an International Forum on Bio Security. Without the initiation of coordinated international measures to prevent the creation, proliferation and potential use of such materials, all international airports and ports are at risk. Such efforts should also include procedures for the dissemination of such information to international agencies tasked with handling an outbreak of any lethal agent. International cooperation for controlling an incident will therefore require the participation of such organizations as the International Organization on Civil Aviation (ICAO) and the International Maritime Organization (IMO).

15.3 History and Potential

Consider the potentiality of the following headline: "Thousands Die as the Result of a Bioterrorist attack at YOUR airport in YOUR city." Every security manager and health practitioner should be aware of the fact that the above potential headline could easily apply to them considering the nation's current state of readiness. All it takes is a basic degree in biology or chemistry. Almost every convenience store proffers for sale aerosol deodorizers that could be adapted as a suitable container. The agents, though harder to acquire than when Saddam Hussein ordered his first batch overnight mail from a U.S. lab, they are still easy enough to acquire in today's global environment. All that would really be needed would be the intense desire to acquire, package and relcasc an agent. Regardless of the West's natural aversion to such an incident, it has happened before and will likely happen again.

Rogue states, such as former Ba'athist Iraq, have already demonstrated the dangers of proliferation of biologic and chemical weapons for governments seeking to use a "poor man's nuke." However, there also exists a new and even more highly disturbing phenomenon. Essentially, the acquisition of such devices is no longer restricted to nation states. Individuals and groups are also capable of targeting the private sector for whatever reason. The vast economic resources of the al-Qa'eda network certainly make the possibility of such an incident feasible if not likely.

Al Q'aeda has been eager to acquire both biological and chemical weapons. Not long ago, U.S. intelligence identified sites in Afghanistan that were suspected of producing such agents. It was believed that they may have already produced small quantities of cyanide gas but concrete evidence has yet to be obtained. In today's "Internet" environment, the potential perpetrator has readily available knowledge pertaining to these weapons. Therefore, private security practitioners and concerned local and state emergency response personnel must become equally educated. Simply put, in today's high tech environment, authorities whom ignore the possibility of a biological or chemical attack, as one that "will never affect" their transportation facility, do so at potentially momentous risk.

A little basic knowledge can go a long way in diminishing the effects of a catastrophic event and responsible officials must renew efforts to expand and update training and information dissemination programs. There are two basic categories of biologicals. First, microorganisms, which consist of living organic germs, like anthrax. The second includes toxins that are the by-product of living organisms such as botulism.

The U.S. Biological Weapons Act of 1989 defines a biological agent as any "microorganism, virus or infectious substance capable of causing detrimental changes in the environment; harming or damaging food, water or equipment supplies; or causing disease in humans, animals or plants or other living organisms." More importantly, officials need to recognize that all biologic and chemical agents need to be weaponized to be effectively used as a tool in a terrorist or hostile situation. "Biowatch," mentioned earlier, is designed to continuously analyze cities' air, and could potentially save thousands of lives in the earliest days of an attack. So far, the network of 500 sensors nationwide has never raised a false alarm.

The Centers for Disease Control have published a listing of pathogens considered prospective current bioterror threats. All of them represent some degree of threat to a transportation environment.[3] These pathogens have been divided into three categories, A through C. Category-A pathogens receive the highest priority. They are also considered the easiest to spread and are capable of inducing high death tolls, trigger panic, and therefore require priority consideration for public health awareness. Anthrax is a classic example of a disease caused by a Category-A pathogen. Category-B pathogens (such as the bacteria that causes brucellosis) are given the second-highest precedence. They are considered fairly simple to spread but could still result in a death toll worthy of significant public health response and would require noteworthy improvement in observation and diagnostic abilities over those currently in use. Category-C pathogens are given the third highest precedence and are considered to be pathogens that may be used as future weapons.

Incidents of biological warfare, as previously stated, have taken place throughout the span of recorded history; however, technological advances of the twentieth century have changed the threat from sporadic to practical. Medical historians define the worst outbreak of anthrax as the "black bane." It swept through Europe in the 1600s and likely killed over 60,000 people. Napoleon even tried to infect residents of Italy with malaria in 1797. The use of disease as a means of warfare and terrorism is an emerging trend on an age-old notion. Previous attempted uses include efforts dating back to the 1500s, when minimal information regarding disease and the process of infection were available. It has been thought that doctors recognized early on that the inhalation of the unpleasant smell of decomposing flesh was a precursor to sickness. With the use of this newfound knowledge, armies began to use dead animals as an unconventional weapon to infect the enemy. Armies would throw dead animals over walls to transmit the disease to opposing forces, as well as the non combatant population. It was anticipated that the unpleasant smell of the decomposing flesh would be so appalling that the defenders of fortresses would want to quickly agree to a cease-fire. However, today, one incident has the potential ability to kill literally millions of travelers or victims in a single incident and terrorists have no intended desire to reach a settlement.

Transportation facility security managers, law enforcement and health practitioners still have one advantage in combating these types of etiologic threats. The user of such a weapon is still most challenged during the manufacturing phase either from unintended exposure or release of the agent. The perpetrator is therefore more vulnerable to discovery at that point in the process than any other. Even the most virulent agent needs to be stabilized and ultimately, at least temporarily, contained by the use of specialized equipment and more than a rudimentary knowledge of microbiology. Such a need for sophistication and equipment acquisition provides clues which can lead authorities to the perpetrators.

The possibility of terrorists, similar to any lab worker, inadvertently infecting themselves is always a reality. But, due to the suicidal and fanatical dedication of many terrorists, they are likely to consider any casualties as reasonable costs or acceptable collateral damage. A more dangerous issue is that of controllability. Release of an agent either during manufacturing or after intended release, better characterized as "uncontrollability", has persisted as an issue since the Middle Ages. For example, in 1346, a Tartar army afflicted with the Bubonic plague used the bodies of deceased and dying soldiers to spread the disease along the Crimean Coast. Survivors of the 1346 attack eventually made their way to Italy where they further transmitted the disease. It has generally been recorded that in the years between 1347 and 1351, nearly half of Europe's population was allegedly eradicated as a result of the Bubonic plague; evidencing the need to control a pathogen when released. The outbreak spread exponentially and dramatically which as stated devastated the population of Europe during the fourteenth century.

An outbreak in a transportation environment has similar potentiality for dissemination. The spatial diffusion of certain agents, in fact, could cause the death of millions. From a prevention and law enforcement perspective, the criminal actor or terrorist is most vulnerable to discovery in this initial acquisition and preparation phase. International efforts, therefore, need to be focused and concentrated in this direction. Unfortunately, in part due to lack of attention for whatever reason to biological and chemical threats, individuals and groups can now rather easily create a workable delivery device filled with a deadly agent relatively free from detection by authorities. Due to the widespread unavailability of appropriate detection equipment, transportation facilities are particularly vulnerable. In spite of recent events, many officials still dismiss the idea as just too horrific to consider and are so overwhelmed by the prospect of such an event, they have proverbially hid their heads in the sand. The threat is clearly out there, even though it is not well-publicized, as evidenced by several fairly recently detected efforts to manufacture such a deadly product in Minnesota, Japan and France.

In 1984, French police raided a safe house of the German Red Army Faction terrorist group and located a bathtub containing flasks which were filled with clostridium botulism, one of the most lethal substances known. More recently, Japanese police confirmed that Aum Shinri Kyo was also stockpiling biological agents. A huge supply of ricin was also discovered in a bathtub in Alexandria, Minnesota in the possession of a white supremacy group. Adding to the seriousness of the situation, the current revolution in biotechnology may well produce other agents that could be even more toxic and resilient than those ever developed before. An event that immediately followed the September 11th attacks introduced the first successful bioterrorism attack in the United States. Envelopes containing spores of anthrax accompanied by hate letters criticizing the United States and Israel were mailed through the United States postal system to different media groups, as well as directly to Senator Tom Daschle.

Fortunately, not all recipients became infected. Regrettably, several forms of anthrax infected many of the people who had handled the letters within the postal system. During the sequence of events, five people were killed and seventeen others were infected.[5] Though small in proportion to the events of 9/11, Americans were killed and subsequently contaminated and the effects could have been much worse. Recent attempts to deliver dangerous material to members of the European Union in 2004 highlight the continued threat. The relatively easy accessibility of such agents remains problematic.

As stated, the acquisition of seed stock does not pose a very significant challenge. For example, some pathogenic organisms are simply endemic to specific geographic regions and are found in natural reservoirs. All that is required is a plane ticket and some basic knowledge of microbiology. The attainment of the Ebola or Marburg virus, for example, could be acquired and transported anywhere upon notification of an outbreak and appropriate collection. Even more frightening, one sick passenger on a flight into a jurisdiction could bring the disease literally anywhere. In addition, some biological agents can still be bought from the American Type Culture Collection or the Microbiological Research Establishment in weakened form or from financially strapped Russian labs. It should be noted that controls in Western labs have been strengthened since the Iraqis bought an initial supply. Those control improvements however do not change the fact that almost anything is probably available on the Russian black market.

On a further scary note, future genetic research may be able to pinpoint the genetic characteristics of both the target population and the potential agent. In other words, the agent would target specific individuals genetically. This could lead to an "ethnic" agent. The ramifications of this are almost unspeakable in the hands of a terrorist group or a deranged individual. Theoretically, terrorists could release an agent in an airport or other transportation environment and only kill individuals of a specific ethnic background.

15.4 Airports, Ports, Railroad Stations and Mass Transit

The threat can emanate from a terminal assault, a hijacking, and the use of an aircraft or ship as a weapon and even the exposure of commercial aircraft to surface-to-air missiles. The Senate joined the House of Representatives in September 2002 in voting overwhelmingly to permit pilots to carry guns in the cockpit. The wisdom of this publicity motivated vote remains to be fully evaluated. A gun can not protect anyone from the release of a pathogen on board an aircraft, cruise ship or commercial shipping vessel. The government has engaged in many false starts over the years in protecting the public transportation system. This is likely one of them.

In another rush to "defend the public," the government should not have lowered the standards for cargo and baggage screeners in an attempt to meet Congressional mandated but arbitrary compliance dates for federal screening within the transportation arena. The fact that twenty-nine people were arrested in fall 2002 on federal charges of lying or offering false papers to get jobs at three Florida airports and the fact that a gentlemen successfully shipped himself makes the point.

At airports, where most of the security effort had previously been placed, the GAO issued a report in June 2000 stating that screeners repeatedly failed to detect threat objects located on passengers and carry-on baggage; missing about 20 percent of the objects which would have posed as threat. The statistics actually showed a decline in the detection rate between the years 1991–1999. Furthermore, when the FAA initiated more realistic tests which closely approximated terrorist tactics, the screeners performed even worse. The potentiality for detecting biological and chemical agents is even more spurious. As is self evident, part of this laxness was due to quality of the employees, training and a huge turnover rate. It was difficult to retain experienced employees due to low pay, poor benefits, repetitive and monotonous work and poor or stressful work environment. The Transportation Security Administration has faced the same problems and news reports of confiscated dangerous articles continue to proliferate today.

In addition, access to the flight-line and to aircraft is relatively easy for someone determined to do so. In tests conducted by the government, agents repeatedly gained access to aircraft and other secure areas. In one test conducted by the Inspector General (IG) in May 2000, seven out of ten agents successfully penetrated the aircraft or had access to cargo. Access control presents unique problems for airport officials. Unlike traditional copper based security systems, fiber optic sensors are clearly required because fiber optic sensors do not emit unwanted signals that might interfere with aircraft transmissions. An airport is a distinctly unique environment warranting special security measures. Other transportation operations simply face the enormity of the task, where for example, U.S. Customs only has personnel sufficient to physical search a miniscule number of cargo containers. The threats are real and the challenges significant, especially in the area of the potential use of biological and chemical weapons.

15.5 Trace Detection Technologies

Tests are continuing to evaluate how lethal agents would disperse during an assault. One conducted in 2000 tested the airflow system over Salt Lake City airport. The Department of Energy used a gas meant to mimic a toxic cloud. The city was chosen due to unique air flows in the areas as well as the impending 2002 Winter Olympics. Similar tests, as well as an incident response exercise were conducted at the Athens airport prior to the 2004 Summer Olympics and were completed at the Las Vegas airport in August 2003. Airflows present a complex problem particularly through the urban canyons of metropolitan cities. New optical equipment can actually determine whether a suspicious cloud quite a distance away contains dangerous material and hand held monitors are also now available that can detect small amounts of biological and chemical agents. In reality, the costs of acquiring sufficient quantities of these tools are often not available.

Detection of an attack may not be instantaneous but be more insidious. In reality, the first signs of an attack are likely to appear in a doctor's office. Because biological agents tend to be odorless and colorless, reported illness might be the first signs an attacked has already occurred. Tracking patients with such symptoms is problematic at best considering the availability of international travel and the mobility of travelers. Theoretically, many doctors can not accurately distinguish between anthrax exposure symptoms and influenza. Public health officials and civil defense directors will need to be interconnected to keep informed about such incidents. The infrastructure in the United States is a long way from effectively coping with such threats.

There are four minimum standards that must be met in order for any future bioterror detection technology to be effective. It is crucial that the device be sensitive, fast, accurate, and capable of detecting a wide array of pathogens. Safety is an additional factor. Sensitivity is also a significant asset for obvious reasons. Many hazardous pathogens are fatal at doses of less than ten organisms, which indicate that even a very small number of organisms in the air can be fatal. If a detection unit cannot identify such a low quantity, it is unproductive and ultimately noneffective. Sensitivity is also noteworthy because of the possibility of large amounts of contamination as the result of "background noise" in any given air sample. There are constantly thousands of particles of such items as sand, smoke, pollen, and dirt present in the air.[6] To be able to isolate, identify and contain organisms is critical to effective use of any system.

The fact that some of these agents are almost impossible to detect further intensifies the problem; especially within the transportation venue. In addition, the technology to detect a biological or chemical agent in transit is not readily available. The inability to detect the agents is only worsened by the fact that once located and identified; medical prophylactic measures might prove to be inadequate. Furthermore, considering the fact that security managers are already fighting tooth and nail for a part of budgetary resources, personal protection equipment has not been considered to be essential additions to private security equipment supplies.

Speed is another vital and essential element. Time will be of the essence should a pathogen be released in a transportation facility. The final objective for any detection equipment should therefore be instant, or at least nearly instant results. In a period of minutes large numbers of people could easily become infected and in turn, spread the pathogen further. Accuracy is also imperative. If an area is believed to be safe, when in fact it is tainted, disastrous results are inevitable. On the other hand, an incorrect positive detection could cost an enormous amount of time, cleanup and evacuation and subsequently lost revenue.

Finally, it is important that the detection unit be able to identify more than one type of pathogen. If a unit only identifies a single type of pathogen, it would require several different units to properly protect any location. This would also mean that any one operator would need to be proficient and qualified in the use of many different protocols; adding to training costs and eventual reliability. As stated before, cost is also a relevant though sometimes distasteful factor.

As mentioned, quick, portable and sensitive sensing systems capable of detecting a wide range of threats are critical to avoiding a major disaster. Significant strides are being made in pathogen detection. For example, a mass spectrometry method known as MALDI-MS (matrix assisted laser desorption/ionization mass spectrometry) sorts and identifies bacterial components. Researchers hope the equipment will eventually be able to isolate agents within five minutes. The equipment's applicability within a transportation scenario is yet to be determined.

Realistically, it is also both expensive and impractical to vaccinate personnel against all agents, equip personnel with individual protection suits or even to have decontamination kits, respirators and the like available as response tools in all transportation facilities. Even if victims are provided with emergency medical care and later hospitalization, it is unclear whether these agencies are up to the enormous task. Clearly, the technical community needs to expend considerably more effort to develop effective detection equipment. Currently, significant viability problems plaque biological trace detection systems specifically in airports; one of the most basic involving basic hygiene, but others persist as well.

In attempting to detect biological agents, personal contact is an obvious vehicle for transmitting various microbial diseases from one individual to another. When x-ray machines were first introduced into airports, passengers expressed concern over exposure to radiation, even though the risks were minimal. Introducing trace detection equipment has once again raised the issue of "passenger acceptability" of new technology. For example, current trace detection devices require the passenger to actually touch the door before entering, which means that they could leave some disease-producing microorganisms behind in sufficient quantity to infect but not to be readily detected with sufficient accuracy and swiftness.

Experts have reasoned that if the transfer of infectious diseases in the passenger screening setting were to occur, it would most likely result from the hand-mediated transfer of disease producing microorganisms. The likelihood of disease transmission during passenger screening is dependent upon numerous disease specific factors but passengers will simply respond to the basic concept that they could get infected. That rationale could once again increase the average passenger's resistance to air travel due to "alleged" intrusive screening methods. The factors which could increase or decrease transmission include the integrity and cleanliness of the skin and other host factors, such as the virulence of the disease causing microorganism and the actual amount of organisms transferred. If it is difficult to explain the limited risk involved to the average traveler. Therefore, use of current biological and chemical trace detection remains challenging.

Some efforts have been made to make improvements in detection capabilities. For example, *New Scientist* revealed in 1998 that Washington's Naval Research team had tested a plane weighing forty-two pounds that is capable of detecting minute quantities of biological agents. The planes were designed to fly into suspected contaminated areas and detect up to four separate bacterial agents.

> An onboard sampling chamber has been designed to allow air to pass through and thus creating a vortex in a pool of water. Every five minutes the water in the chamber washes over a sensor comprised of four optical fibers. The optical fibers have a probe affixed to the core of each fiber. Each of the probes is coated with an antibody for a particular bacterium allowing for the adhesion in water if present of the spore of the particular bacterium to the probe.[7]

15.6 Training

Efforts to train personnel in proper response techniques are essential to a comprehensive anti-bioterrorism program. As with any complicated program, it is the actual performance of the plan that counts and that performance is always dependent on the quality of training conducted. Educating and training personnel requires a rather large investment in terms of time, assets and financial support, but failure to do so will result in far more significant losses.

Sandia National Laboratories[8] has brought virtual reality into the realm of airport security. This particular virtual reality application allows rescue personnel to practice responding to a terrorists attack over and over again without consequence. The simulation involves the release of a biological agent into a small airport. The responding security or health personnel are immersed into a three dimensional computer-simulated setting of virtual patients in a virtual disaster. The program seeks to train medical personnel to make instantaneous and correct decisions and to avoid become victims of the terrorists themselves.

Like video games, the simulation can be run repeatedly. Mistakes can be corrected and appropriate responses ingrained in the student. Such instinctive responses are difficult to teach, especially in a potentially contaminated environment. The computer simulation engages the user's eyes and ears by wearing sensors on the arms, legs and waist. All of the user's actions are fed back into the simulation. Users are also taught the significant lessons of self-protection when the simulation tags them as exposed or deceased. Students learn initial decontamination procedures for themselves and the victims; avoiding the situation where the rescuer needs to be rescued.

The airport used in the simulation is a one-story, simple three-gate facility. The software program recreates the disbursement of the biological agent, in this case Staphylococcal enterotoxin B (SEB), throughout the airport. The program, though simulating a small airport explosion, would be useful for transportation personnel as well first responders. The Defense Advanced Research Projects Agency (DARPA) funded the research. The Department of Energy's Office of Science and Technology Pilot Projects in Biomedical Engineering Program is also working to make the program even more realistic.

The U.S. Department of Energy's Hazardous Materials Management and Emergency Response Training Center is a critical element of the training aspect in the war on bio- and chemical terrorism. The center offers versatile facilities, including classrooms and realistic field training scenarios. Efforts must continue to train military personnel, first responders and other health professionals not only about the impending threat from this type of terrorism, but appropriate procedures to save the lives of as many victims as possible.

15.7 Combating Bioterrorism

As is always the case, it is difficult to identify specific factors, which would increase or decrease the specific biological threat to any commercial organization, governmental institution or public facility. However, advanced preparation is always the key to any successful disaster response or preventive plan. At a minimum, security managers should review all procedures with biologicals and chemicals in mind. For example:

- *Get Outside Help! Review the State and Local Guide 101. Guide for All-Hazard Emergency Operations Planning*. The document was published in 1996. It outlines the preparedness, response and short-term recovery planning components that the Federal Emergency Management Agency (FEMA) recommends to be included in state and local emergency operations plans. It provides the transportation authorities with FEMA's recommendations on how to handle the entire planning process. The document encourages emergency managers to address all the hazards that threaten a jurisdiction in a single operations plan rather than stand alone plans. Planners must also consider the effectiveness of appropriate liaison procedures with authorities such as FEMA, DOD, FBI and the CDC. CDC (404-639-1293).[9]
- In the event of an incident, as much as possible, control and contain any further release of any suspected biologicals. Determine the actual nature and extent of the threat. Contact the federal authorities under the Federal Response Plan. It is a signed agreement between twenty-seven federal departments and agencies and the American Red Cross that provide the mechanisms for coordinating delivery of federal assistance and resources to augment efforts of state and local governments overwhelmed by a natural disaster.[10]
- Evacuate personnel to a safe distance. Ascertain the actual identity of the agent. Both a primary and secondary secured perimeter must be established. Refer to the *Federal Interagency Domestic Terrorism Concept of Operations Plan* (CONPLAN) which provides guidance to federal, state and local agencies concerning how the federal government would respond to a potential or actual terrorist attack, especially involving a weapon of mass destruction.[11]
- Determine whether appropriate procedures for a terrorist type attack include a search plan, an evacuation strategy, a post-incident recovery plan, and a crisis communication strategy. Refer to the *Hazardous Materials Planning Guide 2001 Update*. This document provides guidance on developing state and local emergency response plans for hazardous materials incidents. The team consists of sixteen federal agencies, each with responsibilities and expertise in emergency response to hazardous chemical releases, oil discharges and other toxic spills.

- Be prepared to make a complete after-action report.

In addition, take note that former Secretary of Defense, William S. Cohen, in conjunction with ten state governors, acknowledged the establishment of ten National Guard Rapid Assessment and Initial Detection, RAID teams. The teams are part of the Department of Defense and are available to support local, state and federal authorities in the event of an incident. They are located at Los Alamitos, CA; Aurora, CO; Marietta, GA; Peoria IL; Natick, MA; Fort Leonard Wood, MO; Scotia, NY; Fort Indiantown Gap, PA; Austin, TX; and Tacoma, WA. The teams are prepared to assist emergency first responders upon request for any suspected or actual WMD attack.

Since September 11, Congress has authorized approximately $1.1 billion to help states improve bioterrorism preparedness. The initial bill actually passed the House by a vote of 425-1. The Department of Health and Human Resources allocate the funds which are intended to improve surveillance and investigation of infectious diseases, expand laboratory capacity and improve communications between hospitals and health departments. As a benchmark, states are required to develop plans for regional hospitals to accommodate at lest 500 patients in the event of an attack, be able to process urgent disease reports twenty-four hours a day and provide at least one epidemiologist for each metropolitan area of more than 500,000 people. All of these tasks are critical in developing adequate plans to protect the most likely targets, public transportation systems.

It should be noted that once an airplane is airborne, the risk can become acute. Commercial aircraft carry extremely fine filters to clean recirculating air; catching anything 0.3 micron or larger. However, adequate response would have to be incredibly swift. The death of the pilots would likely cause the aircraft to crash in any case. Terminals, hangers, warehouses and other buildings can not be considered places of refuge in the event of an attack.

Because pathogens can inhabit buildings, effective decontamination techniques are essential. In the past, buildings were decontaminated with bleach, bucket and broom. Researchers are currently testing a system in which a fog of enzymes and chemicals are released that degrades chemical and biological agents. This would provide a much needed response to an incident within a transportation facility, quickly infiltrating the same space as the pathogen.

If an attack occurs outside, ventilation systems inside transportation terminals should be adjusted so that the interior pressure is slightly higher than outside. Intake systems need also to be filtered with high efficiency air (HEPA) filters. Release inside will require the ability to detect the pathogen as quickly as possible. Minimally, all terminals should meet the requirements of the American Society of Heating, Refrigeration and Air Conditioning engineers which recommend filters that can remove even small spores, such as anthrax with considerable efficiency.

Furthermore, it will be important not to overlook the psychological reaction of the public to such an incident. They will certainly react to feelings of being unprotected and helpless. Those reactions could present issues of crowd control, rioting, or outright opportunistic crimes. Consequently, a close working relationship between public affairs officers for both transportation and healthcare officials and the media must be developed. Security managers must have a plan for how they will deal with the panic on the part of the public and maybe even employees. As stated, senior managers must keep local, state and federal officials informed and seek early intervention by experts and government authorities.

15.8 Conclusion

If both private and public security officials take a biologic threat seriously; a major effort will be needed to develop contingency plans and initiate coordinated and mutually supportive programs across a broad spectrum of agencies. Currently, major health professional organizations are a long way from providing adequate training and education to their own healthcare community let alone the rest of the population. Adequate diagnostic and identification of a biologic attack and subsequent disease will require a major push. Plus, last but not least, public health, intelligence, and law enforcement agencies as well as the private sector should recognize the threat for what it is—a national priority considering the potential consequences.

As demonstrated by the September 11th attacks, transportation facilities are major critical infrastructures; affecting not only human life but the global economy. The U.S. has over 400 major international airports, massive seaport operations, and daily operated mass transit systems. All of these environments are frequently used and assist not only in transferring material and people but contribute to the national well-being. A second massive attack, as was apparently planned for the holiday season 2003–2004, would have once again crippled the global economy and devastated a sense of security for millions of Americans.

It needs to be recognized that anything is possible. For example, during the Cold War the Russians designed germs which could be sprayed from low flying aircraft. They intended the planes to fly low in a straight line for hundreds of miles. Even if only some livestock were infected, the contagious disease would wipe out livestock over a huge area for months. The same method of infection could be applied to humans. Additionally, Zacarious Moussaoui, the infamous potential hijacker arrested in Minnesota just prior to September 11, had information in his personal computer relating the renting crop dusting aircraft. Surely, he was not interested in helping farmers to protect the potato crop.

Bioterrorism has been evident throughout history for centuries and is likely to remain a plague on mankind in the hands of terrorists. Unfortunately, the inevitability of the use of biological and chemical agents as a means of warfare and terrorism has developed into a serious dilemma with, realistic scenarios becoming more and more probable within the twenty-first century. The concerns have risen dramatically in recent years. These agents are relatively easy to manufacture, easy to conceal and potentially lethal to millions of people.

Recent events have highlighted the importance of preventing such attacks in the first place to the fullest extent possible and of deploying the means to respond to them should all efforts at prevention fail. The global community must insist that governments vigorously pursue the development of equipment to detect and verify the presence of chemical and biological agents, to protect not only individuals but also critical infrastructures. Better methods to decontaminate people, equipment and places and the capability to adequately provide medical care to victims must also be pursued. Finally, programs to train those that must respond to tragic events needs attention.

Additionally, and because of the acquisition of alarming intelligence about al-Qaeda's progress toward obtaining a nuclear or radiological weapon, the Bush Administration has deployed hundreds of sophisticated sensors at U.S. borders, at some overseas facilities and in and around

Washington. D.C. Ordinary Geiger counters worn on belts have been in use by the Customs Service for years. Newer devices are called gamma ray and neutron flux detectors. They had been carried by Nuclear Emergency Search Teams and are deployed as required. The task is daunting and every effort should be made to pursue more research in combating the nuclear, biological and chemical threat to the nation's transportation systems.

Endnotes

1. The editors. "*SA* perspective: Can biologists be trusted," *Scientific American*, January, 2004, p. 6.

2. Aaron Litner. "U.S. has long studied biological chemical weapon techniques," *Milwaukee Journal*, October 14, 2001.

3. http://www.bt.cdc.gov/agent/agentlist-category.asp.

4. http://www.pbs.org/wgbh/nova/bioterror/hist_nf.html, NOVA, 2001.

5. http://www.cdc.gov/ncidod/EID/vol8no10/02-0353.htm.

6. http://state.gov/www/global/arms/treaties/geneval.html.

7. Lila Guterman. "Death in the air," *New Scientist* 159(2151):11 (1998).

8. Sandia is a multiprogramming laboratory operated by Sandia Corporation, a Lockheed Martin company, for the Department of Energy. With major facilities in Albuquerque, NM and Livermore, CA, the company has major research and development responsibilities in national security, energy and environmental technologies and economic competitiveness. http://www.sandia.gov/media/NewsRel/NR1999/biosim.htm.

9. http://www.fema.gov/rrr/gaheop.shtm.

10. http://www.fema.gov/rrr/frp/.

11. http://www.fema.gov/rrr/conplan/.

Chapter 16

Bioterrorism and the Law: A National Perspective[1]

Lawrence O. Gostin

Synopsis

16.1 Introduction

The United States is engaged in a Homeland Security project of near unprecedented proportions. The project is designed to avert terrorist attacks of every description. This ranges from conventional attacks, say through explosives, to nuclear, chemical, and biological attacks. The terrorist threat has always been present, but it has taken on new meaning and urgency after the attacks on the World Trade Towers in New York and the Pentagon in Washington, D.C. on September 11, 2001. On October 4, 2001, a Florida man named Robert Stevens was diagnosed with inhalational anthrax.[2] The intentional dispersal of anthrax through the U.S. postal system in New York, Washington, Pennsylvania and other locations resulted in five confirmed deaths, hundreds treated, and thousands tested.[3] The potential for new, larger, and more sophisticated attacks have created a sense of vulnerability. National attention has urgently turned to the need to rapidly detect and react to bioterrorism.

The hope, of course, is that new strategies and resources designed to fight terrorism will also improve public protection from naturally occurring or accidental sources. Ancient, constant, and abiding diseases that kill (e.g., malaria, tuberculosis, measles, and acute respiratory or diarrhoeal infections) are still among the greatest causes of mortality globally. Endemic diseases have re-emerged in more virulent, multi-drug resistant forms. Diseases once endemic only in the Third World have arrived in the First World (e.g., West Nile virus and monkeypox). Emerging infections have been newly identified in humans (e.g., hemorrhagic fevers, HIV/AIDS and SARS) and animals (e.g., bovine spongiform encephalopathy and avian influenza), some with devastating consequences for world health, world trade, and tourism.

Much attention has been given to the policies and resources necessary to make the country safer such as improved security at borders, airports, seaports. The country has focused particularly on law enforcement, emergency response, and criminal intelligence. Much less attention has been devoted to the importance of a strong public health infrastructure and modern laws to ensure that public health agencies have all the power necessary.

This chapter describes the nation's lack of preparedness for bioterriorism, explains the need for law reform, briefly describes important law reform initiatives, and discusses the delicate balance between public health and civil liberties in a constitutional democracy.

16.2 Lack of Preparedness for the Threat of Bioterrorism

Bioterrorism can be defined as the intentional use of a pathogen or biological product to cause harm to a human, animal, plant, or other living organism to influence the conduct of government or to intimidate or coerce a civilian population. A report by the National Intelligence Council for the Central Intelligence Agency concluded that infectious disease is not only a public health issue, but also a problem of national security: the U.S. population is vulnerable to bioterrorism as well as emerging and re-emerging infectious diseases.[4] In 1998, the U.S. Commission on National Security in the 21st Century concluded that biological agents are the most likely choice of weapons for disaffected states and groups. Biological weapons are nearly as easy to develop, far more lethal, and will likely become easier to deliver than chemical weapons; and, unlike nuclear weapons, biological weapons are inexpensive to produce and the risk of detection is low.[5] In 1993, the U.S. Congressional Office of Technology Assessment estimated that the aerosolized release of 100 kilograms of anthrax spores upwind of Washington, D.C. could result in approximately 130,000 to 3 million deaths, a weapon as deadly as a hydrogen bomb.[6]

For years, experts have been calling attention to the threat of bioterrorism and the unique problems that arise in modern society.[7] The Internet allows for the widespread dissemination of information on biological agents and technology. Advancements in biotechnology make bioproduction capabilities accessible to individuals with limited experience. The dual use nature of this knowledge and technology—allowing for both legitimate and illicit use—makes tracking and identifying bioterrorists much more difficult. And while certain countries are known or suspected to have biological weapons programs, non-state actors have become important as well.[8] Documents recovered in Afghanistan suggest that al-Qa'eda has conducted extensive research on weapons that can cause mass fatalities, including biological weapons.[9]

Government and public health officials must be able to react quickly and intelligently to a potentially catastrophic disease outbreak, whether intentionally instigated or naturally occurring. Two exercises, Dark Winter (smallpox)[10] and TOPOFF (plague),[11] simulated biological attacks in the United States to test government response and raise awareness of the bioterrorism threat. Both simulations demonstrated serious weaknesses in the U.S. public health system that could prevent an effective response to bioterrorism[12] or severe, naturally occurring infectious diseases.[13] In 2003, the Department of Justice conducted a follow-on exercise, TOPOFF II, which showed some improvement, but still discovered numerous deficiencies in preparedness.

By most accounts the public health infrastructure is weak, leading the Institute of Medicine to conclude that, in many ways, public health agencies are in disarray. Numerous reports have drawn attention to the lack of public health preparedness.[14] The Centers for Disease Control and Prevention (CDC) concludes that, despite recent improvements, the public health infrastructure "is still structurally weak in nearly every area."[15]

Indeed, it is possible to find structural deficiencies in each of the major components of the public health system. First, public health statutes are often outdated, inconsistent, and fail to conform to modern public health and constitutional principles. Law reform is needed to support the mission, functions, and essential services of public health agencies as well as to ensure emergency preparedness.[16] Second, the public health work force lacks appropriate education, training, and leadership skills to perform its role. Of the approximately 500,000 public health professionals, fewer than half have had formal, academic training in public health.[17] Assessing and strengthening competence will require adequate recruitment and compensation, high-level training, and evaluation of quality services.[18] Third, public health agencies do not have state-of-the-art information and communications systems. Harnessing the potential of technology is essential for collection, use, and dissemination of information. It will improve surveillance, outbreak investigations, program evaluations, and interventions. Fourth, laboratory capacity among states and localities is inadequate in terms of availability and quality. Most laboratories need multiple upgrades for their physical facilities, including freezer capacity and specimen receiving capability.[19] The nation's public health laboratories should be assessed and funded to ensure capacity and integrate new technologies as they emerge.

The recent emphasis on bioterrorism preparedness and influx of federal funds could strengthen the public health system if the resources assured dual functionality—enabling agencies to protect both against bioterrorism and the wide variety of health threats. Public health professionals, however, express concern about substitution effects so that bioterrorism funds actually detract from ongoing programs.[20] An independent evaluation using major indicators such as response plans demonstrated continued lack of preparedness for public health emergencies.[21] More troubling still, public health agencies face severe cuts due to the current state budget crisis.[22] Since states provide the majority of funds for public health, preparedness may suffer further deterioration.

16.3 The Need for Law Reform

Law has long been considered an important tool of public health. While federal lawmaking authority is constitutionally limited in scope, as an exercise of their broader police powers states have more flexibility in legislating to protect the public's health. State public health laws create a mission for public health authorities, assign their functions, and specify the manner in which they may exercise their authority.[23] Prior to September 11, 2001, some states had legislatively (e.g., Colorado)[24] or administratively (e.g., Rhode Island)[25] developed public health response plans for a bioterrorism event. However, problems of obsolescence, inconsistency, and inadequacy may render older state laws ineffective, or even counterproductive.[26] Reforming public health law can improve the legal infrastructure to help respond to bioterrorism and other emerging threats.

State public health statutes frequently are outdated, built up in layers during the twentieth century in response to each new disease threat.[27] Consequently, these laws often do not reflect contemporary scientific understandings of disease (e.g., surveillance, prevention, and response) or legal norms for protection of individual rights. When many of these statutes were written, public health sciences such as epidemiology and biostatistics were in their infancy and modern prevention and treatment methods did not exist.

At the same time, many existing public health laws predate the vast changes in constitutional (e.g., equal protection and due process) and statutory (e.g., disability discrimination) law that have transformed social and legal conceptions of individual rights. Failure to reform these laws may leave public health authorities vulnerable to legal challenge on grounds that they are unconstitutional or preempted by modern federal statutes. Even if state public health law is not challenged in court, public health authorities may feel unsure about applying old legal remedies to modern health threats.

Health codes among the fifty states and territories have evolved independently, leading to profound variation in the structure, substance, and procedures for detecting, controlling, and preventing disease. Ordinarily different state approaches are not a problem, but variation could prevent or delay an efficient response in a multi-state public health emergency. Infectious diseases are rarely confined to single jurisdictions, but pose risks within whole regions or the nation itself. Coordination among state and national authorities is vital, but is undermined by disparate legal structures.

Public health laws remain fragmented within states as well as among them. Most state statutes have evolved over time so that, even within the same state, different rules may apply depending on the particular disease in question. This means that necessary authority (e.g., screening, reporting, or compulsory treatment) may be absent for a given disease. For example, when a resurgence of multi-drug resistant tuberculosis swept major metropolitan areas in the 1990s, many statutes did not allow for directly observed therapy.[28] Worse still, state laws can be so complex that they may not be well understood by health practitioners or their attorneys. Laws that are ambiguous prevent agencies from acting rapidly and decisively in an emergency.

Many current laws not only provide insufficient authority to act, but might actually thwart effective action. This is evident when one examines the key variables for public health preparedness: planning and coordination, surveillance, management of property, and protection of people.

State statutes generally fail to require planning or to establish mechanisms. As a result most states have not systematically designed a strategy to respond to public health emergencies. Perhaps the most important aspects of planning are clear communication and coordination among responsible governmental officials and the private sector. As the recent anthrax outbreaks demonstrate, there should be a defined role for public health, law enforcement, and emergency management agencies. So too, should there be coordination among the various levels (e.g., federal, tribal, state, and local) and branches (legislative, executive, and judicial) of government as well as with private actors, particularly the healthcare and pharmaceutical sectors. A systematic planning process that involves all stakeholders improves communication and coordination. The law can require such planning and sharing of information. However, many public health statutes do not facilitate planning and communication and, due to federal and state privacy concerns, may actually proscribe exchange of vital information among public health, law enforcement, and emergency management agencies. Indeed, some statutes even prohibit sharing data with public health officials in adjoining states.[29] Consider the need for coordination that would be necessary if a biological attack were to occur in the tri-state area of New York, New Jersey, and Connecticut. Laws that complicate or hinder data communication among states and responsible agencies would impede a thorough investigation and response to such a public health emergency.

Surveillance is critical to public health preparedness. Unlike most forms of terrorism, the dispersal of pathogens may not be evident. Early detection could save many lives by triggering an effective containment strategy such as vaccination, treatment and, if necessary, isolation or quarantine. However, current statutes do not facilitate surveillance and may even prevent monitoring. For example, many states do not require timely reporting for many dangerous ("Category A") agents of bioterrorism such as smallpox, anthrax, plague, botulism, tularemia, and viral hemorrhagic fevers.[30] In fact, in the aftermath of September 11th, 2001, virtually no state required immediate reporting for all the critical agents identified by the CDC.[31] At the same time, states do not require, and may actually prohibit, public health agencies from monitoring data collected in the health-care system.[32] Private information that might lead to early detection (e.g., unusual clusters of fevers or gastrointestinal symptoms) held by hospitals, managed care organizations, and pharmacies may be unavailable to public health officials. New federal health information privacy protections may unintentionally impede the flow of data from private to public sectors despite regulators' attempts to broadly exempt public health information sharing from nondisclosure rules.[33]

Coercive powers are the most controversial aspects of any legal system. Nevertheless, they may be necessary to manage property or protect people from significant threats to health. There are numerous circumstances that might require management of property in a public health emergency—e.g., shortages of vaccines, medicines, hospital beds, or facilities for disposal of corpses. It may even be necessary to close facilities or destroy property that is contaminated or dangerous. Even in the case of a relatively small outbreak, such as the recent anthrax attacks, the government considered the need to compulsorily license proprietary medications and destroy contaminated facilities. The law must provide authority, with fair safeguards, to manage property that is needed to contain a serious health threat.

There similarly may be a need to exercise powers over individuals to avert a significant threat to the public's health. Vaccination, testing, physical examination, treatment, isolation, and quarantine each may help contain the spread of communicable diseases. These powers have been exercised historically in relation to airborne infections such as smallpox and tuberculosis, and may be necessary to contain a future outbreak.

In summary, existing public health laws are highly antiquated and in need of reform. They fail to achieve fundamental aspects of public health preparedness: mission and functions of agencies, stable sources of funding, active surveillance and data evaluation, and adequate powers over people and property. Public health laws introduce two kinds of error that urgent require correction. On the one hand, many statutes fail to provide adequate powers to deal with the full range of health threats. On the other hand, when they do authorize coercion, statutes rarely provide clear standards and fair procedures for decision-making. Beyond all this, public health laws are inconsistent within states and among them, layered and obtuse (making them hard to understand and follow), and do not conform to modern ideas in the theory and practice of public health.

16.4 The Model State Public Health Act

The Institute of Medicine (IOM), in its foundational 1988 report, *The Future of Public Health*, acknowledged that law was essential to public health, but cast serious doubt on the soundness of public health's legal basis. Concluding that "this nation has lost sight of its public health goals and has allowed the system of public health activities to fall into disarray." The IOM recommended reform of an obsolete and inadequate body of enabling laws and regulations.[34] In its 2002 report, *We the Healthy People: Assuring America's Health in the 21st Century*, the IOM notes that little progress has been made in implementing its proposal. The Committee recommends that "public health law be reformed so that it conforms to modern scientific and legal standards, is more consistent within and among states, and is more uniform in its approach to different health threats." The Department of Health and Human Services' in *Healthy People 2010* similarly argued that strong laws are a vital component of the public health infrastructure and recommended that states reform outdated statutes.[35]

In response to a sustained critique of the crumbling public health infrastructure, the Robert Wood Johnson Foundation, in partnership with the W.K. Kellogg Foundation, initiated the "Turning Point" project in 1996, Collaborating for a New Century in Public Health. Turning Point launched five National Excellence Collaboratives in 2000, including the Public Health Statute Modernization Collaborative. The mission was "to transform and strengthen the legal framework for the public health system through a collaborative process to develop a model public health law."

The Public Health Statute Modernization Collaborative was led by a consortium of states, in partnership with federal agencies and national organizations. The Collaborative contracted with the author to draft the Model Act under the guidance of a national expert advisory committee. The Collaborative has published a comprehensive assessment of state public health laws, demonstrating the inadequacies of existing law to support modern public health functions.[36] The objective is to ensure that state public health legislation is consistent with modern constitutional principles, and reflects current scientific and ethical values underlying public health practice. The Model Act was published in late 2003, and focuses on the mission, functions, essential services, and powers of public health agencies, as well as the rights of people subjected to public health powers.[37]

16.5 The Model State Emergency Health Powers Act

The law reform process took on new urgency in the aftermath of September 11th, 2001. The Center for Law and the Public's Health at Georgetown and Johns Hopkins Universities drafted the Model State Emergency Health Powers Act (MSEHPA)[38] at the request of Centers for Disease Control and Prevention and in collaboration with members of national organizations representing governors, legislators, attorneys general, and health commissioners.[39] Because the power to act to preserve the public's health is constitutionally reserved primarily to the states as an exercise of their police powers,[40] the Model Act is designed for state—not federal—legislative consideration. It provides the responsible state actors with the powers they need to detect and contain a potentially catastrophic disease outbreak and, at the same time, protect individual rights and freedoms. Thirty-two states and the District of Columbia have passed bills or resolutions that include provisions from or closely related to the Act.[41]

The purpose of the MSEHPA is to facilitate the detection, management and containment of public health emergencies while appropriately safeguarding personal and proprietary interests. The Model Act is structured to reflect five basic public health functions to be facilitated by law: preparedness, surveillance, management of property, and protection of people. The Act gives rise to two kinds of powers: Those that exist in the pre-emergency environment (pre-declaration powers) and those that come into effect only after a state's Governor declares a public health emergency (post-declaration powers). Post-declaration powers deliberately are broader and more robust.[42]

A governor may declare a public health emergency only if a series of demanding conditions are met: (1) an occurrence or imminent threat, that (2) is caused by bioterrorism or a new or re-emerging infectious agent or biological toxin previously controlled and that (3) also poses a high probability of a large number of deaths or serious or long-term disabilities. Recognizing the continuing threat of infectious disease, the Model Act as drafted is not limited to bioterrorism emergencies: a mass epidemic could be sufficiently severe to trigger the Act's provisions even if naturally occurring. The MSEHPA requires the governor to consult with the public health authority and other experts prior to declaring an emergency and authorizes the legislature, by majority vote, to discontinue the emergency at any time.

The pre-declaration powers and duties are those necessary to prepare for and promptly identify a public health emergency. The Public Health Emergency Planning Commission (appointed by the governor) must prepare a plan which includes: coordination of services; procurement of necessary materials and supplies; housing, feeding, and caring for affected populations (with appropriate regard for their physical, cultural and social needs); and the proper vaccination and treatment of individuals in the event of a public health emergency.

Pre-declaration powers include measures necessary to detect initially and then to follow a developing public health emergency, including prompt reporting requirements for healthcare providers, pharmacists, veterinarians and laboratories. Public health professionals must interview and counsel exposed people and investigate materials or facilities endangering the public's health. MSEHPA recognizes that exchange of relevant data among lead agencies is essential to assure the public's health and security. Public health, emergency management, and public safety authorities, therefore, are required to share information necessary to prevent, treat, control, or investigate a public health emergency.

The Model Act provides "special powers" that may be used only after a governor declares a state of public health emergency. The article that authorizes the management of property provides that the public health authority may close, decontaminate, or procure facilities and materials to respond to a public health emergency; safely dispose of infectious waste; and obtain and deploy healthcare supplies. The authorities are required to exercise their powers with respect for cultural and religious beliefs and practices, such as observing, wherever possible, religious laws regarding burial. Compensation of private property owners is provided if there is a "taking"—i.e., the government confiscates private property for public purposes (e.g., the use of a private infirmary to treat and isolate patients). No compensation would be provided for a "nuisance abatement"—i.e., the government destroys property or closes an establishment that poses a serious health threat. This comports with the extant constitutional "takings" jurisprudence of the Supreme Court.[43] If the government were forced to compensate for all nuisance abatements, it would significantly chill public health regulation.

The provisions for protection of people deal with some of the most sensitive areas. The Model Act permits public health authorities to: physically examine or test individuals as necessary to diagnose or to treat illness; vaccinate or treat individuals to prevent or ameliorate an infectious disease; and isolate or quarantine individuals to prevent or limit the transmission of a contagious disease. The public health authority also may waive licensing requirements for healthcare professionals and direct them to assist in vaccination, testing, examination, and treatment of patients.

While the Model Act reaffirms the authority over people and property that health agencies have always had, it supplements these traditional public health powers with a modernized, extensive set of conditions, principles, and requirements governing the use of personal control measures that are now often lacking in state public health law. Public health officials are explicitly directed to respect individual religious objections to vaccination and treatment. Officials must follow specified legal standards before utilizing isolation or quarantine, which are authorized only to prevent the transmission of contagious disease to others and must be by the least restrictive means available. This allows individuals, for example, to be confined in their own homes. The Model Act also affords explicit protections to people in isolation or quarantine that go beyond most existing state laws: the public health authority is affirmatively charged with maintaining places of isolation or quarantine in a safe and hygienic manner; regularly monitoring the health of residents; and systematically and competently meeting the needs of people isolated or quarantined for adequate food, clothing, shelter, means of communication, medication, and medical care. Orders for isolation or quarantine are subject to judicial review, under strict time guidelines and with appointed counsel; the Model Act also provides for expedited judicial relief.

Finally, the Model Act provides for a set of post-declaration powers and duties to ensure appropriate public information and communication. The public health authority must provide information to the public regarding the emergency, including protective measures to be taken and information regarding access to mental health support. Experience following September 11th and the anthrax attacks demonstrated the need for an authoritative spokesperson for public health providing comprehensible and accurate information. These events also revealed the significant mental health implications of terrorism on the population.

Taken as a whole, MSEHPA resolves a series of difficult policy debates in which the public health goals of facilitating the detection, management and containment of public health emergencies are balanced against the need to safeguard individuals' civil rights, liberties, and property. MSEHPA is an outgrowth of a process to identify and legitimize critical public health functions against a framework of personal rights protected by law.

16.6 A Defense of the Model Act

An unlikely alliance of the political left (arguing for civil rights) and political right (arguing for property rights) has joined together to critique the Model Act. Often the critiques represent a defense of self-interest, such as the lobbying of a variety of businesses claiming economic loss to the industry (e.g., pharmaceutical, health care, food, and transportation). In other contexts, the critiques are libertarian in nature, rejecting any diminution of personal liberty. Importantly, the critiques often factually mischaracterize the Model Act (overstating the powers afforded and understating the legal safeguards) and misunderstand existing public health law (failing to recognize that the powers in the Act already exist).[44] The most serious objections to MSEHPA are based on federalism, emergency declarations, governmental abuse of power, libertarianism, and personal safeguards.

A. Federalism

Since acts of terrorism are inherently federal matters, critics argue that there is no need for expansion of state authority. It is certainly true that federal authority is extraordinarily important in responding to catastrophic public health events: bioterrorism may trigger national security concerns, require investigation of federal offences, and affect geographic regions or even the entire country. Consequently, the federal government under the national defense and commerce powers of the Constitution often take the lead, as they did in the anthrax outbreak.

The assertion of federal jurisdiction, of course, does not obviate the need for adequate state and local public health power. States and localities have been the primary bulwark of public health in America. From an historical perspective, local and state public health agencies predated federal agencies. Local boards of health were in operation in the late eighteenth century and state agencies emerged after the Civil War. Federal health agencies, however, did not develop a major presence until Franklin Delano Roosevelt's New Deal. From a constitutional perspective, states have "plenary" authority to protect the public's health under their reserved powers. The Supreme Court has made clear that states have a deep reservoir of public health powers, while federal powers are constitutionally limited.[45] From an economic and practical perspective, most public health activities take place at the state and local level—e.g., surveillance, communicable disease control, and food and water safety. States and localities probably would be the first to detect and respond to a health emergency and would have a key role throughout. This requires states to have effective, modern statutory powers that enable them to work along side federal agencies.

B. Declaration of a public health emergency

Critics express concern that the model act could be triggered too easily, creating overly broad power for theoretical or low-level risks. For example, commentators objected to the idea that a governor might declare a public health emergency for an endemic disease such as HIV/AIDS or influenza. Mindful of this concern, the drafters set demanding conditions for a governor's declaration: bioterrorism or a naturally occurring epidemic that poses a high probability of a large number of deaths or serious disabilities. Indeed, the drafters rejected arguments from high-level officials to set a lower threshold for triggering a health emergency. MSEHPA also makes it clear that ordinary endemic diseases would not qualify.

C. Governmental abuse of power

Critics express concern that governors and public health authorities would abuse their powers. This kind of generalized argument could be used to refute the exercise of power in *any* realm, but has never been a reason to deny government authority to avert threats to health, safety, and security. The most effective safeguard against governmental abuse is the separation of powers, so that no branch wields unchecked authority. By adopting the principle of checks and balances, MSEHPA adopts a classic means of preventing abuse.

The Model Act creates several hedges against abuse: (1) the governor may declare an emergency only under strict criteria and with careful consultation with public health experts and the community; (2) the legislature, by majority vote, can override the governor's declaration at any time; and (3) the judiciary can terminate the exercise of power if the governor violates the standards or procedures of the Model Law or acts unconstitutionally. No law can guarantee that the powers it confers will not be abused. But MSEHPA counterbalances executive power by providing a strong role for the legislature and judiciary.

D. Libertarianism

Critics argue that the model law should not confer compulsory power to vaccinate, test, medically treat, isolate, and quarantine. They reason that services are more important than power; that individuals will comply voluntarily with public health advice; and that trade-offs between civil rights and public health are not required and even are counterproductive. Certainly the HIV/AIDS epidemic has demonstrated that public health and civil liberties can be mutually reinforcing—respect for individual freedoms can promote the public's health. Nevertheless, the arguments that law should not confer compulsory power are misplaced.

First, although the provision of services may be more important than the exercise of power, the state undoubtedly needs a certain amount of authority to protect the public's health. Government must have the power to prevent businesses (e.g., sale of contaminated food) or individuals (e.g., traveling while infectious) from endangering others. It is only common sense, for example, that a person who has been exposed to an infectious disease should be required to undergo testing or medical examination and, if infectious, to be vaccinated or avoid public contact.

Second, although most people can be expected to comply willingly with public health measures because it is in their own interests and desire for the common welfare, not everyone will comply. Provided that public health powers are hedged with safeguards, individuals should be required to yield some of their interests to protect the health and security of the community.

Finally, although public health and civil liberties may be mutually enhancing in many cases, they sometimes come into conflict. When government acts to preserve the public's health, it can interfere with property rights (e.g., freedom of contract, to pursue a profession, or to conduct a business) or personal rights (e.g., autonomy, privacy, and liberty).[46]

Even in principle, it would be almost disingenuous to argue that individuals whose movements pose a significant risk of harm to their communities have a "right" to be free of interference necessary to control the threat. Similarly, property rights do not trump the protection of the common good from extreme peril. There simply is no basis for these arguments in constitutional law, and perhaps little more in political philosophy. Even the most liberal scholars accept the harm principle—that government should retain power to prevent individuals from endangering others.[47]

The Supreme Court has been equally clear about the limits of freedom in a constitutional democracy. The rights of liberty, due process, and property are fundamental but not absolute. Justice Harlan in the foundational Supreme Court case of *Jacobson v. Massachusetts* (1905) wrote, "There are manifold restraints to which every person is necessarily subject for the common good. On any other basis organized society could not exist with safety to its members."[48] Similarly, private property was held subject to the restriction that it not be used in a way that posed a health hazard, as Lemuel Shaw of the Massachusetts Supreme Judicial Court observed in 1851: "We think it settled principle, growing out of the nature of well ordered civil society, that every holder of property . . . holds it under the implied liability that it shall not be injurious to the right of the community."[49]

Critics argue, without support from any judicial authority, that the Supreme Court's landmark decision in *Jacobson*, reiterated by the Court over the last Century, is no longer apposite. There is, according to this line of argument, a constitutional right to refuse interventions even if the individual poses a public risk. Yet, the courts have consistently upheld compulsory measures to avert a risk,[50] including the power to compulsorily test,[51] report,[52] vaccinate,[53] treat,[54] and isolate[55] provided there are clear criteria and procedures.

E. Personal safeguards

The real basis for debate over public health legislation should not be that powers are given, but whether they are hedged with appropriate safeguards of personal liberty. As discussed above, there are no plausible grounds for arguing that government should not have the power to avert significant risks to the public. The core of the debate over the Model Act ought to be whether it appropriately protects personal liberties by providing clear and demanding criteria for the exercise of power and fair procedures for decision-making. It is in this context that the attack on MSEHPA is particularly exasperating because critics rarely suggest that the Act fails to provide crisp standards and procedural due process.

It is important to note that compulsory powers for testing, physical examination, treatment, isolation, and quarantine already exist in state public health law. These powers have been exercised since the founding of the Republic. MSEHPA, therefore, does not contain new, radical powers over the individual. Most tellingly, the Model Act contains much better safeguards of individual liberty than appear in communicable disease statutes enacted in the early-to-mid twentieth century.

Unlike older statutes, MSEHPA provides clear and objective criteria for the exercise of powers, rigorous procedural due process, respect for religious and cultural differences, and a new set of entitlements for humane treatment. First, the criteria for the exercise of compulsory powers are based on the modern "significant risk" standard enunciated in constitutional law and disability discrimination law. The Act also requires public health officials to adopt the "least restrictive alternative." Second, the procedures for intervention are rigorous, following the most stringent requirements set by the Supreme Court, including the right to counsel, presentation and cross examination of evidence, and reasons for decisions. Third, the Act shows toleration of groups through its requirements to respect cultural and religious differences whenever consistent with the public's health. Finally, the Act provides a whole new set of rights for the care and treatment of people subject to isolation or quarantine. These include the right to treatment, clothing, food, communication, and humane conditions.

In summary, MSEHPA provides a modern framework for effective identification and response to emerging heath threats, while demonstrating respect for individuals and toleration of groups. Indeed, the Center agreed to draft the law only because a much more draconian approach might have been taken by the federal government and the states acting on their own and responding to public fears and misapprehensions.

16.7 Rethinking the Public Good

American values at the turn of the twenty-first century fairly could be characterized as individualistic. There was a distinct orientation toward personal and proprietary freedoms and against a substantial government presence in social and economic life. The attacks on the World Trade Center and Pentagon and the anthrax outbreaks re-awakened the political community to the importance of public health. Historians will look back and ask whether September 11th, 2001 was a fleeting scare with temporary solutions or whether it was a transforming event.

There are good reasons for believing that resource allocations, ethical values, and law should transform to reflect the critical importance of the health, security and well-being of the populace. It is not that individual freedoms are unimportant. To the contrary, personal liberty allows people the right of self-determination, to make judgments about how to live their lives and pursue their dreams. Without a certain level of health, safety, and security, however, people cannot have well-being; nor can they meaningfully exercise their autonomy or participate in social and political life.

The purpose of this chapter is not to assert which are the more fundamental interests: personal liberty or health and security. Rather, the purpose is to illustrate that both sets of interests are important to human flourishing. The Model State Emergency Health Powers Act was designed to defend personal as well as collective interests. But in a country so tied to rights rhetoric on both sides of the political spectrum, any proposal that has the appearance of strengthening governmental authority was bound to travel in tumultuous political waters.

Disclaimer and Acknowledgment

The Center for Law and the Public's Health is supported by Cooperative Agreement Number U50/CCU319118-02 from the Centers for Disease Control and Prevention (CDC). The contents of this chapter are solely the responsibility of the author and do not necessarily represent the official views of the CDC or the organizations providing assistance in the development of the model act. The Sloan Foundation provided funding for the development of MSEHPA and the Milbank Memorial Fund provided support for technical assistance to the states. MSEHPA grew out of the work of the Public Health Statute Modernization Project of the Robert Wood Johnson Foundation ("Turning").

Endnotes

1. This chapter is based on Lawrence O. Gostin et al., "The Model State Emergency Health Powers Act: Planning and response to bioterrorism and naturally occurring infectious diseases," *JAMA* 288:622 (2002); Lawrence O. Gostin, "Public health law in an age of terrorism: Rethinking individual rights and common goods," *Health Aff.* 21:79 (2002). *See also* Lawrence O. Gostin, *Public Health Law: Power, Duty, Restraint* (Berkeley: University of California, 2000).

2. John A. Jernigan et al. "Bioterrorism-related inhalational anthrax: The first ten cases reported in the United States," *Emerging Infectious Diseases* 7:933 (2001); Larry M. Bush et al. "Index case of fatal inhalational anthrax due to bioterrorism in the United States," *New Eng. J. Med.* 345:1607 (2001).

3. Morton N. Swartz. "Recognition and management of anthrax B: An update," *New Eng. J. Med.* 345:1621 (2001).

4. National Intelligence Council. *The Global Infectious Disease Threat and Its Implications for the United States* (Washington, DC: Central Intelligence Agency, 2000).

5. U.S. Commission on National Security in the 21st Century. *New World Coming: American Security in the 21st Century, Supporting Research and Analysis* (1999), available at http://www.nssg.gov/Reports/reports.htm (last visited May 31, 2002).

6. Thomas V. Inglesby et al. "Anthrax as a biological weapon: Medical and public health management," *JAMA* 281:1735 (1999).

7. Thomas V. Inglesby et al. "Preventing the use of biological weapons: Improving response should prevention fail," *Clin. Infectious Diseases* 30:926 (2000); James M. Hughes. "The emerging threat of bioterrorism," *Emerging Infectious Diseases* 5:494 (1999); Donald A. Henderson. "The looming threat of bioterrorism," *Sci.* 283:1279 (1999); Leonard A. Cole. "The specter of biological weapons," *Sci. Am.* 275:60 (1996); Michael T. Osterholm and John Schwartz. *Living Terrors: What America Needs to Know to Survive the Coming Bioterrorist Catastrophe* (NY: Delacourte, 2002).

8. James M. Hughes. "The emerging threat of bioterrorism," *Emerging Infectious Diseases* 5:494 (1999).

9. Robert Cottrell and Richard Wolffe. "Safe houses yielding documents on weapons of mass destruction," *Fin. Times Limited*, November 23, 2001.

10. Tara O'Toole et al. "Shining light on Dark Winter," *Clin. Infectious Diseases* 34:972 (2002).

11. Thomas V. Inglesby et al. "A plague on your city: Observations from TOPOFF," *Clin. Infectious Diseases* 32:436 (2001).

12. Joseph Barbera et al. "Large-scale quarantine following biological terrorism in the United States: Scientific examination, logistic and legal limits, and possible consequences," *JAMA* 286:2711(2001).

13. Donald A. Henderson, Testimony before the Foreign Relations Committee: Hearing on the Threat of Bioterrorism and the Spread of Infectious Disease, 107th Cong., 1st Sess., September 5, 2001.

14. Institute of Medicine, Public Health Systems and Emerging Infections: Assessing the Capabilities of the Public and Private Sectors: Workshop Summary (2000).

15. U.S. Department of Health and Human Services. *Public Health's Infrastructure: A Status Report* (Atlanta: Centers for Disease Control and Prevention, 2001).

16. U.S. Department of Health and Human Services, *Healthy People 2010* (Washington, DC: Office of Disease Prevention and Health, 2000); Lawrence O. Gostin, "Public health law reform" *Am. J. Pub. Health* 91:1365 (2001); Public Health Statute Modernization National Excellence Collaborative. *Model State Public Health Act: A Tool for Assessing Public Health Laws* (2003; available at http://www.turningpointprogram.org/Pages/MSPHAfinal.pdf); Lawrence O. Gostin et al. "The Model Emergency

Health Powers Act: Planning for and response to bioterrorism and naturally occurring infectious diseases," *JAMA* 2888:622, (2002); Lawrence O. Gostin. "Public health law in an age of terrorism: Rethinking individual rights and common goods," *Health Aff.* 21:79 (2002).

17. Trust for America's Health. *Public Health Preparedness: Progress and Challenges Since September 11th, 2001* (Washington, DC: Trust for America's Health, 2002).

18. Institute of Medicine. *Who Will Keep the Public Healthy? Educating Public Health Professionals for the 21st Century* (Washington, DC: Institute of Medicine, 2002).

19. Association of State Public Health Laboratories. "Core Functions and Capabilities of State Public Health Laboratories," *Morbidity & Mortality Wkly. Rep.* 51:1 (2002).

20. Lawrence K. Altman and Anahad. O'Connor. "Health officials fear local impact of smallpox plan," *N.Y. Times*, January 5, 2003, at A1.

21. Trust for America's Health. *Ready of Not? Protecting the Public's Health in the Age of Bioterrorism* (Washington, DC: Trust for America's Health, 2003).

22. Adam Cohen. "Editorial observer: What Alabama's low-tax mania can teach the rest of the country," *N.Y. Times*, October 20, 2003, at A16.

23. Lawrence O. Gostin. *Public Health Law: Power, Duty, Restraint* (Berkeley: University of California, 2000).

24. Colo. Rev. Stat. Ann. 24-32-2103 (West 2001).

25. Rhode Island Department of Health. *The Emergence of Bioterrorism as a Public Health Threat in the 21st Century*, available at http://www.health.state.ri.us/biot/article.htm.

26. Lawrence O. Gostin. "Public health law reform," *Am. J. Pub. Health* 91:1365 (2001).

27. Lawrence O. Gostin et al. "The law and the public's health: A study of infectious disease law in the united States," *Colum. L. Rev.* 99:59 (1999).

28. Institute of Medicine. *Ending Neglect: The Elimination of Tuberculosis in the United States* (Washington, DC: Institute of Medicine, 2000).

29. Lawrence O. Gostin et al. "The public health information infrastructure: A national review of the law on health information privacy," *JAMA* 275:1921 (1996).

30. Centers for Disease Control and Prevention. *Public Health Assessment of Potential Biological Terrorism Agents* (Atlanta: Centers for Disease Control and Prevention, 2002).

31. Heather Horton et al. "Disease reporting as a tool for bioterrorism preparedness," *J. L. Med. & Ethics* 30:262 (2002).

32. Lawrence O. Gostin et al. "The public health information infrastructure: A national review of the law on health information privacy," JAMA 275:1921 (1996).

33. Jocelyn Kaiser. "Patient privacy: Researchers say rules are too restrictive," *Sci.* 30:262 (2002).

34. Institute of Medicine. *The Future of Public Health* (1988).

35. Department of Health and Human Services. *Healthy People 2010* (2000).

36. Lawrence O. Gostin and James G. Hodge Jr., State Public Health Law Assessment Report, available at http://www.turningpointprogram.org.

37. http://www.turningpointprogram.org. *See* http://www.hss.state.ak.us/dph/deu/turningpoint/nav.htm.

38. Center for Law and the Public's Health at Georgetown and Johns Hopkins Universities, The Model State Emergency Health Powers Act (2001), *available at* http://www.publichealthlaw.net/MSEHPA/MSEHPA2.pdf (last visited April 4, 2004).

39. Justin Gillis. "States weighing laws to fight bioterrorism," *Washington Post*, November 19, 2001, A1.

40. Lawrence O. Gostin. *Public Health Law: Power, Duty, Restraint* (Berkeley: University of California, 2000).).

41. Justin Gillis. "States weighing laws to fight bioterrorism," *Washington Post*, November 19, 2001, A1.

42. Readers should refer to the specific language of the MSEHPA for the most accurate account, available at http://www.publichealthlaw.net/MSEHPA/MSEHPA2.pdf.

43. Lucas v. South Carolina Coastal Council, 505 U.S. 1003 (1992).

44. George J. Annas. "Bioterrorism, public health, and civil liberties," *New Eng. J. Med.* 346:1337 (2001).

45. Gibbons v. Ogden, 22 U.S. (9 Wheat.) 1 (1824) (conceiving state police powers as "an immense mass of legislation . . . Inspection laws, quarantine laws, and health laws of every description . . . are components of this mass.").

46. Lawrence O. Gostin. *Public Health Law: Power, Duty, Restraint* (Berkeley: University of California, 2000).; Lawrence O. Gostin ed., *Public Health Law and Ethics: A Reader* (Berkeley: University of California, 2002).

47. Joel Feinberg. *The Moral Limits of the Criminal Law*, volumes 1–4 (NY: Oxford University, 1987–1990).

48. Jacobson v. Massachusetts, 197 U.S. 11, 26 (1905).

49. Commonwealth v. Alger, 7 Cush.53, 84–85 (1851).

50. Washington v. Harper, 494 U.S. 210, 227 (1990) (upholding forced administration of antipsychotic medication if the inmate is dangerous to himself or others and the treatment is in the inmate's medical interest).

51. Skinner v. Railway Labor Executives' Ass'n, 489 U.S. 601 (1989).

52. Whalen v. Roe, 429 U.S. 589 (1977).

53. Zucht v. King, 260 U.S. 174 (1922).

54. McCormick v. Stalder, 105 F.3d 1059, 1061 (5th Cir. 1997) (finding that the state's compelling interest in reducing the spread of tuberculosis justifies involuntary treatment).

55. Greene v. Edwards, 263 S.E.2d 661 (1980).

Chapter 17

The Truth about Bioterrorism

Dr. Amnon Birenzvige and Charles H. Wick, Ph.D., LTC (Ret.)

Synopsis

17.1 Introduction

Since the event of 9-11 the threat of bioterrorism and other weapons of mass destruction (WMD) in this country increased significantly. Unfortunately, this threat is poorly understood and, at times, greatly exaggerated. We frequently see and read in the news media "expert" opinion that is either not very realistic or, on the other hand, minimizes the threat. This greatly increases the public confusion in this matter. In this chapter we try to put this threat in its proper perspective and present various existing problems and issues that need to be solved in order to combat this threat and provide the American public with best possible protection.

Early in World War II Japan investigated the possible use of biological warfare materials for the purpose of sabotage.[1] Mr. Merck emphasized in his report that any country without large expenditure can develop BW. In 1960 the House of Representatives reported that the U.S. infrastructure is particularly vulnerable to a CBR attack[2] and recommended that more research be done on how to protect these facilities.

In this report we attempt to put this threat in its proper perspective. We evaluate some of the "popular" stories, we review under what circumstances this threat can produce mass casualties, and we report on recent activities of potential threat groups (all taken from open sources). Finally we evaluate the state of our preparedness to face this threat and make some recommendations to enhance it.

17.2 The Fiction

A. Fiction #1

Many of us heard and saw on one or the other news program a statement that "a handful" of biological agent or a test tube full of nerve agent can poison every person in New York City.

This statement is only partly true. True, a handful of certain biological agents or a test tube of the nerve agent VX contains probably enough material to kill the whole population of New York City, providing everybody will line up and be injected with the agent. However, dropped from the top of a tall building it is unlikely that many, if any, casualties will result. At this point it is interesting to note that it was reported that Aum Shiri Kyo launched at least nine bio attacks on Tokyo without producing casualties.[3]

We can make a rough calculation on the amount of material required to contaminate an area 1 km × 1 km with anthrax that will provide a person in this area with a LD50.

If we assume the anthrax spore to be spherical with a diameter of 1 μm and a density of 1 gr/cm^3, then the total weight of 10,000 spores—LD50 for anthrax[4] is 5.2×10^{-9} gr. Normal breathing rate for a person is 10 L/min or 10,000 cm^3/min. Thus the concentration of anthrax should be 5.2×10^{-13} gr/cm^3 for a person to receive LD50 dose in ten minutes exposure. Assuming the mixing layer over a city extend to 1 km (from the heat island effect and the increased surface roughness of the urban area), then to contaminate a volume of 1 km^3 or 1,015 cm^3 to the LD50 concentration will require 520 grams. If we assume that dispersion further reduces the concentration by at least two or three orders of magnitude we can conclude that to achieve a lethal concentration one will require close to 50 kg of anthrax spores. If we further assume that during the day the mixing layer extends to 10–15 km and that the anthrax preparation is almost 100 percent active the task of contaminating a city to a level that will cause very large number of casualties (LD50) becomes nontrivial at all and might be very hard to accomplish covertly. Even dispersed from low altitude, like from a moving car, the effect is not at all clear. Probably people in the immediate vicinity of the dissemination will receive a lethal dose, however farther away from the dispersion point the agent concentration will decrease quickly. This, however should be verified by actual testing.

Note that the most appropriate time (to achieve maximum effect) to disperse BW agents is during a period when the atmosphere is stable and dispersion is limited to a shallow boundary layer. This is demonstrated in Figure 17.1. As can be seen, during stable conditions the contamination disperses as a narrow plume and stays close to the ground. This results in much higher concentrations. However, when the atmosphere is unstable the plume disperses very quickly. Stable conditions occur during the night under clear skies. Most people are in their homes that provide further protection from outdoor contaminants.[5] We should also note that the urban heat island effect and the increase surface roughness of the urban area have a significant effect on the depth of the mixing height and result in a much deeper boundary-mixing layer.[6] Epstein expressed similar views in his presentation in 1997.[7]

B. Fiction #2

We frequently hear from "experts" that our municipal water supply is vulnerable to contamination by bio terrorists. Let us examine this scenario.

Per capita use of water in the U.S. (c. 1995) is 1,280 gallons of fresh water per day.[8] Of these 350 gallons per day are used in urban and suburban areas per household.[9] If we assume that distribution of urban water

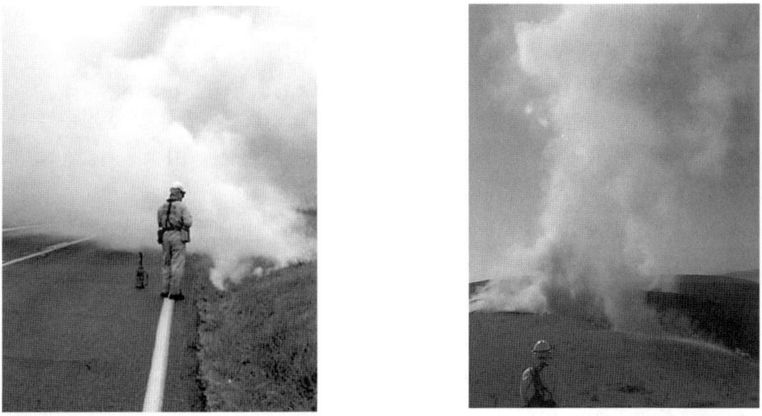

stable unstable

Figure 17.1 *Effect of atmospheric stability on dispersion (photos from www.nps.gov)*

use in the U.S. is similar to the one in Europe, then only 1.3 percent or 4.5 gallons are used for cooking and drinking.[10] The authors estimates that at least 80 percent of these are used for cooking and preparation of hot beverages (coffee or tea) and are boiled. This leaves about one gallon per day per household for direct consumption (less than 0.3 percent of the total water used). Assuming an average household is comprised of four people (two adults and two children) average daily water consumed per person is one quart (about one litter), or less. This is close to the EPA's estimate of a daily per capita consumption of about two liters a day.[11]

A city of 1,000,000 population, or 250,000 households consumes 87.5 millions gallons a day. To contaminate the water supply to a ppm concentration with active biological material requires 87.5 gallons of active material for a day's supply. Assuming the suspension has about 10 percent active material that means 875 gallons of suspension. A water reservoir for a metropolitan area normally holds several months' worth of water.[12] Assuming, conservatively, that the reservoir holds only a one-year supply (365 days), over 300,000 gallons of suspensions will be required to contaminate it to a ppm level. We also need to remember that municipal water passes through water purification and chlorination before being distributed to the consumer. In an unscientific survey conducted by the authors, they determined that most Americans who are connected to the municipal water supply prefer to drink bottled water. Most complaints are that the water tastes like chlorine. We also need to remember that most traditional BW agents are much more effective when inhaled than when ingested.

17.3 The Threat of Bioterrorism

The discussion above does not mean to imply that BW agents do not present a threat. Under certain circumstances that will be discussed bellow BW agent present a real danger and can cause mass casualties. BW agents can, probably, be dispersed by an individual or from a moving car. However, the effect of such an attack is not at all clear. In the opinion of the author such an attack will result in few casualties, but will not cause casualties numbered in the hundreds or thousands. The main effect of such an attack will likely be psychological. A similar effect was seen with the recent dissemination of anthrax through the mail. Even though it produced only few casualties (five fatalities) it did cause major disruption. Similarly, a terrorist can, possibly, tap into the water supply of a public building or a small neighborhood. However, even in this case the task will not be trivial and, probably, will not result in a large number of casualties since, as discussed above, a very small portion of the water used daily are ingested directly without any treatment.

The threat of bioterrorism, however is real. The proliferation of BW capabilities is increasing and at least ten nations now, some of which are known to support terrorist organizations, have the capabilities to produce biological agents.[13] In 1995 Aum Shinri Kyo broke fresh ground by using WMD as a weapon of terror. Since then there had been reports by some news organizations that there have been indications that Palestinian terrorists have tried to use cyanide and probably some nerve agents during several homicide bombings in Israel.[14] Terrorists have shown their willingness to commit mass murder. The knowledge on how to prepare BW agents is now available over the Internet. Recent news reports on CNN and other news organizations showed al-Qa'eda experimenting with chemical agents and possibly biological agents. And finally, scientists from the former Soviet Union are potentially up for grab for the highest bidder.

Enclosed spaces are particularly vulnerable to bioterrorism attack due to the limited volume in which the biological material needs to disperse. Areas like shopping centers, and other large buildings that contain central HVAC systems for air circulation are vulnerable. The agent can either be dispersed inside or introduced into the building through the HVAC system. Subway systems are also vulnerable since the agent can be dispersed throughout the system by the moving train which pushes the air ahead of them (piston action).[15] This vulnerability was recognized in 1948 in a special report on BW activities of the Research and Development Board of the national military establishment who recommended to test the vulnerability of ventilation systems of key building and the vulnerability of the subway system to a bioterrorist attack.[16] This vulnerability was again recognized by the 86th Congress in 1960.[2] In 1966, the U.S. Army demonstrated this vulnerability during a test in the New York City subway. A nonpathogenic biological material—*Bacillus globigii* (known as BG)—was dispersed inside the subway tunnel. The BG spread very quickly throughout the subway line.[17–21]

A sea breeze is a predictable meteorological phenomenon that occurs on the sea-land interface. Figure 17.2 is a pictorial explanation to this phenomenon. It usually starts in early afternoon as a result from the uneven heating of the land and the sea. This predictable phenomenon can be exploited to contaminate large areas on the seashore. In 1950 the U.S. Army demonstrated that when they sprayed *Serratia marcescens*—a non-pathogenic bacteria—from ships off the coast of San Francisco. Air samples that were collected indicated that the bacteria were spread over a very large area of the San Francisco bay.[17-21,22] Of course, the reverse phenomena, or the land breeze that occurs at night can be used to attack ships from the shore.

It is interesting to note that according to news reports al-Qa'eda owns more than twenty commercial seagoing ships.[23] Commercial ships carry ballast water for stability. These ballast water are released as they get closer to shore and shallow water. A commercial ship can hold up to 60,000 tons of ballast water.[24] If the ballast water were contaminated with BW agents they could be used to contaminate large areas along the sea shore. We strongly recommend that the possibility of this threat be investigated.

17.4 Issues and Problems in Protecting Against Bioterrorism

Chemical warfare agents act immediately. Hence the effect of a chemical terrorist attack will be immediately evident by presence of immediate casualties. The place and time of the attack will be immediately identified and recognize and will allow the first-responders to react in order (i.e., evacuate victims, secure the immediate location of the attack and take other measured to minimize casualties, and, finally, to decontaminate and restore the site of the attack).

Conversely, the effect of biological agents is not immediately evident. Onset of symptoms can start days to weeks after exposure. Given the mobile nature of the American society an onslaught of patients with similar symptoms in hospitals all across the country can be the first indication that a biological terrorist attack had occurred. It will be very hard, or impossible to pinpoint the time and place where the attack took place without a reliable detection system.

At the present time all biological agents detectors suffer from the malady of false alarms. The reason for these false alarms is not due to malfunction of the detectors but is the result of the great sensitivity that

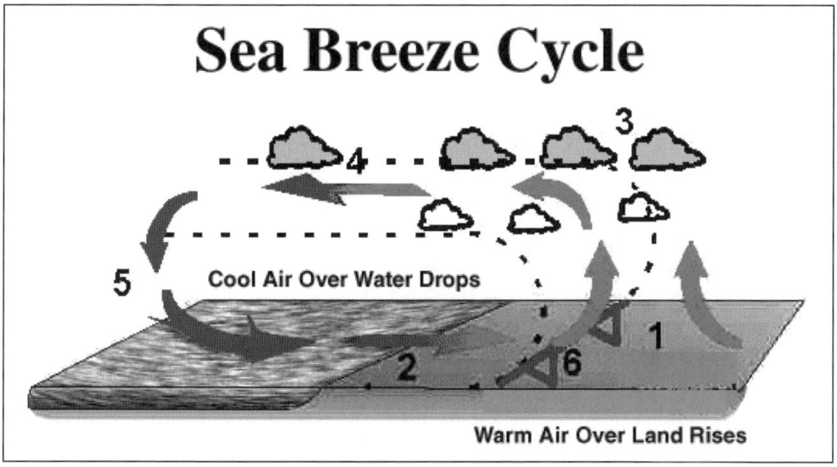

Figure 17.2 *A pictorial explanation for sea breeze*

any bio detector is required to have. The reason for the large number of false alarms is that the atmosphere contains large number of biological and non-biological aerosols. The bioaerosols can range in size from sub μm to several tens of μm. The concentration of the bioaerosols varies greatly in time and space and depends on the time of day, season, land use, meteorology, human activity and other, yet unknown, factors. The short-term variability is often within order of magnitude of the threat that needs to be detected. Hence a detection strategy needs to be based on a two tier approach: (1) quick (within a matter of minutes) detection indicating that an unnatural (man-released) biological event occurred followed by (2) sampling and quick analysis for verification and identification. Only after confirmation that indeed a bioterrorism event occurred can public action (such as cordoning of the area, activation of first responders and public announcement) take place.

Statistical theory predicts that by fusing information from orthogonal sensors, over all data reliability increases. Hence a reliable biological detection system should consist of a combination of multiple orthogonal technologies.

Once a detection system has indicated that a bioterrorist attack is underway, there is a need for quick confirmation and identification of the biological agent that was deployed. For that purpose there is a need for an air sampler that will be triggered automatically by the detection system. Since, as was discussed before, the main threat of bioterrorism is in enclosed spaces such a sampler can be placed in the return air duct of the HVAC system and could be retrieved without causing panic in the general populace.

Theoretical studies show that by circulating the air of an enclosed space through a disinfecting device the overall exposure of the occupants can be significantly reduced.[25,26] At least two current technologies can have this effect: (1) the pulse light device,[27] and (2) the TiO_2-UVA device.[28] Serious consideration should be given to the possibility of installing these types of devices in the return air duct of the ventilation systems of key buildings.

17.5 Recommendations

1. As was discussed earlier, detection is the key to bioterrorism defense. At the present time the background bio-aerosols result in an excessive rate of false alarms of any bio-detectors. We recommend that a bio-detection system that takes background variability into account be developed. Such a system will likely be comprised of multiple orthogonal technologies and data fusion algorithm.
2. Develop a suitable sampler-collector that can be automatically activated when an unnatural event is detected.
3. In enclosed system, develop and evaluate a system to disinfect the air when an unnatural event is detected.

Authors' disclaimer. This information is not to be construed as an official Department of the Army position unless so designated by other authorizing documents. The Public Affairs Office number is PAO-04-478. This is the clearance for public release.

References

1. House report No 815 "Research on CBR" – a report of the committee on science and aeronautics, the House of representative 86th congress, first session 1960. In US Army activities in the United States Biological Warfare and Programs 1942-1977 Volume 2 Annexes (1994).

2. William J. Broad and Judith Miller, "The Threat of Germ Weapons Is Rising. Fear too",Week in Review, December 27, 1998 Quoted from the *New York*

Times. Reviewed on line http://www.nytimes.com/library/122798germ-warfare-review.html. Last reviewed December 29, 1998.

3. Theodore J. Cieslak and Edward M. Eitzen, Jr. "Bioterrorism": Agents of Concern" USAMRIID technical report, August 2000.

4. "Assessment of Human Exposure to Air Pollutants - a Literature Survey", A. Birenzvige, EPA Contract 68-02-2843, Progress report, October 1979.

5. Hashem Akbari, LBL, Heat Islang Group, Berkeley, CA, Personal communications August, 2002.

6. Gerald L. Epstein "Chemical/Biological Terrorism: No Longer Hypothetical", Department of Energy/White House Office of Science and Technology Policy, delivered at the International Conference on Aviation Safety and Security in the 21st Century January 13-15, 1997, reviewed on line http://www.gwu.edu/~cms/aviation/track_ii/epstein.htm Last reviewed September 6, 2002.

7. Wayne B. Solley, Robert R. Pierce and Howard A. Perlman, "Estimated Use of Water in the United States in 1995", U. S. Geological Survey Circular 1200, U. S. Geological Survey, U. S. Department of the Interior, United States Government Printing Office: 1998, http://water.usgs.gov/watuse/pdf1995/html/ lasr reviewed 5 August 2002.

8. http://www.parthnet.org/search/tips/081302.html last reviewed 19 August 2002.

9. European Environment Agency, Indicator Fact Sheet Signals 2001 - YIRo1HHO7 water Consumption http://themes.eea.eu.int/Sectors_and_ activities/households/indicators/energy/hh07household.pdf last reviewed 20 August 2002.

10. "Drinking Water and Health Advisories, Estimated Per Capita Water Ingestion in the United States" April 2000. Reviewed on line at http://www.epa.gov/waterscience/drinking/percapita/ last reviewed September 3, 2002.

11. Elizabeth N. O'Brien, "Per Capita Consumption,"reviewed on line, http://whale.wheelock.edu/DeerIsland/PerCapitaConsumption.html. Last reviewed September 3, 2002

12. Dr. Ivan Eland, director of defense policy studies at the Cato Institute, "Protecting the Homeland: The Best Defense Is to Give No Offense," Cato Policy

Analysis No. 306, May 5, 1998, reviewed on line http://www.cato.org/pubs/pas/pa-306.html last reviewed September 6, 2002.

13. http://www.debka.com/Hebrew/body_index.html August 6, 2002

14. C.L. Staten, "Questions and Answers on Bio-Warfare / Bio-Terrorism with Dr. Alibek," July 14, 1999. Reviewed on line http://www.emergency.com/1999/alibek99.htm.

15. In U.S. Army activities in the United States Biological Warfare and Programs 1942-1977 Volume 2 Annexes (1994), annex E.

16. U.S. Army activities in the United States Biological Warfare and Programs 1942–1977 Volume 2 Annexes (1994).

17. http://www.fas.org/nuke/guide/usa/cbw/bw.htm.

18. Libertarian Party Press release October 26, 2001 report on testimony before the subcommittee on Health, U.S. Senate in 1977.

19. LTC George W. Christopher et al., "Biological Warfare: A historical Perspective," JAMA Special communication 278 No 5 (1997) reviewed on line http://jama.ama-assn.org/issues/v278n5/ffull/jsc7044.html.

2. "Biological Testing Involving Human Subjects by the Department of Defense, 1977," Hearing before the subcommittee on health and scientific research of the committee on human resources, United State Senate, 95th congress, first session (1977).

21. J. Mills et al., "Serratia marcescens Endocarditis: A Regional Illness Associated with Intravenous Drug Abuse," *Ann. Int. Med.* 18:29–35 (1976).

22. Commander Vijay Sakhuja, Marine Security Analyst, Institute of Peace and Conflict Studies Article # 679 "Challenging Terrorism at Sea," January 19, 2002, reviewed online http://www.jpcs.org/issues/newarticles/679-ter-sakhuja.html

23. Dr. Steve Raaymakers, Global Ballast Water Management Program, a cooperative initiative of the Global Environmental Facility and the International Maritime Organization, personal communication August 23, 2002.

24. Amnon Birenzvige, "On the Protection Provided from Exposure to Chemical Warfare Agents by Enclosed Spaces," CRDEC-TR-86026

25. A. Birenzvige, “A Model Calculate the Indoor Concentration of a Chemical Contaminant—Sensitivity Analysis,” Presented at the 49th MORS, Albuquerque, N.M., June 1982.

26. Charles Wick et al., “Pulsed Light Device for Deactivating Biological Aerosols,” ERDEC-TR-456 (1982).

27. Dr. Robert Bair, Director Industry-University consortiums on Bio-surfaces (IUCB), State University of NY at Buffalo, Buffalo, NY, Personal communication (2002).

About the Editor

Cyril H. Wecht, M.D., J.D. received his M.D from the University of Pittsburgh, and his J.D. from the University of Maryland. He is certified by the American Board of Pathology in anatomic, clinical, and forensic pathology, and is a Fellow of the College of American Pathologists, the American Society of Clinical Pathologists and the National Association of Medical Examiners. Dr. Wecht was formerly Chairman of the Department of Pathology and President of the Medical Staff at St. Francis Central Hospital in Pittsburgh, and is actively involved as a medical-legal and forensic science consultant, author, and lecturer. He also serves as the elected Coroner of Allegheny County (Pittsburgh, Pennsylvania).

He is a Clinical Professor at the University of Pittsburgh Schools of Medicine, Dental Medicine, and Graduate School of Public Health; an Adjunct Professor at Duquesne University Schools of Law, Pharmacy, and Health Sciences; a Distinguished Professor at Carlow College; and Chairman of the Advisory Board of the Cyril H. Wecht Institute of Forensic Science and Law at Duquesne University School of Law. He has served as President of the American College of Legal Medicine and the American Academy of Forensic Sciences, and also as Chairman of both the Board of Trustees of the American Board of Legal Medicine and the American College of Legal Medicine Foundation.

He is the author of more than 475 professional publications; an editorial board member of eighteen national and international medical-legal and forensic scientific publications; and editor of thirty-five books, including a five-volume set, *Forensic Sciences* (Matthew Bender), and two three-volume sets, *Handling Soft Tissue Injury Cases* and *Preparing and Winning Medical Negligence Cases* (both published by Michie).

Dr. Wecht has organized and conducted postgraduate medical-legal seminars in more than fifty countries throughout the world in his capacity as Director of the Pittsburgh Institute of Legal Medicine. He has personally performed approximately 15,000 autopsies, and has supervised, reviewed, or been consulted on approximately 35,000 additional post-mortem examinations, including cases in several foreign countries.

Dr Wecht has testified in more than 1,000 civil, criminal, and workers compensation cases in state and federal courts in more than thirty states and several foreign countries.

Dr. Wecht has appeared as a frequent guest on numerous national TV and radio shows, discussing various medical-legal and forensic scientific subjects, including medical malpractice; alcohol and drug abuse; assassinations of President John F. Kennedy, Senator Robert F. Kennedy, and Reverend Martin Luther King; death of Elvis Presley; Sheppard case; O.J. Simpson case; JonBenet Ramsey case; Diallo case; Chandra Levy death investigation; and Laci Peterson homicide. These cases, as well as those involving Mary Jo Kopechne, Sunny von Bulow, Jean Harris, Dr. Jeffrey McDonald, the Waco Branch Davidian fire, Vincent Foster, and many others, are discussed from the perspective of Dr. Wecht's own professional involvement in his books, *Cause of Death*, *Grave Secrets*, *Who Killed JonBenet Ramsey?* and *Mortal Evidence*.

Dr. Wecht and his wife, Sigrid, have four children, and eleven grandchildren, all of whom reside in Allegheny County. He has received numerous awards and honors from various professional, community, and governmental organizations, including County Detectives' Association of Pennsylvania, Deputy Sheriffs' Association of Pennsylvania, Vectors, New York Society of Forensic Sciences, American College of Legal Medicine, National Junior Chamber of Commerce, and the American Legion.

He has been invited as a Distinguished Professor to lecture in several foreign countries, and is an Honorary Life Member of the National Academies of Legal Medicine of France, Spain, Belgium, Yugoslavia, Mexico, Columbia, and Brazil.

Dr. Wecht has lectured at numerous medical, law, and other graduate schools, as well as many colleges and universities, and numerous professional organizations and governmental agencies, including Harvard Law School, Yale Medical School, the FBI Academy, and the Medical Division of the CIA.

About the Authors

Michael P. Allswede, D.O., is Director of the Strategic Medical Intelligence (SMI) initiative, which he brought to the Center for Biosecurity in 2004. Based on a prototype program in operation in Pittsburgh for five years, SMI employs locally accessible volunteer doctors to improve early warning and detection of bioterrorism so as to prevent its occurrence and improve the medical community's response if it occurs. SMI is the nation's first attempt at creating partnerships between local clinical medical leaders, public health officials, and the Federal Bureau of Investigation.

Dr. Allswede holds concurrent appointments as Assistant Professor in the Department of Emergency Medicine and at the Graduate School of Public Health at the University of Pittsburgh. In this position, he serves as Medical Toxicologist and Chief of the Special Emergency Response Section. In addition, Allswede is Medical Task Force Chair of the University of Pittsburgh Medical Center Bioterrorism Response Executive Committee.

Allswede's fluency in bridging both academic emergency medicine and real-life hospital and crisis response operations is reflected in both his teaching and government appointments. His academic career includes a posting as Associate Residency Director for the University of Michigan's program in emergency medicine. Allswede is principal investigator and creator of the "Pittsburgh Matrix," a hospital planning tool for use in addressing various bioterror challenges according to the scope of the threat and the timeline of detection. Allswede is also a collaborator on a syndromic detection and biosurveillance project. He also teaches a bioterrorism course at Sandia National Laboratory sponsored by the University of New Haven. His numerous academic and popular publications focus on bioterrorism detection, response, and treatment.

Allswede's public service includes developing a prototype State-level training and management system for use in responding to incidents involving the use of weapons of mass destruction. Dubbed RaPiD-T (for recognition, protection, decontamination—triage and treatment), the program offers a multi-disciplinary approach to crisis management for emergency response practitioners. Allswede developed RaPiD-T by drawing on his experience as an instructor in the U.S. Department of Defense Domestic Preparedness Program, authorized by the Nunn-Lugar-Domenici legislation of 1996; in this role he has trained Metropolitan Medical Strike Team members in Detroit, New York, Chicago, and Boston. In recognition of this work, Allswede was appointed by Attorney General Janet Reno to the National Domestic Preparedness Office (NDPO) State and Local Advisory Board. (The NDPO was the precursor to the Department of Homeland Security.) Allswede has also represented the U.S. Secret Service in a NATO technology development project and is a consultant on emergency response technologies.

Concurrent with his medical career, Dr. Allswede served eight years in the U.S. Army Reserve, volunteering for duty in Desert Storm with the 24th Mech Inf BDE, and again in South American to support ongoing anti-drug interdiction activities. Dr. Allswede retired a Captain, and Commanding Officer of the 408th Clearing Company, a front line medical unit tasked for management of chemical, biological, radiation, and traumatic casualties.

Allswede received his D.O. at the College of Osteopathic Medicine and Surgery in 1988 and served a rotating internship at Detroit Osteopathic Hospital. He was a post-graduate Emergency Medicine Resident at Chicago Osteopathic Medical Center and completed a critical care fellowship at Chicago Medical School and Cook County Hospital.

Lindsey R. Baden, M.D., is an infectious diseases specialist at Brigham and Women's Hospital and an Assistant Professor of Medicine at Harvard Medical School, both in Boston, Massachusetts.

Michael M. Baden, M.D. Former Chief Medical Examiner, New York City, Chief Forensic Pathologist, New York State Police.

John G. Bartlett, M.D., is Stanhope Baynes Jones Professor of Medicine and Chief of the Division of Infectious Diseases at Johns Hopkins University School of Medicine. He received his undergraduate degree at Dartmouth in 1959 and his medical degree at Upstate Medical Center in Syracuse in 1963. Training in internal medicine was done at the Brigham Hospital in Boston and the University of Alabama, he then received his fellowship training in infectious diseases at UCLA. In 1970, he joined the faculty of UCLA, and then joined the faculty of Tuft's University School of Medicine where he served as Associate Chief of Staff for Research at the Boston VA Hospital. In 1980, he moved to Hopkins to assume his current position. Dr. Bartlett has worked in several areas of research, all related to his specialty in infectious diseases. Major research interests have dealt with anaerobic infections, pathogenic mechanisms of *Bacteroides fragilis*, anaerobic pulmonary infections, and *Clostridium difficile*-associated colitis. Since moving to Hopkins in 1980, his major interests have been HIV/AIDS, managed care of patients with HIV infection and, most recently, bioterrorism. Dr. Bartlett has authored 470 articles, 282 book chapters and sixty-one editions of fourteen books.

Dr. Amnon Birenzvige, Ph.D., received his B.S.C and M.S.C. from the Technion, Israel Institutes of technology in physical chemistry and his Ph.D. from the State University of New York at Albany, NY in Aerosol and Atmospheric physics and chemistry. He has over thirty-five years' experience in studying the behavior of vapors and aerosols in the atmosphere. He conducted pioneering research on the exchange of air contaminants between the outdoor atmosphere and the indoor and on human exposure to air contaminants as they move about their daily activities. For the past twenty-five years Dr. Birenzvige had been employed by the Edgwood Chemical and Biological Center of the U.S. Army. There he conducted research on various aspects of CB defense. Some of his most notable accomplishments is to developed recommendations for protecting the civilian population for CB agent, which was adopted by the office of Homeland Security and the Israeli Defense Forces, study the problems of CB defense in cold weather, develop a field expedient test for testing face mask integrity, and conduct a study on the background biological aerosol in the background environment. During the cold war he also served as an advisor to the Berlin Brigade and assisted them in developing their tactics and strategy in the event of a chemical or biological attack on the city. He served on several FEMA workshops on "sheltering in place" in the event of an accidental or deliberate release of hazardous material and participated in writing in writing FEMA guidelines on the subject. He has over 150 publications in the forum of open literature publications, technical reports and presentations at technical meeting

Major John J. Buturla, Director, State of Connecticut, Department of Public Safety, Division of Homeland Security.

Bruce W. Dixon, M.D., received his B.S. in chemistry from the University of Pittsburgh and his M.D. from the University of Pittsburgh School of Medicine. He completed his residency at Duke University and served in Professional and Academic capacities there before returning to the University of Pittsburgh in 1975. Currently, Dr. Dixon is an Associate Professor of Medicine at the University of Pittsburgh School of Medicine, a position he has held since 1979.

Since 1992, in addition to his teaching duties, Dr. Dixon has been the Director of the Allegheny County Health Department. Dr. Dixon manages all Health Department programs, which impact air quality, environmental quality, and human health areas. He personally directs the Sexually Transmitted Diseases/HIV/AIDS Program, which provides diagnosis, treatment, and patient care, including social services case management, to residents of Allegheny County.

In October, 2000, Dr. Dixon was instrumental in forming a new nonprofit corporation, Allegheny Correctional Health Services, Inc., which is responsible for inmate medical services at the Allegheny County Jail. Dr. Dixon is serving as Chief Executive Officer and Chair of the Board of Directors.

Raymond Fish, M.D., received his B.S. and M.S. degrees in electrical engineering from the UIUC (University of Illinois in Urbana-Champaign). He received a Ph.D. in biomedical engineering from Worcester Polytechnic Institute and Clark University, and an M.D. from the University of Chicago. Dr. Fish is board-certified in emergency medicine, which he has practiced for twenty-five years. Before entering medical practice he worked for three and a half years in electrical engineering and research, most of which was at the National Institute of Neurological Diseases and Stroke. Dr. Fish has appointments at the University of Illinois at Urbana-Champaign in biomedical engineering, the Medical School and in electrical and computer engineering.

Lawrence O. Gostin, J.D., LL.D (Hon.) is the John Carroll Research Professor at Georgetown University Law Center; Professor of Public Health at the Johns Hopkins University; and Director of the Center for Law & the Public's Health at Johns Hopkins and Georgetown Universities (CDC Collaborating Center "Promoting Public Health Through Law"). He is a Research Fellow at the Centre for Socio-Legal Studies, Oxford University. Professor Gostin is an elected lifetime Member of the Institute of Medicine and serves on the IOM Board on Health Promotion and Disease Prevention. Professor Gostin also consults for the World Health Organization and UNAIDS. Professor Gostin has lead major law reform initiatives for the U.S. government including the Model Emergency Health Powers Act (MEHPA) to combat bioterrorism and other emerging health threats. Professor Gostin received the Rosemary Delbridge Memori "who has most influenced Parliament and government to act for the welfare of society." He also received the Key to Tohoko University (Japan) for distinguished contributions to human rights in mental health.

Professor Gostin's latest books are *The AIDS Pandemic: Complacency, Injustice, and Unfulfilled Expectations* (University of North Carolina Press, 2004); *The Human Rights of Persons with Intellectual Disabilities: Different but Equal* (Oxford University Press, 2003); *Public Health Law and Ethics: A Reader* (University of California Press and Milbank Memorial Fund, 2002); *Public Health Law: Power, Duty, Restraint* (University of California Press and Milbank Memorial Fund, 2000).

Dr. Henry C. Lee is one of the world's foremost forensic scientists. Dr. Lee's work has made him a landmark in modern-day criminal investigations. He has been a prominent player in many of the most challenging cases of the last forty-five years. Dr. Lee has worked with law enforcement agencies in helping to solve more than 6,000 cases. In recent years, his travels have taken him to England, Bosnia, China, Brunei, Bermuda, Middle East, South America and other locations around the world.

Dr. Lee's testimony figured prominently in the O.J. Simpson trial, and in convictions of the "Woodchipper" murderer as well as hundreds of other murder cases. Dr. Lee has assisted local and state police in their investigations of other famous crimes, such as the murder of Jon Benet Ramsey in Boulder, Colorado, the 1993 suicide of White House Counsel Vincent Foster, the murder of Chandra Levy, the kidnapping of Elizabeth Smart and the reinvestigation of the Kennedy assassination.

Dr. Lee is currently the Chief Emeritus for the Scientific Services and was the Commissioner of Public Safety for the State of Connecticut from 1998 to 2000 and served as Chief Criminalist for the State of Connecticut from 1979 to 2000. Dr. Lee was the driving force in establishing a modern State Police Forensic Science Laboratory in Connecticut.

In 1975, Dr. Lee joined the University of New Haven, where he created the school's Forensic Sciences program. He has also taught as a professor at more than a dozen universities, law schools, and medical schools. Though challenged with the demands on his time, Dr. Lee still lectures throughout the country and world to police, universities and civic organizations. Dr. Lee has authored hundreds of articles in professional journals and has co-authored more than thirty books, covering the areas, such as DNA, fingerprints, trace evidence, crime scene investigation and crime scene reconstruction. His recent books; *Famous Crimes Revisited*, *Cracking Cases* and *Blood Evidenc*e have been well received by the public.

Dr. Lee has been the recipient of numerous medals and awards, including the 1996 Medal of Justice from the Justice Foundation, and the 1998 Lifetime Achievement Award from the Science and Engineer Association. He has also been the recipient of the Distinguished Criminalist Award from the American Academy of Forensic Sciences; the J. Donero Award from the International Association of Identification, and in 1992 was elected a distinguished Fellow of the AAFS.

Dr. Lee was born in China and grew up in Taiwan. Dr. Lee first worked for the Taipei Police Department, attaining the rank of Captain. With his wife, Margaret, Dr. Lee came to the United States in 1965, and he earned his B.S. in forensic science from John Jay College in 1972. Dr. Lee continued his studies in biochemistry at NYU where he earned his masters degree in 1974 and Ph.D. in 1975. He has also received special training from the FBI Academy, ATF, the RCMP, and other organizations. He is a recipient of seven honorary doctorate degrees from Universities in recognition of his contributions to law and science. Dr. And Mrs. Lee have been married for forty years and have two grown children, a daughter, Sherry, and a son, Stanley.

Ashraf Mozayani, Pharm D., Ph.D., D-ABFT, is a nationally recognized board-certified forensic toxicologist. Dr. Mozayani is the Laboratory Director and the Chief Toxicologist for the Harris County Medical Examiner's Office in Houston, Texas. Before this position, she was the Chief Toxicologist for the District of Columbia at the Office of the Chief Medical Examiner. Dr. Mozayani is an Assistant Clinical Professor in the Department of Medicine at the University of Texas in Houston, an Adjunct Assistant Professor in the Department of Pharmacy at Texas Southern University and an Adjunct Assistant Professor in the Department of Pathology at University of Texas Medical Branch, Galveston.

Dr. Mozayani has published and presented numerous articles related to forensic toxicology (cocaine, marijuana, amphetamines, drug testing in hair, inhalants, and opiates, GHB, alcohol, and several prescription drugs). She is also editor of the book *Drug-Facilitated Sexual Assault: A Forensic Handbook* and *Handbook of Drug Interaction: A Clinical and Forensic Guide*. She is the U.S. editor of the new forensic journal *Forensic Science, Medicine and Pathology*. Dr. Mozayani serves as a consultant in toxicology to government and private industry and has been qualified as an expert witness in forensic toxicology and pharmacology in the federal, state and numerous military courts of the United States.

Major Timothy Palmbach, M.S., J.D., received his M.S. in forensic science from the University of New Haven in New Haven, CT and his J.D. from the University of Connecticut School of Law in Hartford, CT. He is the director of the Connecticut Division of Scientific Services and works with Dr. Henry Lee in crime scene reconstruction. He is an adjunct instructor at the University of New Haven and Central Connecticut State University and has been a guest lecturer at University of Connecticut School of Law, Western Connecticut University, Saint Joseph College and Northwestern Connecticut Community College.

He has processed more than 200 crime scenes and is a qualified expert witness in crime scene processing, blood spatter pattern interpretation and digital enhancement of forensic photographs.

Dr. Fredric Rieders founded National Medical Services in 1970, and served as its Chair and Laboratory Director. For fourteen years he was Chief Toxicologist at the Office of the Medical Examiner for the City of Philadelphia. Dr. Rieders is a Professor of Pharmacology and Toxicology, Jefferson Medical College, and holds a Ph.D. in pharmacology-toxicology from the Thomas Jefferson University and diplomates in forensic toxicology and toxicological chemistry, and is certified as a laboratory director by Pennsylvania, New York, and the Federal Centers for Disease Control. Author of over 100 publications, he was the 1987 recipient of the A.O. Gettler Award of the American Academy of Forensic Sciences and, in 1992, the recipient of the Thomas Jefferson University College of Graduate Studies Distinguished Alumnus Award.

Dr. Michael F. Rieders is a forensic toxicologist and Laboratory Director at National Medical Services where he is Chief Executive Officer. Dr. Rieders is a member of the Society of Forensic Toxicologists, the International Association of Forensic Toxicologists, and is a Fellow of the American Academy of Forensic Sciences, where he has given numerous presentations including, "Death Dealing Caregivers" and "Has Anyone Seen My Eyeball: An LSD Experience." Rieders earned his B.A. in chemistry in 1980 from Arcadia University, and a Ph.D. in pharmacology-toxicology in 1985 at Thomas Jefferson University, where he is a lecturer in the masters program in molecular pharmacology. Dr. Rieders is an active member of the Vidocq Society, which is a crime-solving organization of forensic professionals who donate their time and talents toward resolving unsolved, cold homicides. Dr. Rieders has also published numerous articles in professional journals.

Dr. Maurice Rogev (formerly Rogoff) was born in Cape Town, South Africa in 1927. After completing high school at the South African College Schools (1933–1944), he studied medicine at the University of Cape Town Medical School, graduating in December, 1950 with the degree M.B.Ch.B. (equivalent to the M.D. awarded by Israeli universities)

In 1951, he entered the British Colonial Service in Livingstone, Northern Rhodesia (since renamed Zambia) as an intern in the African and European Hospitals.

While waiting for a career .appointment in the Colonial service Dr. Rogev joined the staff of the City Deep Consolidated Mine Hospital in Johannesburg South Africa (1952–1953) as a medical and surgical intern. His duties included casualty, heat-stroke and pulmonary disease patients.

He joined the British Colonial service in 1954 as a medical officer in Kenya where he was certified as a specialist in forensic medicine by the Kenya government in 1959, after training in London hospitals and institutions selected by the Colonial Crown Agents on behalf of the Kenya government.

During his service in Kenya he was promoted to the rank of Assistant Director of Laboratory Services and Director of the Medical Research Laboratories of the Kenya Ministry of Health in Nairobi, serving in that capacity from 1960–1971. His duties included clinical pathology, morbid anatomy, forensic clinical medical examinations, autopsies, testifying in legal proceedings, public health administration, epidemic prevention and teaching laboratory professional and technical staff.

Dr. Rogev immigrated to Israel in 1972 where he achieved recognition and registration as a specialist in forensic medicine and morbid pathology by the Scientific Board of the Israel Medical Association and recognized by the Ministry of Health of the Government of Israel 1979–1980. In Israel he spent two years at the Leopold Greenberg Institute of Legal Medicine, subsequently joining the Department of Pathology at the Chaim Sheba Medical Center, Tel Hashomer Hospital

He joined the Israel Defence Force in 1978 as Chief Forensic Pathologist and Chief of the Medical Legal Bureau from where he was later seconded to the pathology laboratory.

In 1985, at the urgent request of the Israel Minister of Health, Dr. Rogev accepted appointment as head of the Leopold Greenberg Institute of Legal Medicine and remained in that post until 1988

Dr. Rogev retired from active duty in 1991 with the rank of Leutenant Colonel and continues in private practice as a forensic consultant. He also contributes occasional medical presentations at international forensic meetings and to forensic publications.

William D. Stanhope, P.A., received his M.S. in physician assistant studies from the University of Nebraska College of Medicine. He completed his surgical residency for physician assistants at Montefiore Medical Center. Currently he is the Associate Director for Special Projects at the Center for the Study of Bioterrorism and Emerging Infections at the Saint Louis University School of Public Health.

Lt. Col. Kathleen M. Sweet, M.A., J.D. (USAF Ret.), CEO and President of Risk Management Security Group, is certified by the U.K. and Irish Department of Transport to teach airport cargo security and has also been certified in homeland security (CHS-III) by the American College of Forensic Examiners International. Lt. Col. Sweet received her undergraduate degree from Franklin and Marshall College in Lancaster, Pennsylvania in Russian area studies and she has a master's degree in history from Temple University. She also has been admitted to the bar in Pennsylvania and Texas after graduating from Temple School of Law in Philadelphia, Pennsylvania in 1976. She is a graduate of numerous Air Force and civilian training programs.

After graduating from law school, Dr. Sweet joined Wyeth International Pharmaceuticals as a legal specialist focused on licensing agreements between Wyeth and international agencies. She later joined the US Air Force and initially was a member of the Judge Advocate General's Department. She frequently served as Director of Military Justice at the base and Numbered Air Force level. After fifteen years as a JAG and generally engaged in prosecuting cases on behalf of the military, she transferred to the 353rd Special Operations Wing as a military political affairs officer. She was later an intelligence officer assigned to HQ AMC as an executive officer and command briefer. In 1995 she became an Assistant Air Attaché to the Russian Federation. As an attaché she was engaged in liaison work not only with the Russian Air Force but also the Federal Security Bureau at which time she became interested in counter-terrorism efforts.

Her final military assignment was as an instructor at the Air War College where she taught in the International Security Studies division. She later became an Associate Professor at St. Cloud State University teaching in the Department of Criminal Justice and an Associate Professor at Embry Riddle Aeronautical University; teaching security and intelligence related courses. She is the author of two books, *Terrorism and Airport Security* (Edwin Mellen Press, 2002) and *Aviation and Airport Security* (Prentice Hall Publishers, 2003.) Her third book, *Transportation Security* is pending publication by Prentice Hall and a *Transportation Security Directory* is pending publication by Grey House Publishers. She is considered an expert in the field of airport, aviation and air cargo security and has been well published in the fields of international space programs and associated treaties, space based offensive weapons, bio-terrorism, and aviation security.

She is currently, CEO and President of Risk Management Security Group doing business in Ireland as RMSG Ireland, Ltd. The company engages in all aspects of consulting in transportation-related security including preparation of threat and vulnerability assessments and security awareness training. She is also a contributing consultant with International Risk Control, Ltd. based in London, England.

Louis C. Tripoli, M.D. His many interests include bioterrorism and emerging infectious diseases, forensic and correctional medicine. At the time of this writing, he has been deployed as a Public Health expert working with the U.S. Marines 4th Civil Affairs Group, with the rank of Commander in the U.S. Navy.

As a civilian, Dr. Tripoli holds the titles of Senior Vice-President of Correctional Medical Services, Chairman of Correctional Medicine Institute, Adjunct Assistant Professor of Medicine in the Infectious Diseases Division of Johns Hopkins University, and Adjunct Associate Professor at St. Louis University School of Public Health. He is board-certified in internal medicine and received a certificate in forensic medicine from the American College of Forensic Examiners.

Dr. Tripoli obtained his undergraduate degree from Harvard and his doctorate of medicine from the University of Pittsburgh, where he also completed residency in internal medicine.

Michael Welner, M.D., is responsible for a number of groundbreaking innovations in psychiatry. As founder of the Forensic Panel, he devised and implemented the first peer-reviewed protocols in the United States for forensic consultation. Under Dr. Welner's leadership, the Forensic Panel has achieved his vision of presenting "the last word" to retaining attorneys, opposing counsel, and the courts. This has consistently helped to resolve cases without appearance at trial.

Dr. Welner's casework has spanned numerous areas of the criminal, civil, employment, and family law, often focusing on frontier issues. Through respect for the science, and dogged investigation, Dr. Welner has promoted and embodied diligence and objectivity as a staple of the forensic examination. He has lectured on numerous forensic and clinical issues as an invited speaker of, among others, the American Bar Association, American Society of Clinical Psychopharmacology, International Bar Association, Pennsylvania State Senate Judiciary Committee, and various medical center Grand Rounds, at venues around the world.

In 1996, he introduced the *Forensic Echo*, and originated the format of a cutting-edge, practitioner-written forensic journal that combined commentary with case and science updates with investigative reporting. More recently, Dr. Welner has pioneered the effort toward establishing a forensic definition of evil. The Depravity Scale is a history-driven forensic assessment instrument that will standardize the definition of "heinous," "atrocious," and "cruel" in for purposes of fair and consistent application in criminal sentencing.

In his New York City based clinical practice, Dr. Welner specializes in patients who fail to respond to treatment. Dr. Welner's inquisitive and independent mindset, clinical foundation, and tenacious reliance on evidence-based forensics guide the members of the Forensic Panel and their efforts in each case they examine

Dr. Charles H. Wick, Ph.D., is a research physical scientist with more than 28 years of technical and managerial experience within the Department of Defense and Private Industry. After obtaining four degrees from the University of Washington, Dr. Wick first practiced managerial and technical skills in the civilian sector from 1971-1983. This successful career resulted in several publications, international participation, a patent, and the application of basic research to industry. Dr. Wick joined the Vulnerability/Lethality Division of the US Army Ballistic Research Laboratory in 1983 and won immediate acceptance as an organizer, principal investigator and team leader. A result of his efforts was the first effort to advance the modeling of sublethal chemical, nuclear and biological agents using fundamental knowledge. This was a major advancement.

This work was incorporated into DOD, NATO, and other international applications and helped solve this important and pressing Army problem. Dr. Wick became an international authority on individual performance for operations conducted on an NBC battlefield during this period. Dr. Wick has given numerous briefings to many members with DOD, DoE, industry, and academia. Recent achievements include the invention of a filterless biological protection system, and the basic research leading to the invention of the Integrated Virus Detection System (IVDS). This system is the first instrument of its kind and represents a fundamental breakthrough and major advance in virus analysis technology.

Dr. Wick served with distinction as a Chemical Corps Lieutenant Colonel (USAR) during a twenty-eight-year career including twelve years as a unit commander, six years as a staff officer (twice an ARCOM Staff Chemical Officer), deputy Program Director Biological Defense Systems and his last assignment before retirement on April 1, 1999 as commander, 485th CML BN.

Dr. Wick has more than forty-five publications, both government and open literature, and is recognized by his peers for his research and leadership skills having received numerous citations and awards, including two U.S. Army Achievement Medals for Civilian Service, the Commander's Award for Civilian Service, the Technical Cooperation Achievement Award, and twenty-five other decorations and awards for his contributions to both the community and the nation.

Present Assignment: Team Leader, Point Detection Team, Principal Investigator and Research Physical Scientist, U.S. Army Edgewood Chemical Biological Center (ECBC), U.S. Army Soldier and Biological Chemical Command (SBCCOM), ATTN: AMSSB-RRT-DS, Aberdeen Proving Ground, MD 21010.

Index

A

chest pain, 9, 13, 18, 20, 112, 155, 180

cyanide, 2, 7, 24–25, 39, 144, 172, 174, 179, 184, 191, 195–196, 229, 234, 376, 425, 467

cyanogen chloride, 7, 24, 174, 195–196

D

E

F

G

H

I

M

N

O

P

phosgene, 2, 7, 23, 25, 35, 39, 173–174, 194, 198–199, 202, 204, 229

Q

R

S

T

U

V

Physical Evidence in Forensic Science, #5563

Henry C. Lee and Howard A. Harris

This new classic by America's leading forensic scientists will give you an insider's grasp of physical evidence at the crime scene.

Written in an easy-to-understand format, this outstanding guide by the nation's foremost forensic scientists will introduce to you the basics of crime scene evaluation. This extensive resource is packed with valuable information about the details of collecting, storing, and analyzing all types of physical evidence. You'll learn how to connect the victims and suspects to the crime scene and to the physical evidence left behind to provide convincing testimony based on scientific facts.

Discover if the police and prosecution have done their jobs properly to process all crime scene materials.

Part I offers an overview of forensic science and discusses the future path of forensic science and its applications in the courtroom and society. Part II gives you an exhaustive list of physical evidence typically left behind at crime scenes and explains the correct method to process this evidence. In part III, you'll learn about the current issues in search and seizure. A discussion of common blood screening test reagents and the druggist's fold is treated in the appendices.

Details often make the difference between winning and losing that important case. This in-depth reference also provides you with the details regarding: light and smoke at the crime scene, bullet identification, the difference between transient and pattern evidence, noting post-mortem lividity marks and other special imprints and indentations, how odors offer clues to the crime, studying dry versus wet blood samples, how to do a crime scene reconstruction, and most importantly how to recognize and co-ordinate all the elements of the crime scene.

Written by the foremost experts in the field of forensic science, you will learn from the best how to make your investigation solid and successful. 6 1/8" × 9 1/4", softbound, 297 pages. Casebound edition also available (#5564).

Advanced Forensic Criminal Defense Investigations, #5554

Edited by Grace Elting Castle, Compiled by Paul J. Ciolino

Written by veteran investigators known for their professional expertise, this book is packed with information on every aspect of the criminal forensic investigation. Whether you represent the defense or prosecution, this is the ideal resource to consult when working with an investigator. What avenues or possible leads have not been considered? What new techniques are being employed for the other side?

How can you implement or challenge these new technical advances in medicocriminal entomology, GSR tests, or voice identification? For example, what's the difference between an atomic absorption GSR test and and a scanning electron microscope test? How does blowback challenge the threshold levels for GSR established by crime labs? Why do some workers, like plumbers and electricians, lend themselves to incriminating GSR tests?

Conducting thorough background checks often leads to the tip which cracks the case. However, do you adequately know the background of your expert? Do you know how to prevent unwelcome surprises in the courtroom regarding your own expert's credibility? Similarly, establishing a comfortable and productive rapport when investigating the backgrounds of potential informants and witnesses in various cases including white-collar crime is also discussed. Investigating a case yourself? What possible defense strategies should be considered?

Chapter 15, Homicide Defense Investigations, offers advice on the classic and alternative defenses usually used in trial. What about the defendant accused of sexual assault? Mentally handicapped defendants? All this and more are treated to an in-depth analysis to help decipher even the most complex of cases.

This book details case examples and many sample interview questions to ask various experts when soliciting critical information. 6 1/8" × 9 1/4", casebound, 322 pages.